First Edition of Mind Maps In Biochemistry

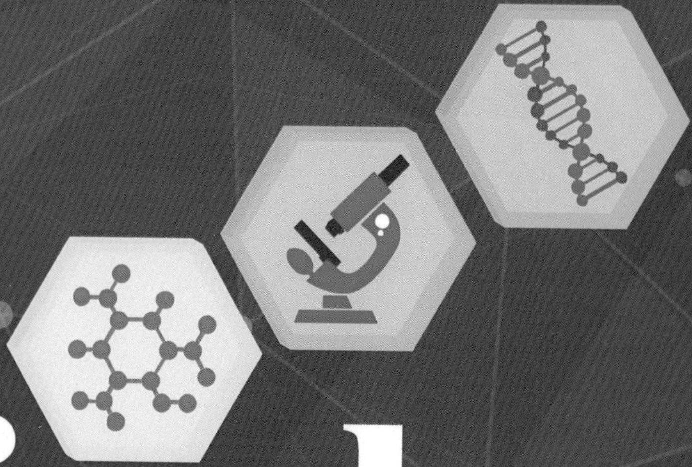

Biochemistry
Mind Maps

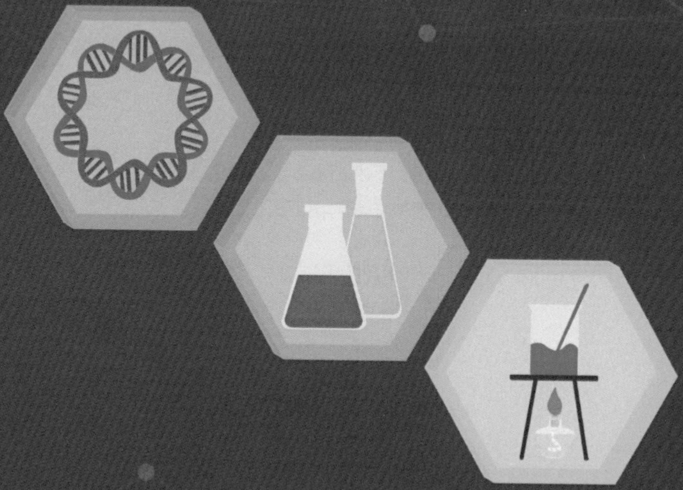

Mohamed J. Saadh

Hala M. Sbaih

5' A U G A C C A C G U G G G U G A 3'

To order additional copies of this book, contact:
Xlibris
0800-056-3182
www.xlibrispublishing.co.uk
Orders@ Xlibrispublishing.co.uk

ISBN: Softcover   978-1-9845-9314-6
         EBook   978-1-9845-9315-3

Print information available on the last page

Rev. date: 01/07/2020

Table of contents

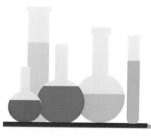

Table of contents

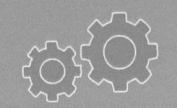

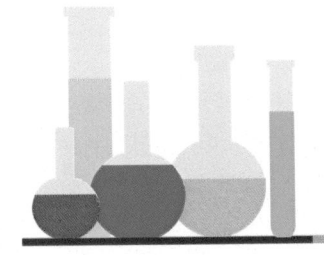

Preface of the first edition

A student who has entered the portals of colleges finds it difficult to understand the subjects taught to him. This book is written in a very simple and easy style. It is up-to-date and exhaustive in covering the core topics of biochemistry.

The first book of mind maps in biochemistry that covered the fundamentals of biochemistry to gain a clear understanding, providing detailed, specific information on the principles of chemical processes within and relating to living organisms.

This book aims to address new change in a variety of biochemical disturbance using diagramming tools, to generate, visualize structure, and classify ideas, and as an aid studying and organizing information, solving problems, making decisions and writing.

We continue to welcome constructive comments from all students who use our book as part of their studies and academics who adopt the book to complement their teaching.

Mohamed J. Saadh

Hala M. Sbaih

2019

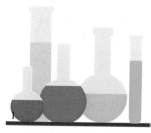

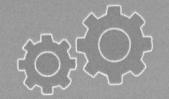

At the beginning, thanks to Allah who gave me the chances to live and learn for everything done to me and for giving me more and more than I deserve. Thanks for your endless kindness and your generous courtesy and please accept this work.

Gratefully, I would like to thank the author Hala M. Sbaih, Pharmacist, for not only suggesting the idea for this book, but also for her invaluable assistance, comments, and continuous kind cooperation.

Finally, I wish to express our gratitude to all my colleagues at Middle East University-Jordan who have been supportive in the production of this new first edition, especially, Associate Professor. Ammar Almaaytah, Dean of Faculty of Pharmacy for their kind help.

Mohamed J. Saadh

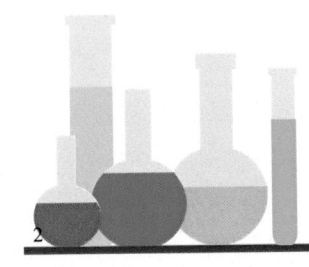

Mohamed J. Saadh, BSc. MSc. PhD Biochemistry
Assistant Professor of Biochemistry, Faculty of Pharmacy, Middle East University, Jordan
P.O. Box. 383 Amman 11831 Jordan
Mobile: +962 78 6945883
Email: mjsaadh@yahoo.com

Hala M. Sbaih , BSc. Pharmacy
P.O. Box: 383 Amman 11831 Jordan
Mobile: +962 796811942
Email: hala_isbahe@yahoo.com

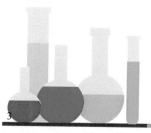

OVERVIEW

Proteins are the most abundant and functionally diverse molecules in living systems. Virtually every life process depends on this class of molecules. For example, enzymes and polypeptide hormones direct and regulate metabolism in the body, whereas contractile proteins in muscle permit movement. In bone, the protein collagen forms a framework for the deposition of calcium phosphate crystals, acting like the steel cables in reinforced concrete. In the bloodstream, proteins, such as hemoglobin and plasma albumin, shuttle molecules essential to life, whereas immuno globulins fight infectious bacteria and viruses. In short, proteins display an incredible diversity of functions, yet all share the common structural feature of being linear polymers of amino acids.

Animal Cell Structure

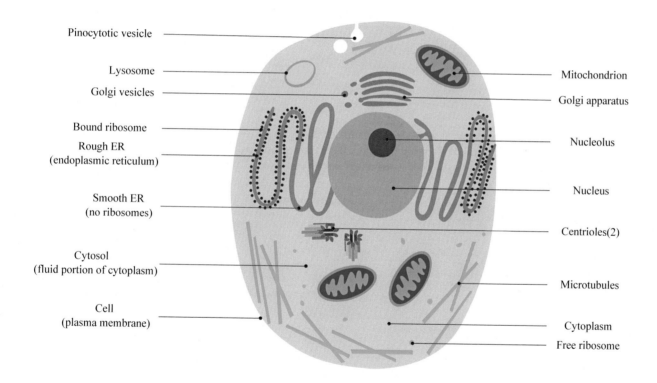

Pinocytotic vesicle

Lysosome

Golgi vesicles

Bound ribosome

Rough ER
(endoplasmic reticulum)

Smooth ER
(no ribosomes)

Cytosol
(fluid portion of cytoplasm)

Cell
(plasma membrane)

Mitochondrion

Golgi apparatus

Nucleolus

Nucleus

Centrioles(2)

Microtubules

Cytoplasm

Free ribosome

Proteins are molecules made of amino acids. They are coded for by our genes and form the basis of living tissues. They also play a central role in biological processes. For example, proteins catalyse reactions in our bodies, transport molecules such as oxygen, keep us healthy as part of the immune system and transmit messages from cell to cell.

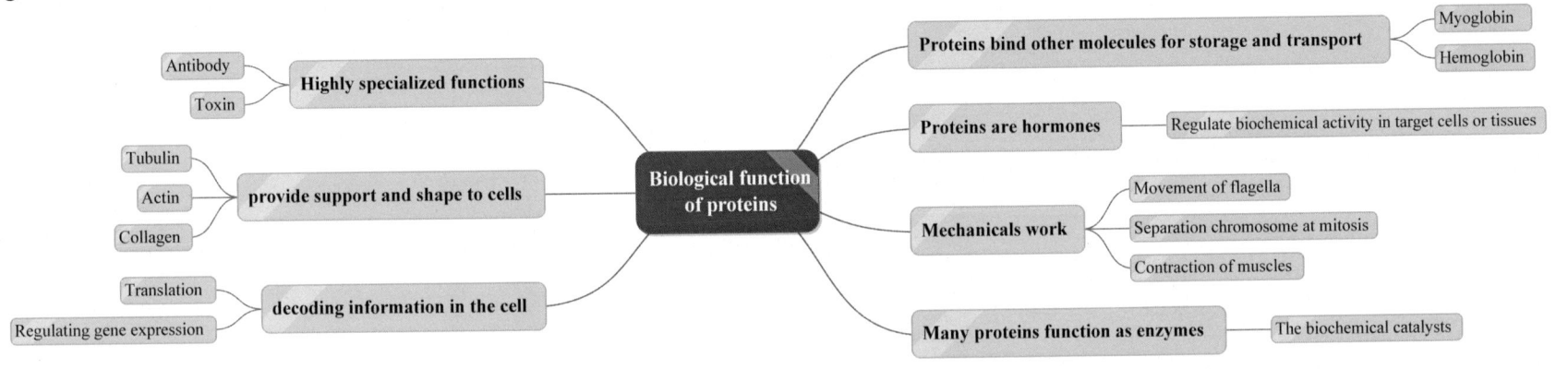

1.1.General structure of Amino acids

Amino acids are a crucial, yet basic unit of protein, and they contain an amino group and a carboxylic group bonded with alpha carbon.

The α-carbon is chiral or asymmetric except the glycine. The side chains (R) of amino acids that determine their role in the proteins behavior.

They play an extensive role in gene expression processes, which includes the adjustment of protein functions that facilitate messenger RNA (mRNA) translation.

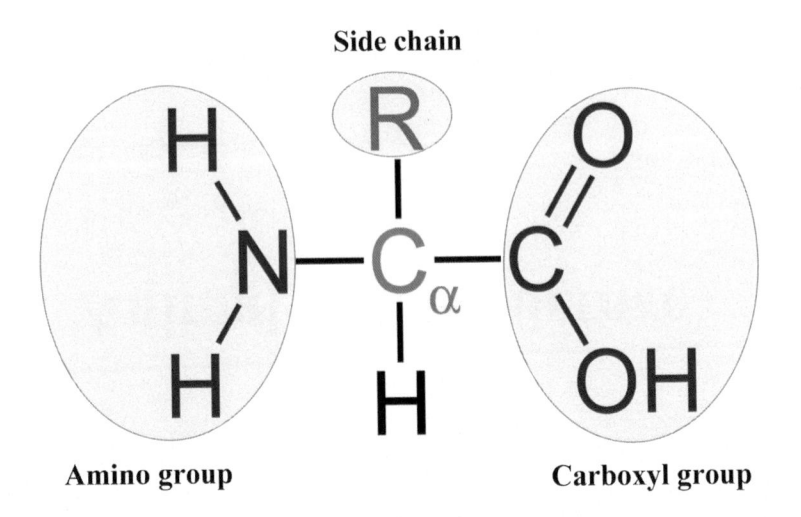

Hydropath is important in protein chain folding because hydrophobic side chains to be clustered in the interior of a protein and hydrophilic residue are usually found on the surface. In addition hydropathy used to predict which segments of membrane-spanning proteins are likely to be embedded in hydrophobic lipid bilayer.

Inside the cell, under normal physiological conditionPH = 6.8-7.4
• The amino group are protonated (-NH3+),Pka≈9
• Carboxyl is ionize (-coo-), Pka≈3
• So amino acid are zwitterions or dipolar ions, even though their net charge may be zero

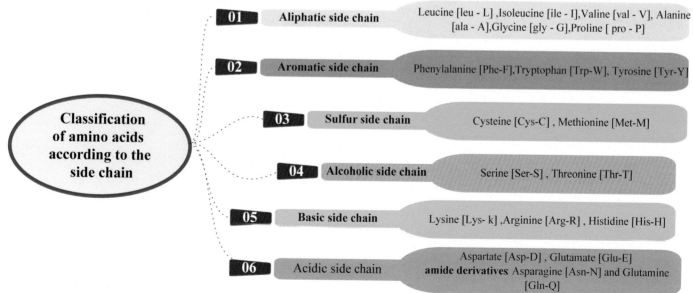

1.2.Classification of amino acids according to the side chain

Amino acids also exist in free form. In particular, 20 standard amino acids are crucial for life as they contain peptides and proteins and are known to be the building blocks for all living things. In nature, over 700 types of amino acids have been uncovered. Almost all of them are α-amino acids. They have been discovered in: bacteria, fungi, algae, various other plants. Amino acids can be classified according the side chain group type (aliphatic, aromatic, sulfur, alcohol, basic, acidic and their amide derivatives. In the form of proteins, amino acid residues form the second-largest component (water is the largest) of human muscles and other tissues. in addition, amino acids participate in a number of processes such as neurotransmitter transport and biosynthesis.

Classification of amino acids according to the side chain

01 Aliphatic side chain — Leucine [leu - L] ,Isoleucine [ile - I],Valine [val - V], Alanine [ala - A],Glycine [gly - G],Proline [pro - P]

02 Aromatic side chain — Phenylalanine [Phe-F],Tryptophan [Trp-W], Tyrosine [Tyr-Y]

03 Sulfur side chain — Cysteine [Cys-C] , Methionine [Met-M]

04 Alcoholic side chain — Serine [Ser-S] , Threonine [Thr-T]

05 Basic side chain — Lysine [Lys- k] ,Arginine [Arg-R] , Histidine [His-H]

06 Acidic side chain — Aspartate [Asp-D] , Glutamate [Glu-E] **amide derivatives** Asparagine [Asn-N] and Glutamine [Gln-Q]

1.2.1 Aliphatic side chain of amino acids

Aliphatic amino acids (glycine, alanine, valine, leucine. Isoleucine, proline) are non-polar and hydrophobic. Hydrophobicity increases as the number of carbon atoms on the hydrocarbon chain increases. Most aliphatic amino acids are found within protein molecules. However, alanine and glycine may be found either inside or outside a protein molecule.

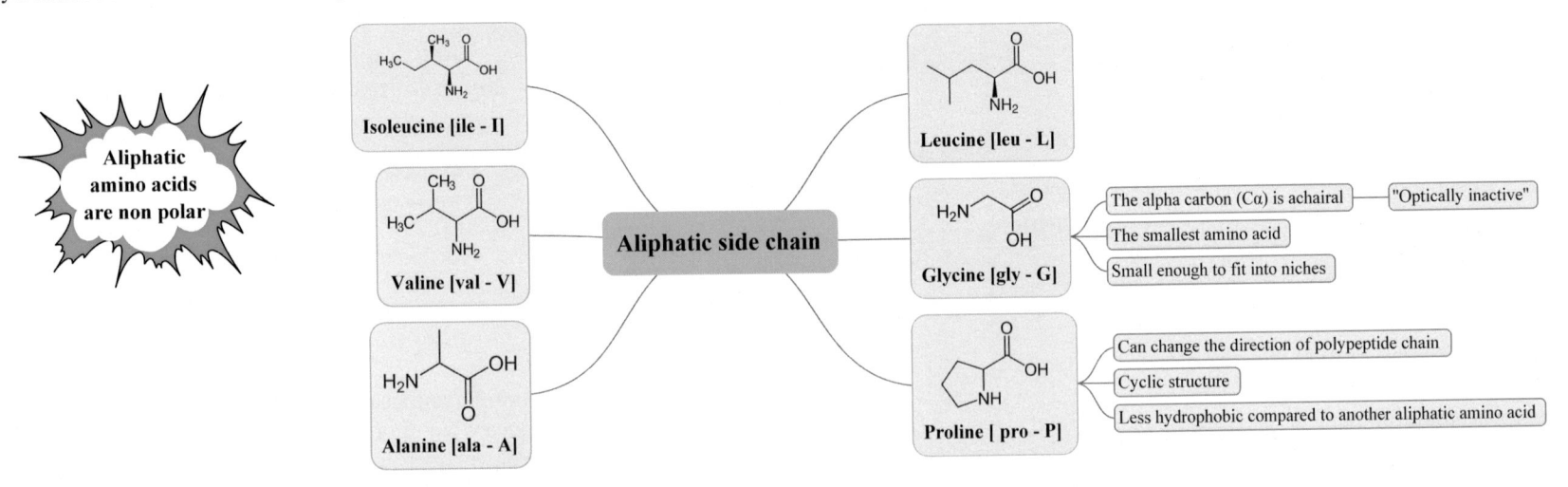

1.2.2.Aromatic side chain of amino acids

Aromatic amino acids are able to absorb light due to their conjugated double bonds. This characteristic of aromatic amino acids is used to quantify the concentration of proteins in an unknown sample. Tyrosine and tryptophan absorb light at 280 nm more than phenylalanine (260 nm). tryptophan is responsible for most of the absorbance of ultraviolet light (ca. 280 nm) by proteins.

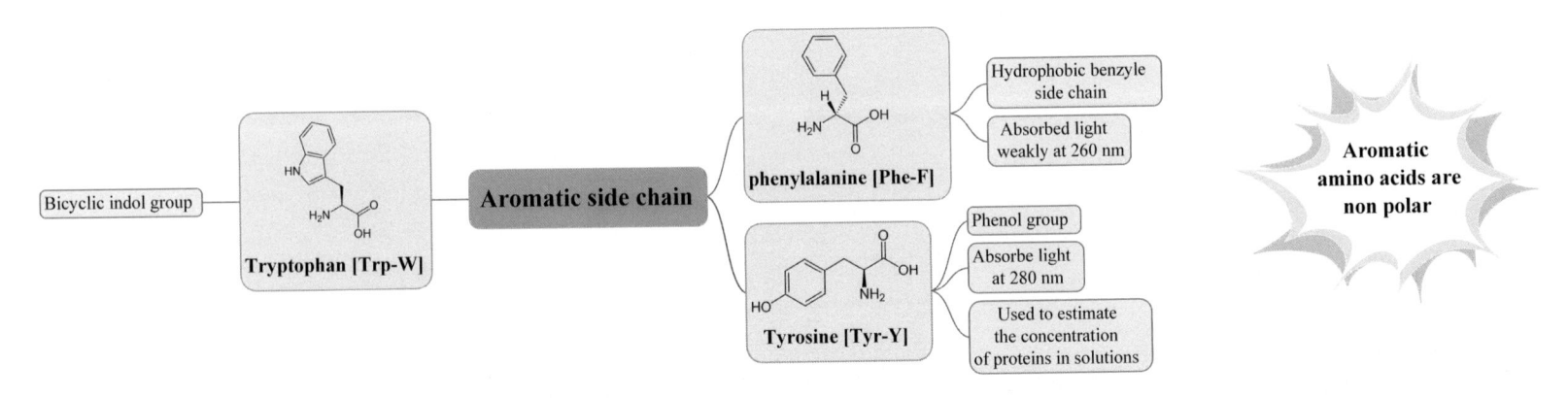

1.2.3.Sulfur containing side chain of amino acids

The sulfur-containing amino acids (cysteine and methionine) are generally considered to be nonpolar and hydrophobic. In fact, methionine is one of the most hydrophobic amino acids and is almost always found on the interior of proteins. Cysteine on the other hand does ionize to yield the thiolate anion. Even so, it has sulfhydryl group of cysteine can react with other sulfhydryl groups in an oxidation reaction that yields a disulfide bond.

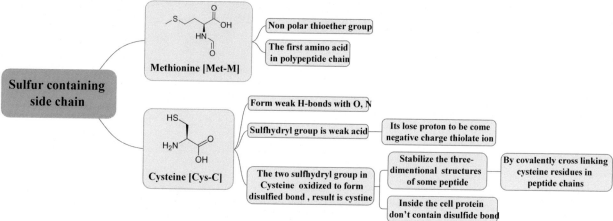

1.2.4.Alcoholic groups in side chain

serine and threonine have uncharged polar side chains (β-hydroxyl groups). These give hydrophilic character to aliphatic side chains.

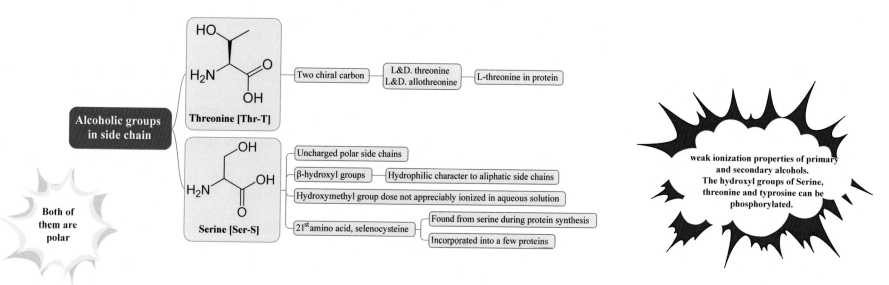

1.2.5.Basic side chain of amino acids

There are three amino acids that have basic side chainsat neutral pH. These are arginine (Arg), lysine (Lys), andhistidine (His).Their side chains contain nitrogen and resemble ammonia, which is a base. Their pKa's are high enough that they tend to bind protons, gaining a positive charge at physiological pH.

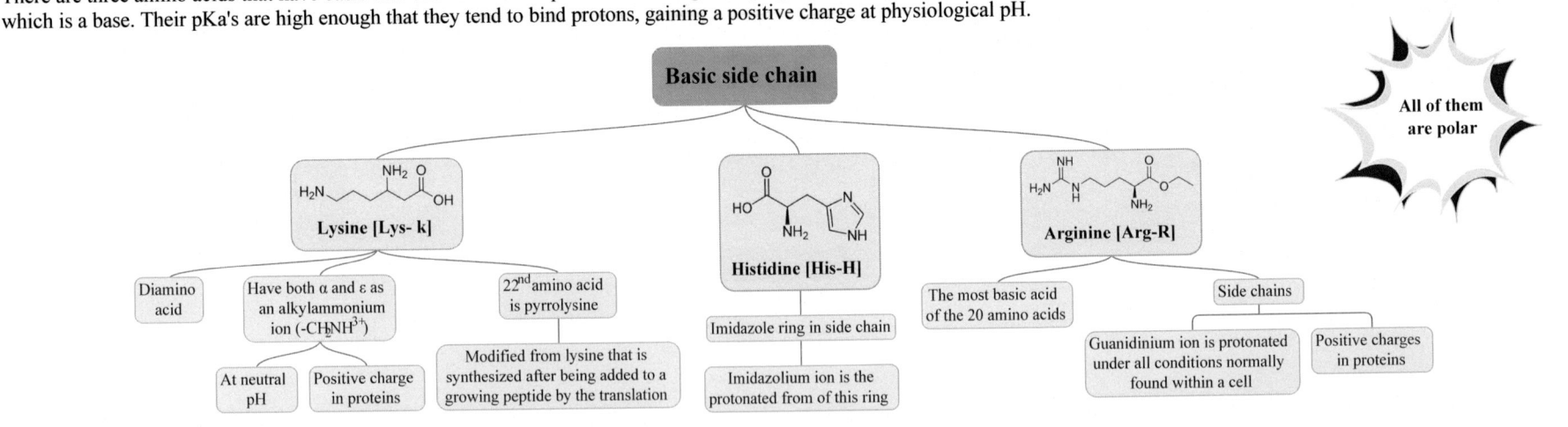

1.2.6.Acidic side chain and their amide derivatives

Two amino acids have acidic side chains at neutral pH. These are aspartic acid or aspartate (Asp) and glutamic acid or glutamate (Glu). Their side chains have carboxylic acid groups whose pKa's are low enough to lose protons, becoming negatively charged at physiological pH. Furthermore, Asparagine(Asn, N) and glutamine (Gln, Q) are amides of aspartic acid or glutamic acid. The side chains of Asparagine and glutamine are uncharged, highly polar and found on the surface on proteins therefore, The polar amide groups of Asparagine and glutamine can form H-bonds with side chains of other polar amino acids.

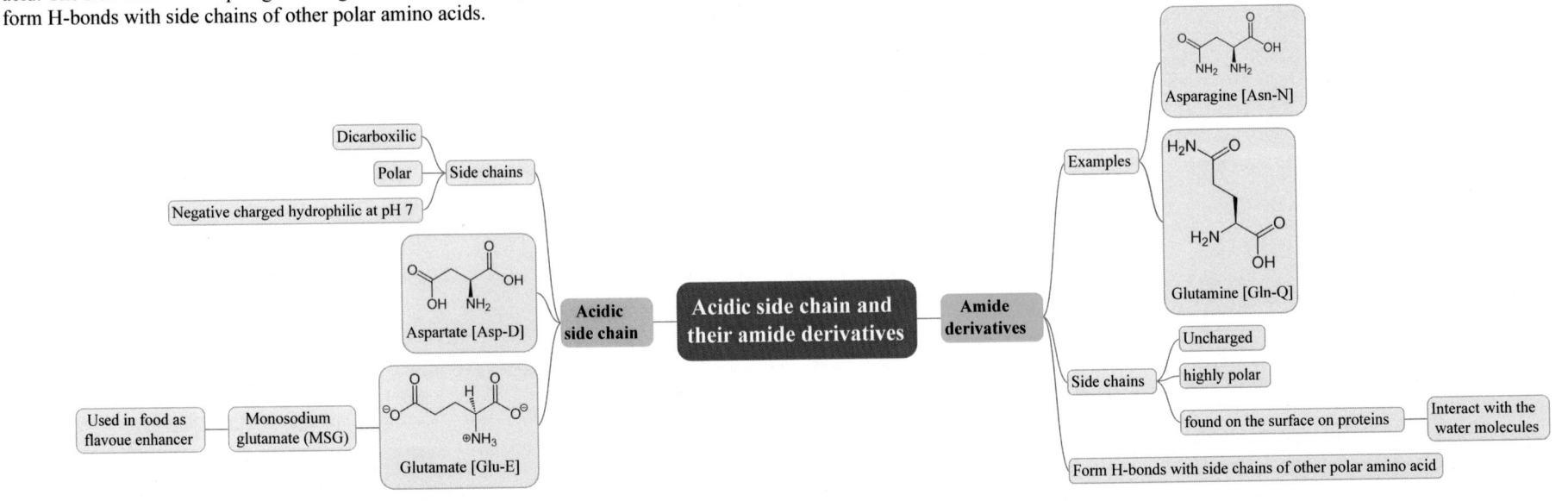

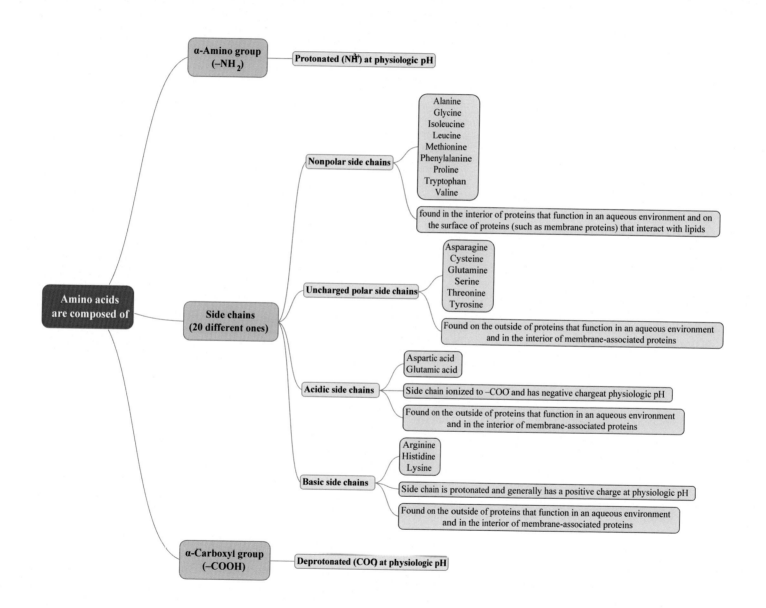

Amino acids are composed of

α-Amino group (–NH₂) — Protonated (NH₃⁺) at physiologic pH

Side chains (20 different ones)

Nonpolar side chains
- Alanine
- Glycine
- Isoleucine
- Leucine
- Methionine
- Phenylalanine
- Proline
- Tryptophan
- Valine

found in the interior of proteins that function in an aqueous environment and on the surface of proteins (such as membrane proteins) that interact with lipids

Uncharged polar side chains
- Asparagine
- Cysteine
- Glutamine
- Serine
- Threonine
- Tyrosine

Found on the outside of proteins that function in an aqueous environment and in the interior of membrane-associated proteins

Acidic side chains
- Aspartic acid
- Glutamic acid

Side chain ionized to –COO⁻ and has negative charge at physiologic pH

Found on the outside of proteins that function in an aqueous environment and in the interior of membrane-associated proteins

Basic side chains
- Arginine
- Histidine
- Lysine

Side chain is protonated and generally has a positive charge at physiologic pH

Found on the outside of proteins that function in an aqueous environment and in the interior of membrane-associated proteins

α-Carboxyl group (–COOH) — Deprotonated (COO⁻) at physiologic pH

Amino acids : Exercises

Q 1: Circle the best correct answer:

1. Which one of the following statements about amino acids is false?
a. Threonine and Isoleucine has two chiral carbons
b. Tyrosine; at neutral pH absorb light strongly at 700 nm
c. Methionine, is amino acid contain sulphur atom
d. isoleucine; is non-polar and found buried in the centre of **proteins**

2. Protein contain only:
a. L-amino acids
b. D-amino acids
c. DL-Amino acids
d. All of these

3. The amino acid that causes a kink and change the direction of polypeptide chain is:
a. Proline
b. Methionine
c. Arginine
d. Leucine

4. The Ip of Histidine is:
a. 9.17
b. 6
c. 7.55
d. 3.91

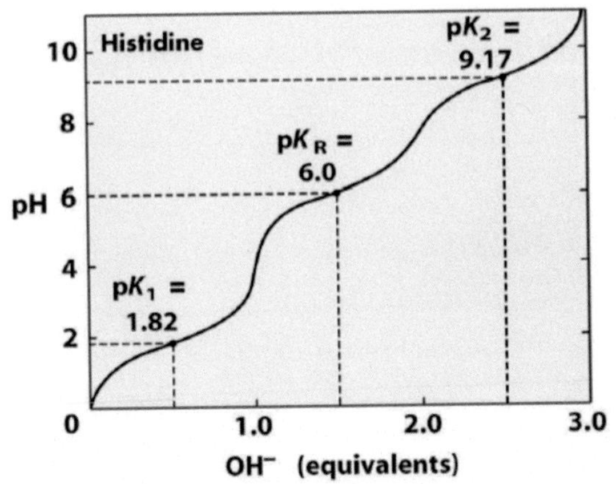

5. Which of the following amino acids are optically inactive and is having achiral carbon atom?
a. Proline
b. Glutamate
c. Arginine
d. Glycine

6. An uncommon amino acid that is found in collagen is:
a. Lysine
b. Taurine
c. Proline
d. 5-hydroxylproline

7. Which of the following statements about cystine is true?
a. Cystine is an example of a nonstandard amino acid, derived by linking two standard amino acids.
b. Cystine forms when the —CH_2—SH R group is oxidized to form a —CH_2— S—S—CH_2— disulfide bridge between two cysteines.
c. Cystine is formed through a peptide linkage between two cysteines .
d. Cystine is formed by the oxidation of the carboxylic acid group on cysteine

8. Which of the following amino acids is dicarboxylic amino acids?
a. Proline
b. Glutamate
c. Arginine
d. Glycine

9. Which of the following amino acids is diamino amino acids?
a. Proline
b. Glutamate
c. Lysine
d. Glycine

10. At isoelectric pH, an amino acid exists as
a. Anion
b. Cation
c. Zwitterion
d. None of these

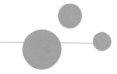

Q 1: Circle the best correct answer:

11. Which of the following aromatic amino acids that absorb light at 280 nm at neutral pH?
a. Phenylalanine and methionine
b. Tyrosine and tryptophan
c. Alanine and serine
d. Arginine and asparagine

12. Amino acid that has sulphur and plays a special role in protein synthesis since almost always the first amino acid in a polypeptide chain:
a. Methionine
b. cysteine
c. Valine
d. Asparagine

13. Which of the following amino acids has a positive charge at pH 7?
a. Alanine & valine
b. Tyrosine proline
c. Arginine & lysine
d. Asparagine & glutamate

14. Amino acids are:
a. building block of carbohydrate
b. building block of nucleic acids
c. building block of lipids
d. building block of proteins

15. The simplest and smallest amino acid is:
a. Glycine
b. Serine
c. Valine
d. Asparagine

16. The 21 st amino acid is:
a. Lysine
b. hydroxyl proline
c. selenocysteine
d. Citrulline

17. The amino acid with a nonpolar side chain is:
a. Serine
b. Valine
c. Asparagine
d. Threonine

18. An example of polar amino acid is:
a. Alanine
b. Leucine
c. Arginine
d. Valine

19. Side chains of all amino acids contain aromatic rings except
a. Pheynl alanine
b. Alanine
c. Tyrosine
d. Tryptophan

20. An aromatic amino acid is
a. Lysine
b. Tyrosine
c. Taurine
d. Arginine

21. A disulphide bond can be formed between
a. Two methionine residues
b. Two cysteine residues
c. A methionine and a cysteine residue
d. All of these

22. Sulphur containing amino acid is
a. Methionine
b. Leucine
c. Valine
d. Asparagine

23. Which amino acid side chains can be phosphorylated?
a. Serine
b. Threonine
c. Tyrosine
d. All of these

Q 2. Write short note on:

a.Essential amino acids.
b.Isoelectric pH.
c.General structure of standard amino acids.
d.The amino acid side chains can be phosphorylated.

OVERVIEW

Proteins are polymers formed from sequences of amino acids, the monomers of the polymer. Proteins form by 20 standard amino acids undergoing condensation reactions, in which the amino acids lose one water molecule per reaction in order to attach to one another with a peptide bond. The linear sequence of the linked amino acids contains the information necessary to generate a protein molecule with a unique three-dimensional shape to be able to perform their biological function, proteins fold into one or more specific spatial conformations driven by a number of non-covalent interactions such as hydrogen bonding, ionic interactions, hydrophobic interaction, and disulfide bridge. To understand the functions of proteins at a molecular level, it is often necessary to determine their three-dimensional structure. The complexity of protein structure is best analyzed by considering the molecule in terms of four organizational levels, namely, primary, secondary, tertiary, and quaternary structures.

Chapter 2 : Structure of proteins

2.1. Primary structure

The primary structure of a protein refers to the sequence of amino acids in the polypeptide chain. The primary structure is held together by peptide bonds that are made during the process of protein biosynthesis. The two ends of the polypeptide chain are referred to as the carboxyl terminus (C-terminus) and the amino terminus (N-terminus).

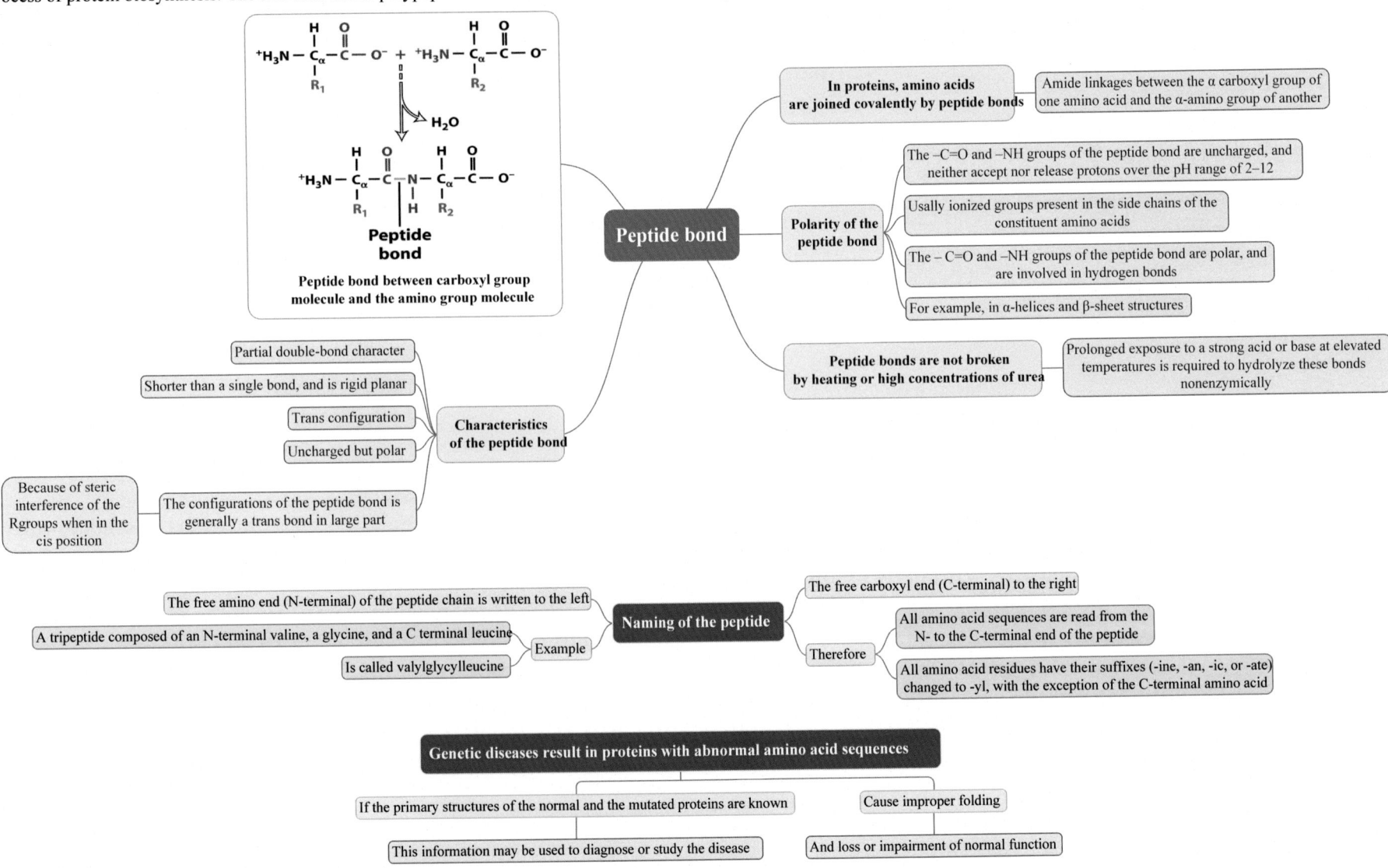

2.2.Secondary structure

Refers to highly regular structures. Two main types of secondary structure, the α-helix and the β-strand or β-sheets, These secondary structures are defined by patterns of hydrogen bonds between the main-chain peptide group**Examples of secondary structure:**

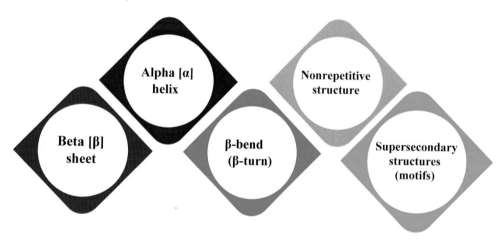

2.2.1. α helix

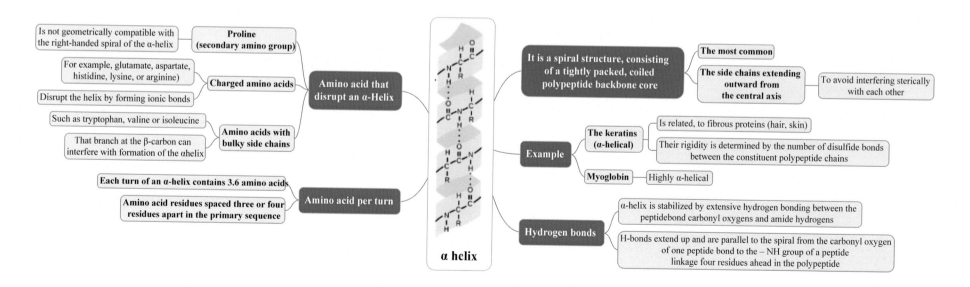

2.2.2.β-sheet

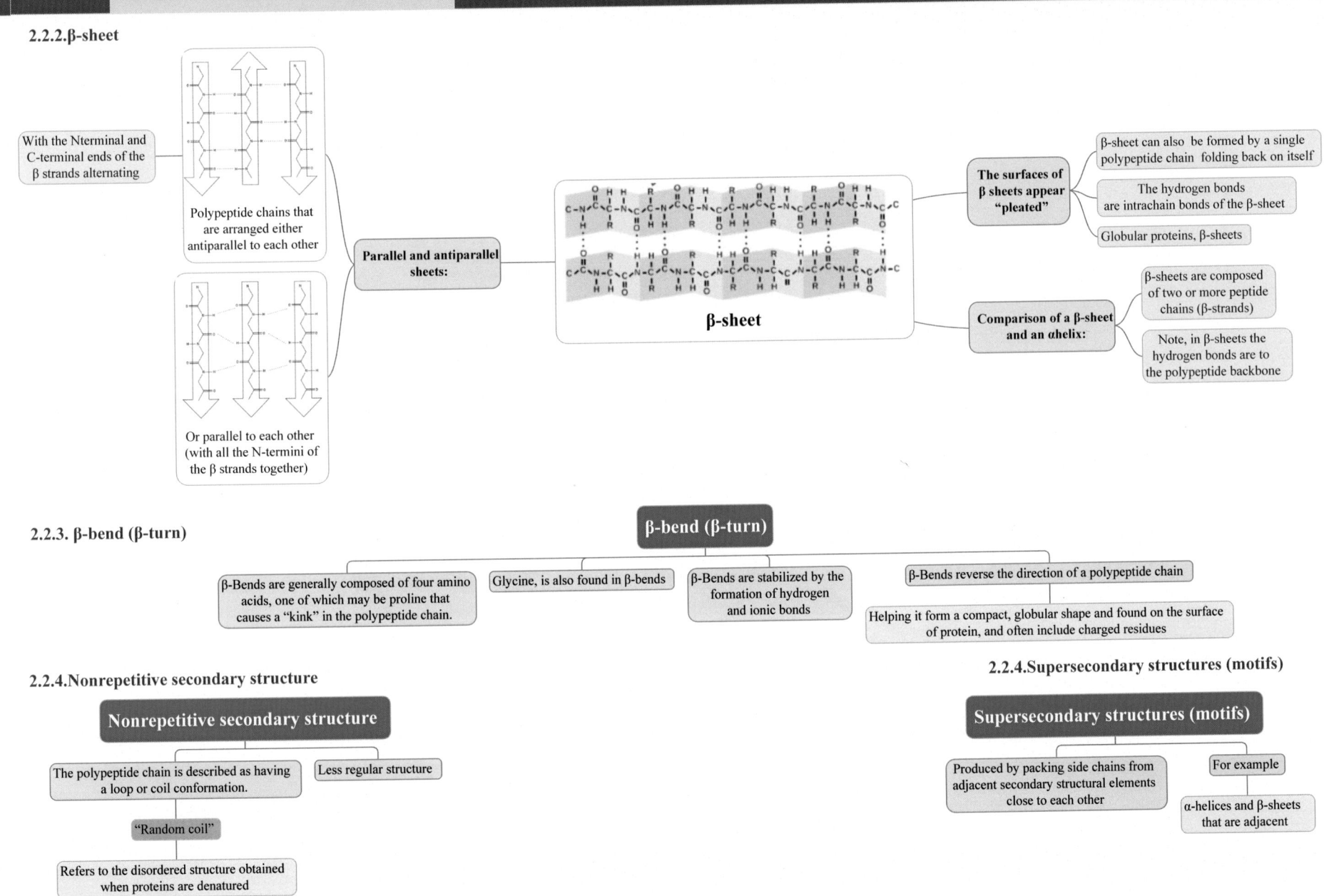

With the Nterminal and C-terminal ends of the β strands alternating

Polypeptide chains that are arranged either antiparallel to each other

Parallel and antiparallel sheets:

Or parallel to each other (with all the N-termini of the β strands together)

β-sheet

β-sheet can also be formed by a single polypeptide chain folding back on itself

The surfaces of β sheets appear "pleated"

The hydrogen bonds are intrachain bonds of the β-sheet

Globular proteins, β-sheets

β-sheets are composed of two or more peptide chains (β-strands)

Comparison of a β-sheet and an αhelix:

Note, in β-sheets the hydrogen bonds are to the polypeptide backbone

2.2.3. β-bend (β-turn)

β-bend (β-turn)

β-Bends are generally composed of four amino acids, one of which may be proline that causes a "kink" in the polypeptide chain.

Glycine, is also found in β-bends

β-Bends are stabilized by the formation of hydrogen and ionic bonds

β-Bends reverse the direction of a polypeptide chain

Helping it form a compact, globular shape and found on the surface of protein, and often include charged residues

2.2.4.Nonrepetitive secondary structure

Nonrepetitive secondary structure

The polypeptide chain is described as having a loop or coil conformation.

Less regular structure

"Random coil"

Refers to the disordered structure obtained when proteins are denatured

2.2.4.Supersecondary structures (motifs)

Supersecondary structures (motifs)

Produced by packing side chains from adjacent secondary structural elements close to each other

For example

α-helices and β-sheets that are adjacent

2.3.Tertiary structure

The tertiary structure will have a single polypeptide chain with one or more protein secondary structures, the protein domains. Amino acid side chains may interact and bond in a number of ways. The interactions and bonds of side chains within a particular protein determine its tertiary structure. The folding and the stabilizing of Tertiary structure by Disulfied bond, Hydrophobic intersections,Hydrogrn bond, and Ionic bonds.

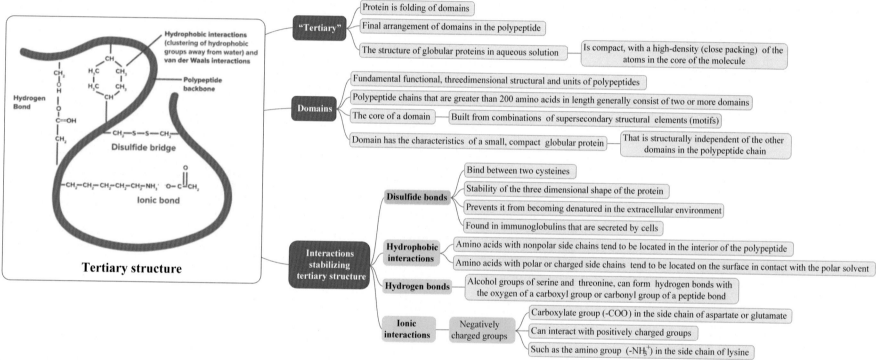

2.4. Quaternary structure

Quaternary structure is the three-dimensional structure consisting from two or more individual polypeptide chains (subunits) held together by non-covalent (Hydrophobic intersections, Hydrogen bond, and Ionic bonds) that operate as a single functional unit. For example, such as the two alpha and two beta chains of hemoglobin.

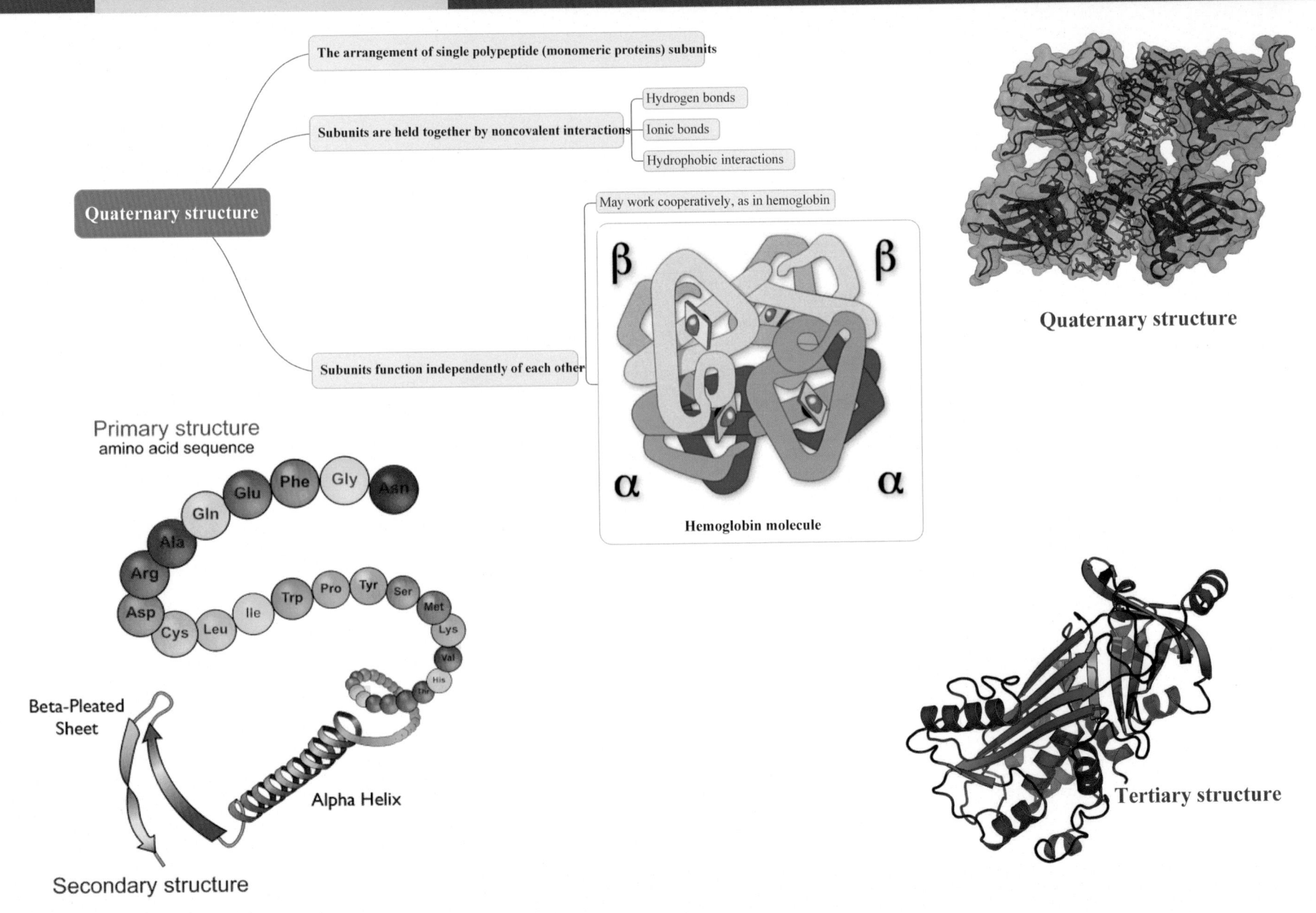

The arrangement of single polypeptide (monomeric proteins) subunits

Subunits are held together by noncovalent interactions
- Hydrogen bonds
- Ionic bonds
- Hydrophobic interactions

May work cooperatively, as in hemoglobin

Quaternary structure

Subunits function independently of each other

β   β

α   α

Hemoglobin molecule

Quaternary structure

Primary structure
amino acid sequence

Glu Phe Gly Asn
Gln
Ala
Arg
Asp   Cys Leu Ile Trp Pro Tyr Ser Met Lys Val His Thr

Beta-Pleated
Sheet

Alpha Helix

Secondary structure

Tertiary structure

20

2.5. Protein folding

Protein folding is the process by which a proteinstructure assumes its functional shape or conformation. All protein molecules are heterogeneous unbranched chains of amino acids. By coiling and folding into a specific three-dimensional shape they are able to perform their biological function.

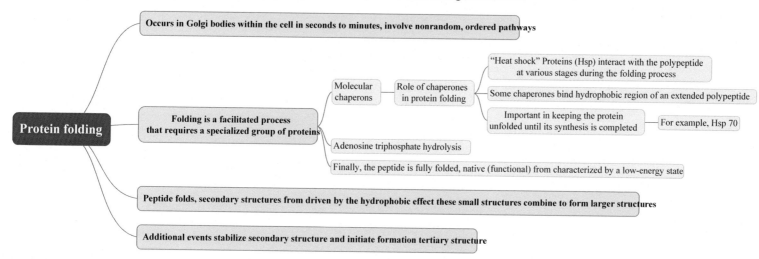

Protein folding

- Occurs in Golgi bodies within the cell in seconds to minutes, involve nonrandom, ordered pathways
- Folding is a facilitated process that requires a specialized group of proteins
  - Molecular chaperons
    - Role of chaperones in protein folding
      - "Heat shock" Proteins (Hsp) interact with the polypeptide at various stages during the folding process
      - Some chaperones bind hydrophobic region of an extended polypeptide
      - Important in keeping the protein unfolded until its synthesis is completed — For example, Hsp 70
  - Adenosine triphosphate hydrolysis
  - Finally, the peptide is fully folded, native (functional) from characterized by a low-energy state
- Peptide folds, secondary structures from driven by the hydrophobic effect these small structures combine to form larger structures
- Additional events stabilize secondary structure and initiate formation tertiary structure

2.6.Denaturation of proteins

Denaturation of proteins involves the disruption and possible destruction of both the secondary, tertiary, and quaternary structures. Since denaturation reactions are not strong enough to break the peptide bonds, the primary structure (sequence of amino acids) remains the same after adenaturation process.

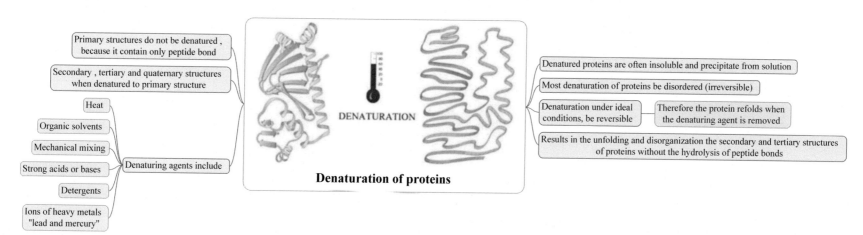

- Primary structures do not be denatured , because it contain only peptide bond
- Secondary , tertiary and quaternary structures when denatured to primary structure
- Denaturing agents include
  - Heat
  - Organic solvents
  - Mechanical mixing
  - Strong acids or bases
  - Detergents
  - Ions of heavy metals "lead and mercury"

DENATURATION

Denaturation of proteins

- Denatured proteins are often insoluble and precipitate from solution
- Most denaturation of proteins be disordered (irreversible)
- Denaturation under ideal conditions, be reversible — Therefore the protein refolds when the denaturing agent is removed
- Results in the unfolding and disorganization the secondary and tertiary structures of proteins without the hydrolysis of peptide bonds

2.7. Protein misfolding disease / Prion disease

In medicine, protein misfolding disease refers to a class of diseases in which certain proteins become structurally abnormal, and thereby disrupt the function of cells, tissues and organs of the body. Often the proteins fail to fold into their normal configuration. In addition misfolded proteins can become toxic in some way or they can lose their normal function. The protein misfolding diseases include such diseases as Creutzfeldt–Jakob disease and other prion diseases, Alzheimer's disease, and Parkinson's disease.

2.8. Protein misfolding disease / Amyloid disease

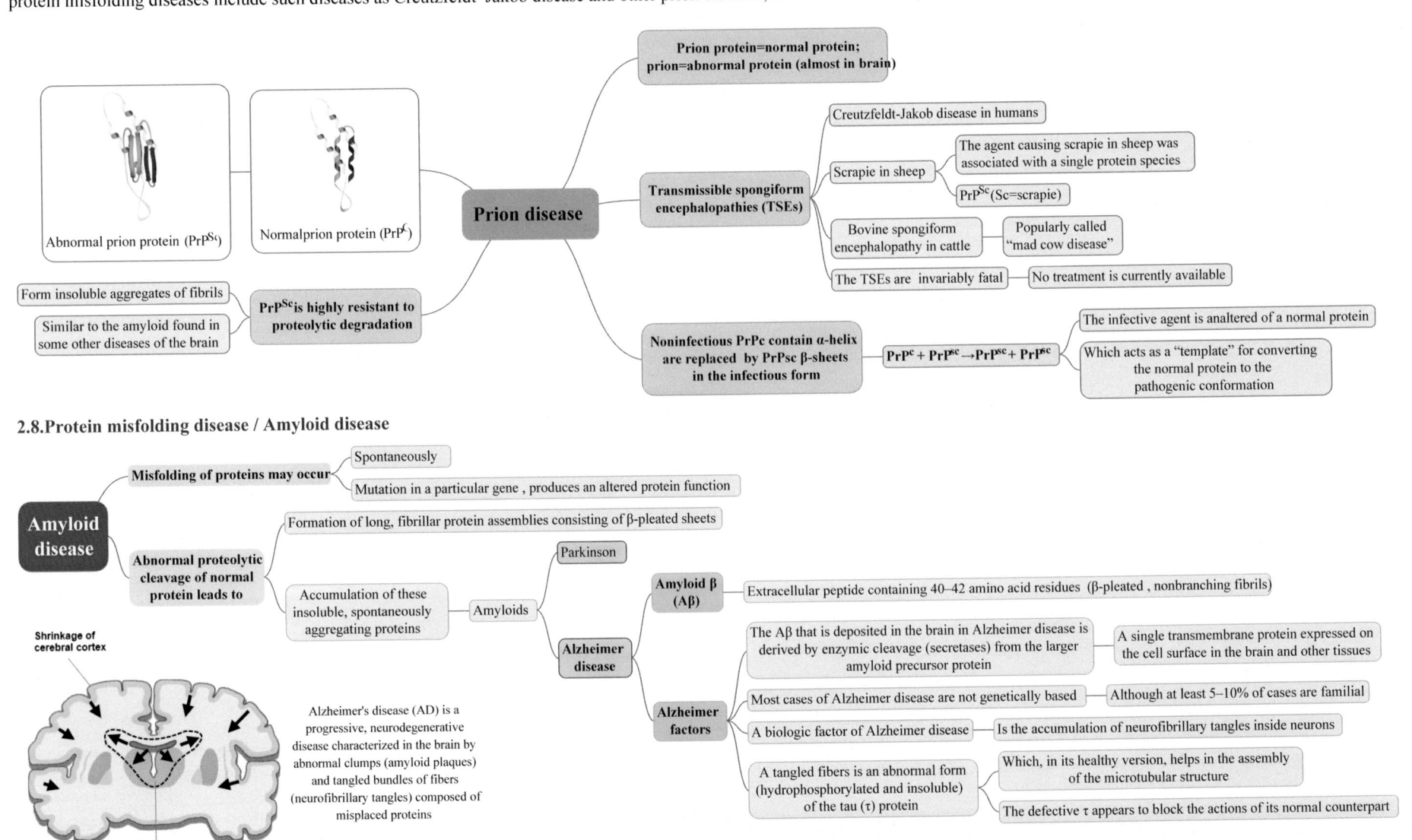

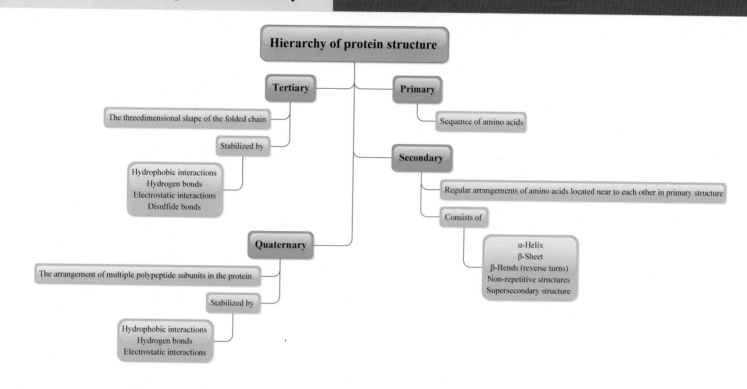

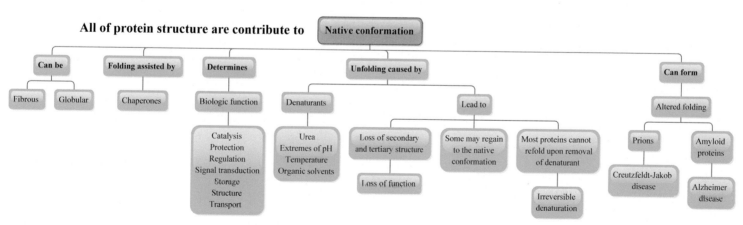

Q 1: Circle the best correct answer:

1. Which of the following statements is true about a peptide bond (RCONHR')?
a. It is non-planar.
b. It is capable of forming a hydrogen bond.
c. The Cis configuration is favoured over the trans configuration.
d. Single bond rotation is permitted between nitrogen and the carbonyl group.

2. Which of the following statements is false about protein secondary structure?
a. The alpha helix, beta pleated sheet and beta turns are examples of protein secondary structure.
b. The ability of peptide bonds to form hydrogen bonds is important to secondary structure.
c. The steric influence of amino acid residues is important to secondary structure.
d. The hydrophilic/hydrophobic character of amino acid residues is important to secondary structure.

3. In the α-helix the hydrogen bonds:
a. are roughly parallel to the axis of the helix.
b. are roughly perpendicular to the axis of the helix.
c. occur mainly between electronegative atoms of the R groups.
d. occur only between some of the amino acids of the helix.
f. occur only near the amino and carboxyl termini of the helix.

4. In an α-helix, the R groups on the amino acid residues:
a. alternate between the outside and the inside of the helix.
b. are found on the outside of the helix spiral.
c. cause only right-handed helices to form.
d. generate the hydrogen bonds that form the helix.
g. stack within the interior of the helix.

5. Thr and/or Leu residues tend to disrupt an α-helix when they occur next to each other in a protein because:
a. an amino acids like Thr is highly hydrophobic.
b. covalent interactions may occur between the Thr side chains.
c. electrostatic repulsion occurs between the Thr side chains.
d. steric hindrance occurs between the bulky Thr side chains.

6. If lysine and arginine are adjacent together that is cause disrupt an α-helix because:
a. forming H-bond
b. Isoleucine change the direction of polypeptide chain
c. electrostatic repulsion
d. steric hindrance

7. Which of the following statements about β-turn is incorrect?
a. β-Bends reverse the direction of a polypeptide chain
b. found on the surface of protein
c. isoleucine and leucine also found in β-turn
d. stabilize by hydrogen and ionic bond

8. Which of the following amino acid residues is commonly found in the middle of β-turn?
a. Ala and Gly.
b. hydrophobic.
c. Pro and Gly.
d. those with ionized R-groups.
e. two Cys.

9. Which of the following terms refers to the arrangement of different protein subunits in a multiprotein complex?
a. primary structure
b. secondary structure
c. tertiary structure
d. quaternary structure

10. Which of the following terms refers to the overall three dimensional shape of a protein?
a. primary structure
b. secondary structure
c. tertiary structure
d. quaternary structure

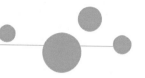

Q 1: Circle the best correct answer:

11. Which of the following terms refers to 'regions of ordered structure within a protein'?
a. primary structure
b. secondary structure
c. tertiary structure
d. quaternary structure

12. Which type of bonding is responsible for stabilize the secondary structure of proteins?
a. Disulphide bridges between cysteine residues.
b. Hydrogen bonding between the C=O and N-H groups of peptide bonds.
c. Peptide bonds between amino acids.
d. Salt bridges between charged side chains of amino acids.

13. Which of the following amino acids that disrupt an α-helix?
a. Proline within protein
b. Leucine and isoleucine adjacent to gather
c. Glycine
d. both a and b

14. Which of the following most accurately describes how secondary structures in proteins are stabilised?
a. Through ionic bonds operating between oppositely charged amino acid side chains.
b. Through covalent bonds joining different parts of the peptide backbone
c. Through hydrogen bonds between different amino acid side chains.
d. Through hydrogen bonds joining different parts of the peptide backbone

15. Which of the following statements is the best describes a protein domain?
a. The α-helical portion of a protein.
b. A discrete region of polypeptide chain that has folded into a self-contained three-dimensional structure.
c. The β-pleated sheet portion of a protein.
d. A feature that rarely occurs in globular proteins.

16. Proteins often have regions that show specific, coherent patterns of folding or function. These regions are called:
a. domains.
b. oligomers.
c. peptides.
d. sites.
e. subunits

17. Which of the following statements is the best describes a secondary structure?
a. spiral structure, consisting of a tightly packed, coiled polypeptide backbone core.
b. The side chains extending outward from the central axis.
c. stabilized by extensive hydrogen bonding between the peptide-bond & Each turn of an α-helix contains 3.6 amino acids
d. all of these

18. Which of the following statements is true about the β-Bends reverse the direction of a polypeptide chain?
a. found on the interior of protein, and often include charged residues.
b. found on the surface of protein, and often include charged residues.
c. found on the glycoproteins.
d. Found on lipid and carbohydrate

19. Which one of the following secondary structures of protein is stabilized by hydrogen bond and ionic bond?
a. β-sheet
b. α-Helix
c. Supersecondary structures (motifs)
d. β-Bends

20. The structure of Helix-loop helix and β-α-β unit is
a. β-sheet
b. α-Helix
c. Supersecondary structures (motifs)
d. β-Bends

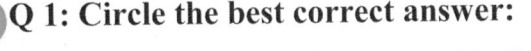

Q 1: Circle the best correct answer:

21. The core of a domain is built from combinations of
a. α-Helix
b. β-Bends
c. α-sheet
d. supersecondary

22. Folding protein is a facilitated process that requires a specialized group of proteins such as:
a. only, chaperons
b. chaperons and adenosine triphosphate hydrolysis.
C. Charcoal and adenosine triphosphate hydrolysis.
d. Only, Adenosine triphosphate hydrolysis only

23. Folding process depends on:
a. chaperones bind hydrophobic region of an extended polypeptide until its synthesis is completed.
b. chaperones bind hydrophilic region of an extended polypeptide until its synthesis is completed.
c. chaperones cause unfolding of protein.
d. Denatured proteins are often insoluble and precipitate from solution.

24. The factors that cause Alzheimer disease is:
a. Accumulation amyloid β (Aβ) and neurofibrillary tangles.
b. a. Accumulation amyloid β (Aβ) and neurofibrillary tau (τ) protein
c. a. Accumulation of abnormal prion.
d. virus infection

25. Non-infectious prion (PrPc) contain α-helix are replaced with…… in the infectious prion form:
a. β-sheets
b. β-turns
c. Supersecondary structures
d. Nonrepetitive secondary structure

26. The Prion disease in human is called:
a. bovine spongiform encephalopathy (mad cow disease)
b. Creutzfeldt-Jakob
c. scrapie
d. Parkinson disease

27. After Denaturation the tertiary structure proteins, It will be converted to:
a. Primary structure
b. Secondary structure
c. Tertiary structure
d. Quaternary structure

28. The differences between the Noninfectious PrPc and the infectious form PrPsc is:
a. PrPc contain α-helix are replaced by β-sheets in PrPsc
b. PrPc contain α-helix are replaced by Nonrepetitive secondary in PrPsc
c. PrPc contain supersecondary are replaced by β-bends in PrPsc
d. PrPc contain tertiary structure are replaced by quaternary structure in PrPsc

27. After Denaturation the tertiary structure proteins, It will be converted to:
a. Primary structure
b. Secondary structure
c. Tertiary structure
d. Quaternary structure

28. The differences between the Noninfectious PrPc and the infectious form PrPsc is:
a. PrPc contain α-helix are replaced by β-sheets inPrPsc
b. PrPc contain α-helix are replaced by Nonrepetitive secondary inPrPsc
c. PrPc contain supersecondary are replaced by β-bends inPrPsc
d. PrPc contain tertiary structure are replaced by quaternary structure inPrPsc

Q 1: Circle the best correct answer:

29. α-helix is stabilized by
a. Hydrogen bonds
b. Disulphide bonds
c. Salt bonds
d. Non-polar bonds

30. Each turn of α-helix contains……… amino acid residues:
a. 3.6
b. 3.0
c. 4.2
d. 4.5

31. The α-helix and β-pleated sheet are examples of:
a. Primary structure
b. Secondary structure
c. Tertiary structure
d. Quaternary structure

32. The a-helix of proteins is
a. A pleated structure
b. Made periodic by disulphide bridges
c. A non-periodic structure
d. Stabilised by hydrogen bonds between NH and CO groups of the main chain

33. An amino acid that does not take part in α helix formation is:
a. Histidine
b. Tyrosine
c. Proline
d. Glycine

34. During denaturation of proteins, all of the following are disrupted except :
a. Primary structure
b. Secondary structure
c. Tertiary structure
d. Quaternary structure

35. Denaturation of proteins involves breakdown of
a. Secondary structure
b. Tertiary structure
c. Quaternary structure
d. All of these

36. In quaternary structure, subunits are linked by
a. Peptide bonds
b. Disulphide bonds
c. Covalent bonds
d. Non-covalent bonds

37. The bond in proteins that is not hydrolyzed under usual conditions of denaturation:
a. Hydrophobic bond
b. Hydrogen bond
c. Disulphide bond
d. Peptide bonds

38. The glycyltyrosylleucine has………….peptides bond:
a. 2
b. 3
c. 4
d. 4

Q 2: Write short notes on:

a. Characteristics of the peptide bond.
b. α-Helix
c. B. β-sheet
d. Chaperone
e. Domains
f. Quaternary structure of proteins
g. Denaturation of proteins
h. Prion disease
i. Alzheimer factors
j. Amino acid that disrupt an α-Helix
k. The interactions that stabilize the tertiary structure

Q 3: Explain

a. Most denaturation of proteins are irreversible
b. Primary structure of proteins are not denatured
c. Proline cause disrupt an α-Helix

OVERVIEW

Widely diverse proteins can be constructed that are capable of various specialized functions. This chapter examines the relationship between structure and function for the clinically important globular hemeproteins, as example globular proteins are one of the common protein types . Globular proteins are somewhat water-soluble (forming colloids in water), unlike the fibrous or membrane proteins. There are multiple fold classes of globular proteins, since there are many different architectures that can fold into a roughly spherical shape. The term globin can refer more specifically to proteins including the globin fold.

3.1. Globular hemeproteins

Heme of hemoglobin protein is a prosthetic group of heterocyclic ring of porphyrin of an iron atom; the biological function of the group is for delivering oxygen to body tissues, such that bonding of ligand of gas molecules to the iron atom of the protein group changes the structure of the protein by amino acid group.

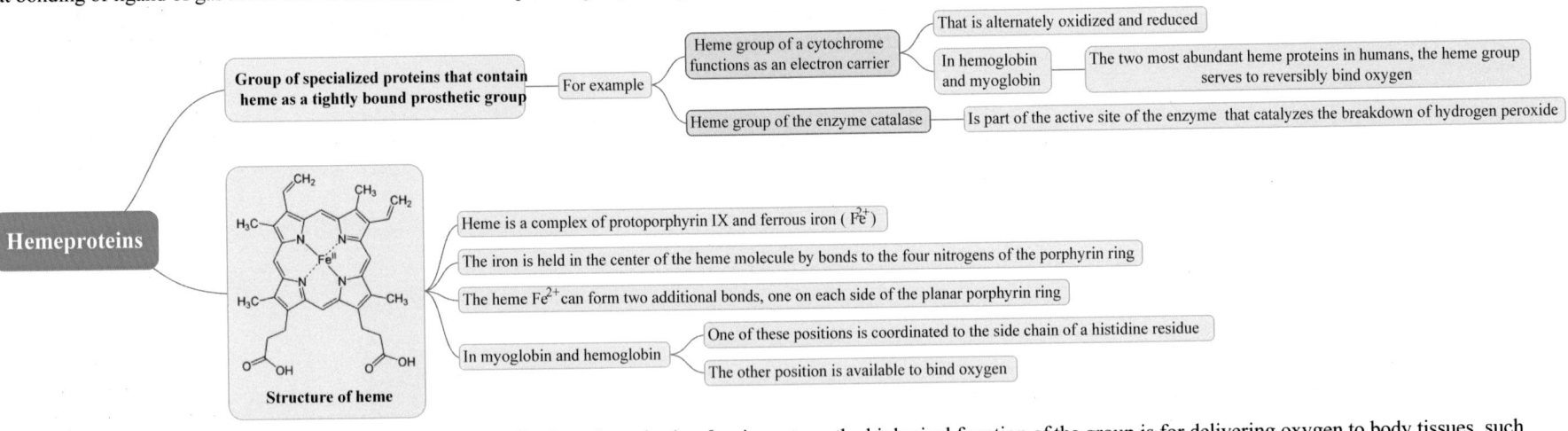

Hemeproteins

Group of specialized proteins that contain heme as a tightly bound prosthetic group

For example

Heme group of a cytochrome functions as an electron carrier — That is alternately oxidized and reduced

In hemoglobin and myoglobin — The two most abundant heme proteins in humans, the heme group serves to reversibly bind oxygen

Heme group of the enzyme catalase — Is part of the active site of the enzyme that catalyzes the breakdown of hydrogen peroxide

Heme is a complex of protoporphyrin IX and ferrous iron (Fe^{2+})

The iron is held in the center of the heme molecule by bonds to the four nitrogens of the porphyrin ring

The heme Fe^{2+} can form two additional bonds, one on each side of the planar porphyrin ring

In myoglobin and hemoglobin
- One of these positions is coordinated to the side chain of a histidine residue
- The other position is available to bind oxygen

Structure of heme

Heme of hemoglobin protein is a prosthetic group of heterocyclic ring of porphyrin of an iron atom; the biological function of the group is for delivering oxygen to body tissues, such that bonding of ligand of gas molecules to the iron atom of the protein group changes the structure of the protein by amino acid group.

Quaternary structure of hemoglobin

The hemoglobin composed of two identical dimers, $(\alpha\beta)1$ and $(\alpha\beta)2$

α-subunits and β-subunits within each dimer are held together by hydrophobic interactions in both interior and surface of each subunit

The two dimer held together by polar bonds (hydrogen an ionic bonds)

The weaker interactions between dimers result in the two dimers occupying different relative positions in deoxyhemoglobin (T form) as compared with oxyhemoglobin (R form)

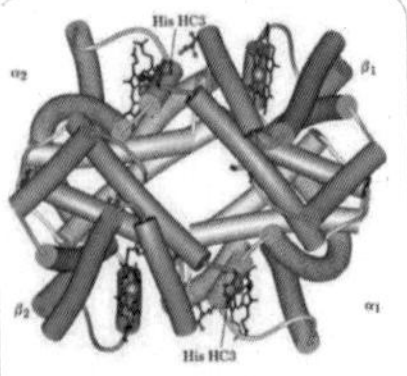

T or taut (tense) form
- The deoxy form of hemoglobin
- the two $\alpha\beta$ dimers interact through a network of ionic bonds and hydrogen bonds that constrain the movement of the polypeptide chains
- The T form is the low oxygen affinity form of hemoglobin

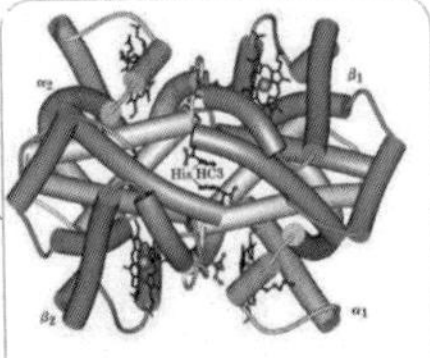

R or relaxed form
- The binding of oxygen to hemoglobin causes the rupture of some of the ionic bonds and hydrogen bonds between the $\alpha\beta$ dimers
- In R form the polypeptide chains have more freedom of movement
- The R form is the high oxygen affinity form of hemoglobin

Chapter 3 : Globular proteins

A hemeprotein is a protein that contains a heme prosthetic group. They are a large class of metalloproteins. The heme group confers functionality, which can include oxygen carrying, oxygen reduction, electron transfer, and other processes. Hemoglobin is the protein molecule in red blood cells that carries oxygen from the lungs to the body's tissues and returns carbon dioxide from the tissues back to the lungs. Hemoglobin is made up of four protein molecules (globulin chains) that are connected together by non-covalent bond.

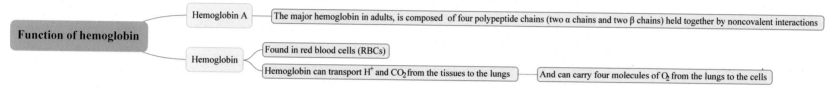

Function of hemoglobin
- Hemoglobin A — The major hemoglobin in adults, is composed of four polypeptide chains (two α chains and two β chains) held together by noncovalent interactions
- Hemoglobin
  - Found in red blood cells (RBCs)
  - Hemoglobin can transport H^+ and CO_2 from the tissues to the lungs — And can carry four molecules of O_2 from the lungs to the cells

Myoglobin is an iron and oxygen-binding protein found in the muscle tissue of vertebrates in general and in almost all mammals. It is distantly related to hemoglobin which is the iron- and oxygen-binding protein in blood, specifically in the red blood cells.

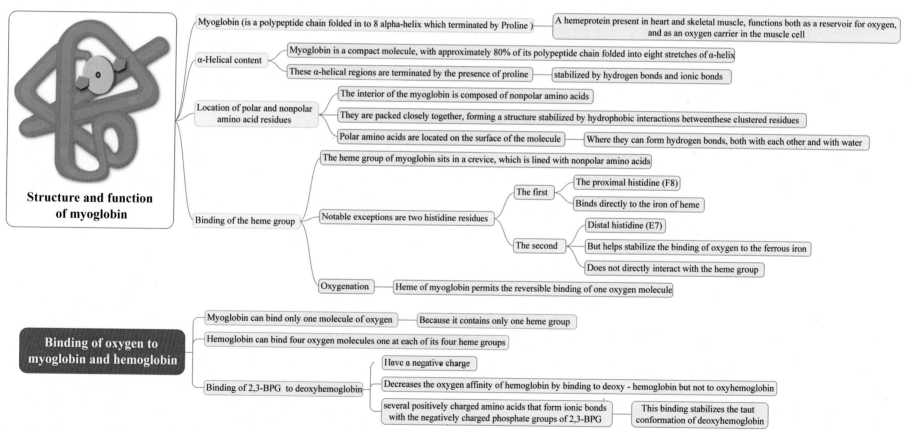

Structure and function of myoglobin
- Myoglobin (is a polypeptide chain folded in to 8 alpha-helix which terminated by Proline) — A hemeprotein present in heart and skeletal muscle, functions both as a reservoir for oxygen, and as an oxygen carrier in the muscle cell
- α-Helical content
  - Myoglobin is a compact molecule, with approximately 80% of its polypeptide chain folded into eight stretches of α-helix
  - These α-helical regions are terminated by the presence of proline — stabilized by hydrogen bonds and ionic bonds
- Location of polar and nonpolar amino acid residues
  - The interior of the myoglobin is composed of nonpolar amino acids
  - They are packed closely together, forming a structure stabilized by hydrophobic interactions betweenthese clustered residues
  - Polar amino acids are located on the surface of the molecule — Where they can form hydrogen bonds, both with each other and with water
- Binding of the heme group
  - The heme group of myoglobin sits in a crevice, which is lined with nonpolar amino acids
  - Notable exceptions are two histidine residues
    - The first
      - The proximal histidine (F8)
      - Binds directly to the iron of heme
    - The second
      - Distal histidine (E7)
      - But helps stabilize the binding of oxygen to the ferrous iron
      - Does not directly interact with the heme group
  - Oxygenation — Heme of myoglobin permits the reversible binding of one oxygen molecule

Binding of oxygen to myoglobin and hemoglobin
- Myoglobin can bind only one molecule of oxygen — Because it contains only one heme group
- Hemoglobin can bind four oxygen molecules one at each of its four heme groups
- Binding of 2,3-BPG to deoxyhemoglobin
  - Have a negative charge
  - Decreases the oxygen affinity of hemoglobin by binding to deoxy - hemoglobin but not to oxyhemoglobin
  - several positively charged amino acids that form ionic bonds with the negatively charged phosphate groups of 2,3-BPG — This binding stabilizes the taut conformation of deoxyhemoglobin

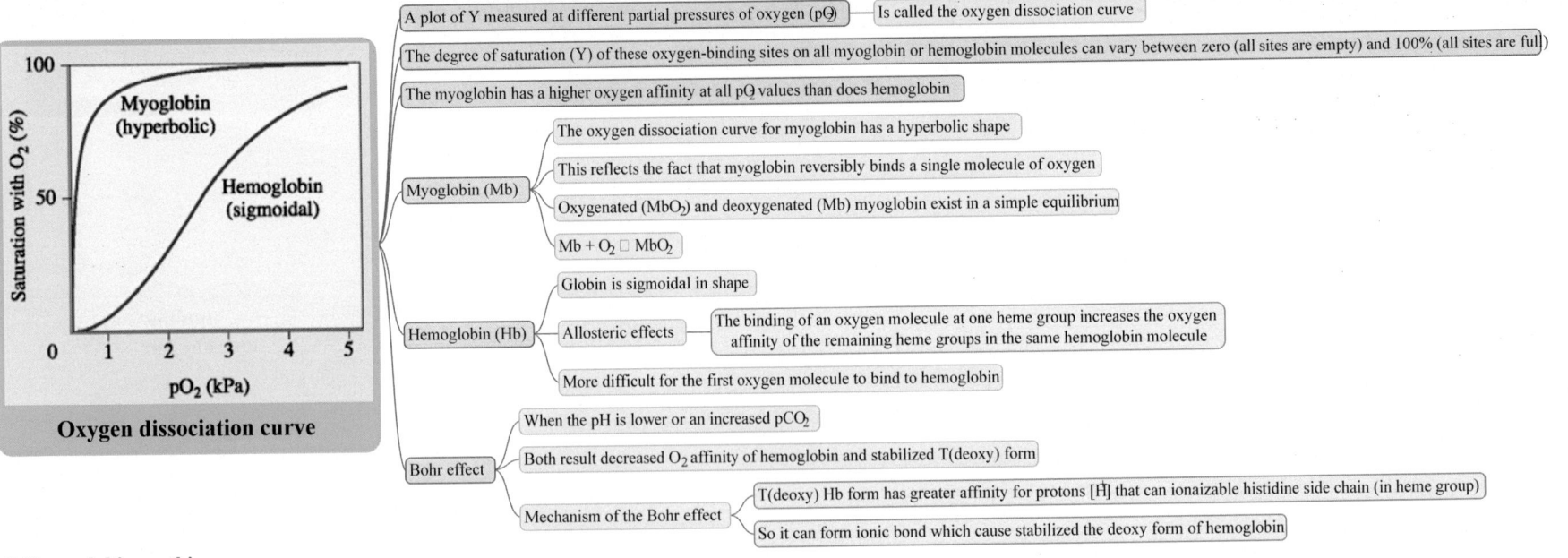

A plot of Y measured at different partial pressures of oxygen (pO$_2$) — Is called the oxygen dissociation curve

The degree of saturation (Y) of these oxygen-binding sites on all myoglobin or hemoglobin molecules can vary between zero (all sites are empty) and 100% (all sites are full)

The myoglobin has a higher oxygen affinity at all pO$_2$ values than does hemoglobin

Myoglobin (Mb)
- The oxygen dissociation curve for myoglobin has a hyperbolic shape
- This reflects the fact that myoglobin reversibly binds a single molecule of oxygen
- Oxygenated (MbO$_2$) and deoxygenated (Mb) myoglobin exist in a simple equilibrium
- Mb + O$_2$ ⇌ MbO$_2$

Hemoglobin (Hb)
- Globin is sigmoidal in shape
- Allosteric effects — The binding of an oxygen molecule at one heme group increases the oxygen affinity of the remaining heme groups in the same hemoglobin molecule
- More difficult for the first oxygen molecule to bind to hemoglobin

Bohr effect
- When the pH is lower or an increased pCO$_2$
- Both result decreased O$_2$ affinity of hemoglobin and stabilized T(deoxy) form
- Mechanism of the Bohr effect
  - T(deoxy) Hb form has greater affinity for protons [H] that can ionaizable histidine side chain (in heme group)
  - So it can form ionic bond which cause stabilized the deoxy form of hemoglobin

Oxygen dissociation curve

3.2.Hemoglobinopathies

Hemoglobinopathies defined as a family of genetic disorders caused by production of a structurally abnormal hemoglobin molecule

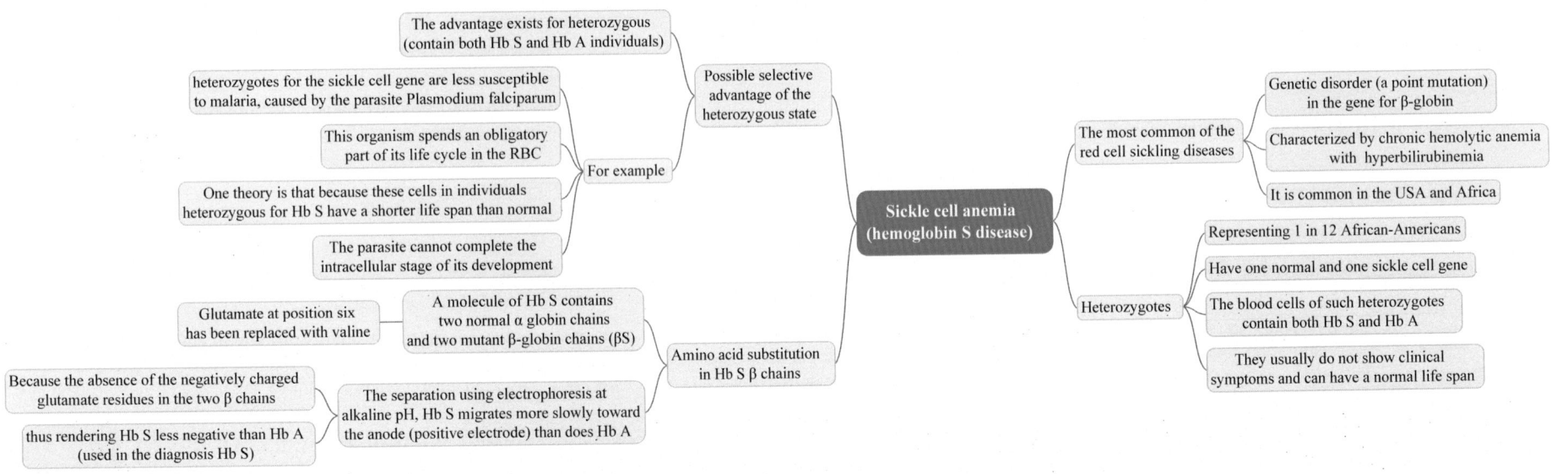

Sickle cell anemia (hemoglobin S disease)

Possible selective advantage of the heterozygous state
- The advantage exists for heterozygous (contain both Hb S and Hb A individuals)
- For example
  - heterozygotes for the sickle cell gene are less susceptible to malaria, caused by the parasite Plasmodium falciparum
  - This organism spends an obligatory part of its life cycle in the RBC
  - One theory is that because these cells in individuals heterozygous for Hb S have a shorter life span than normal
  - The parasite cannot complete the intracellular stage of its development

Amino acid substitution in Hb S β chains
- A molecule of Hb S contains two normal α globin chains and two mutant β-globin chains (βS)
  - Glutamate at position six has been replaced with valine
- The separation using electrophoresis at alkaline pH, Hb S migrates more slowly toward the anode (positive electrode) than does Hb A
  - Because the absence of the negatively charged glutamate residues in the two β chains
  - thus rendering Hb S less negative than Hb A (used in the diagnosis Hb S)

The most common of the red cell sickling diseases
- Genetic disorder (a point mutation) in the gene for β-globin
- Characterized by chronic hemolytic anemia with hyperbilirubinemia
- It is common in the USA and Africa

Heterozygotes
- Representing 1 in 12 African-Americans
- Have one normal and one sickle cell gene
- The blood cells of such heterozygotes contain both Hb S and Hb A
- They usually do not show clinical symptoms and can have a normal life span

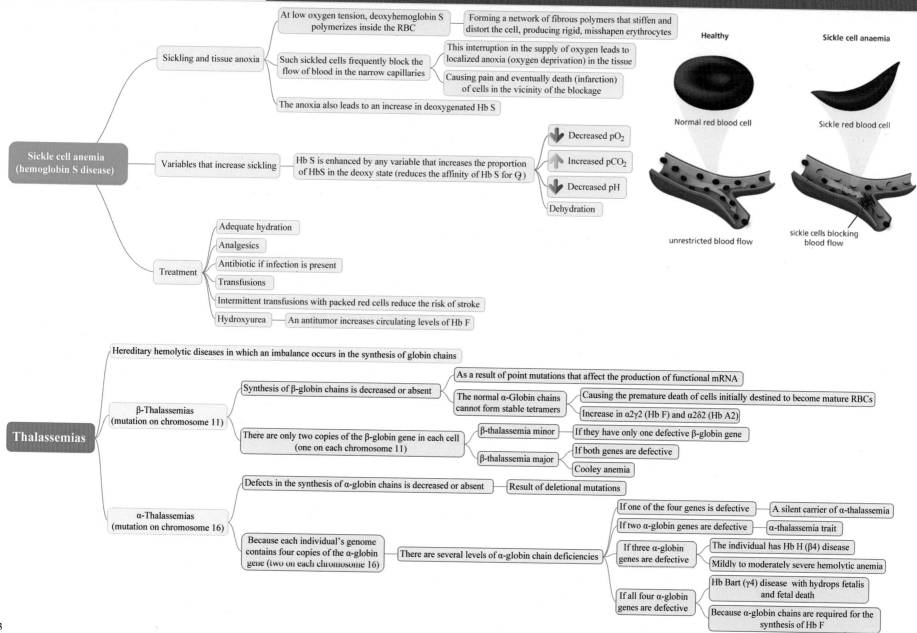

Sickle cell anemia (hemoglobin S disease)

Sickling and tissue anoxia
- At low oxygen tension, deoxyhemoglobin S polymerizes inside the RBC
  - Forming a network of fibrous polymers that stiffen and distort the cell, producing rigid, misshapen erythrocytes
- Such sickled cells frequently block the flow of blood in the narrow capillaries
  - This interruption in the supply of oxygen leads to localized anoxia (oxygen deprivation) in the tissue
  - Causing pain and eventually death (infarction) of cells in the vicinity of the blockage
- The anoxia also leads to an increase in deoxygenated Hb S

Variables that increase sickling
- Hb S is enhanced by any variable that increases the proportion of HbS in the deoxy state (reduces the affinity of Hb S for O_2)
  - ↓ Decreased pO_2
  - ↑ Increased pCO_2
  - ↓ Decreased pH
  - Dehydration

Treatment
- Adequate hydration
- Analgesics
- Antibiotic if infection is present
- Transfusions
- Intermittent transfusions with packed red cells reduce the risk of stroke
- Hydroxyurea — An antitumor increases circulating levels of Hb F

Thalassemias

- Hereditary hemolytic diseases in which an imbalance occurs in the synthesis of globin chains

β-Thalassemias (mutation on chromosome 11)
- Synthesis of β-globin chains is decreased or absent
  - As a result of point mutations that affect the production of functional mRNA
- The normal α-Globin chains cannot form stable tetramers
  - Causing the premature death of cells initially destined to become mature RBCs
  - Increase in α2γ2 (Hb F) and α2δ2 (Hb A2)
- There are only two copies of the β-globin gene in each cell (one on each chromosome 11)
  - β-thalassemia minor — If they have only one defective β-globin gene
  - β-thalassemia major
    - If both genes are defective
    - Cooley anemia

α-Thalassemias (mutation on chromosome 16)
- Defects in the synthesis of α-globin chains is decreased or absent — Result of deletional mutations
- Because each individual's genome contains four copies of the α-globin gene (two on each chromosome 16)
  - There are several levels of α-globin chain deficiencies
    - If one of the four genes is defective — A silent carrier of α-thalassemia
    - If two α-globin genes are defective — α-thalassemia trait
    - If three α-globin genes are defective
      - The individual has Hb H (β4) disease
      - Mildly to moderately severe hemolytic anemia
    - If all four α-globin genes are defective
      - Hb Bart (γ4) disease with hydrops fetalis and fetal death
      - Because α-globin chains are required for the synthesis of Hb F

In Hb C mutantion in β-globin chains, in which glutamate at position six has been replaced with lysine

Patients homozygous for hemoglobin C generally have a relatively mild, chronic hemolytic anemia

Hemoglobin C disease

β-globin chains have the two sickle cell mutation, β-globin chains carry the mutation found in Hb S and Hb C disease

Hemoglobin levels tend to be higher in Hb SC disease than in sickle cell anemia — May even be at the low end of the normal range

3.3.Diagram of the shape of the hemoglobin molecule found in r ed blood cells that carries the oxygen

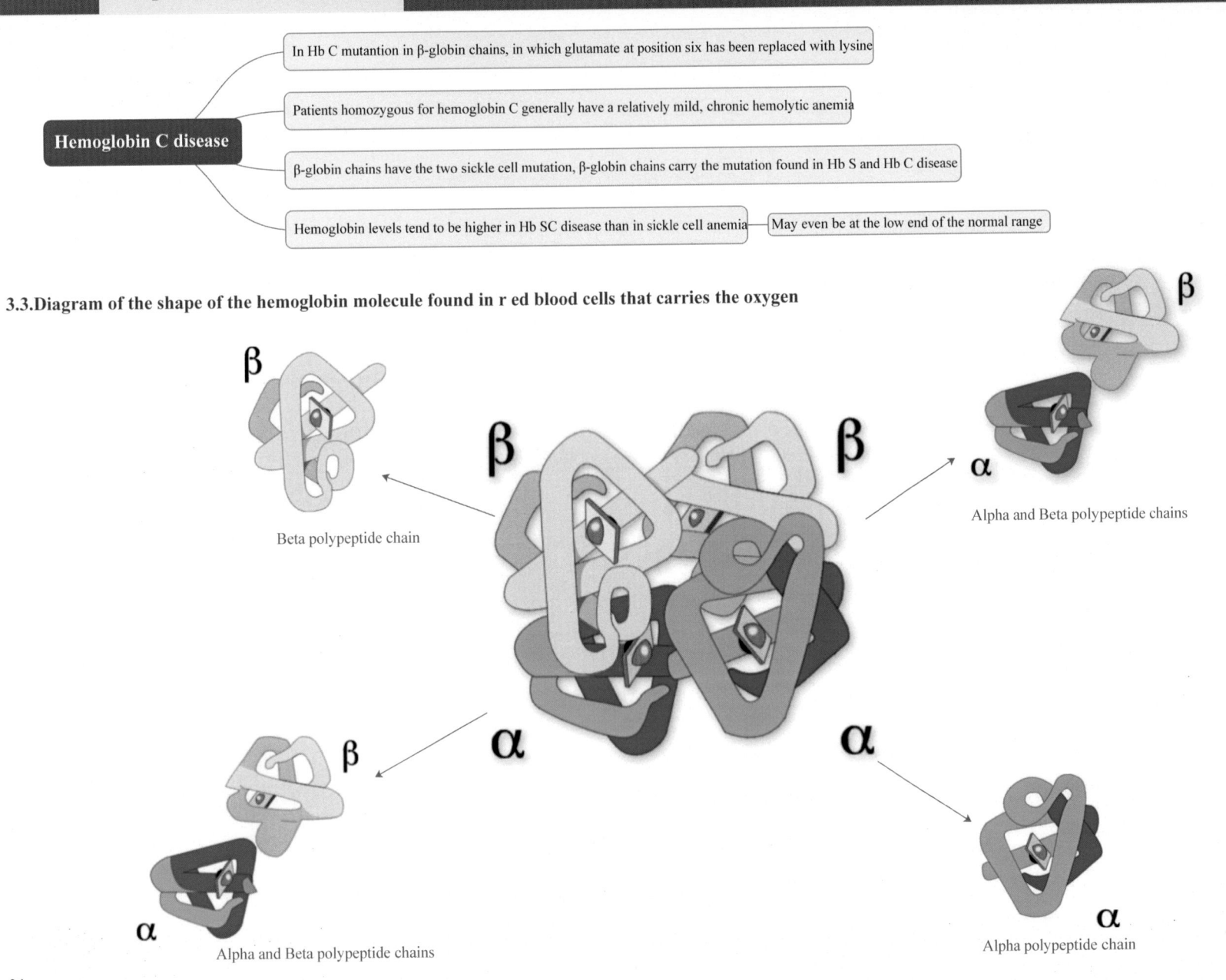

Beta polypeptide chain

Alpha and Beta polypeptide chains

Alpha and Beta polypeptide chains

Alpha polypeptide chain

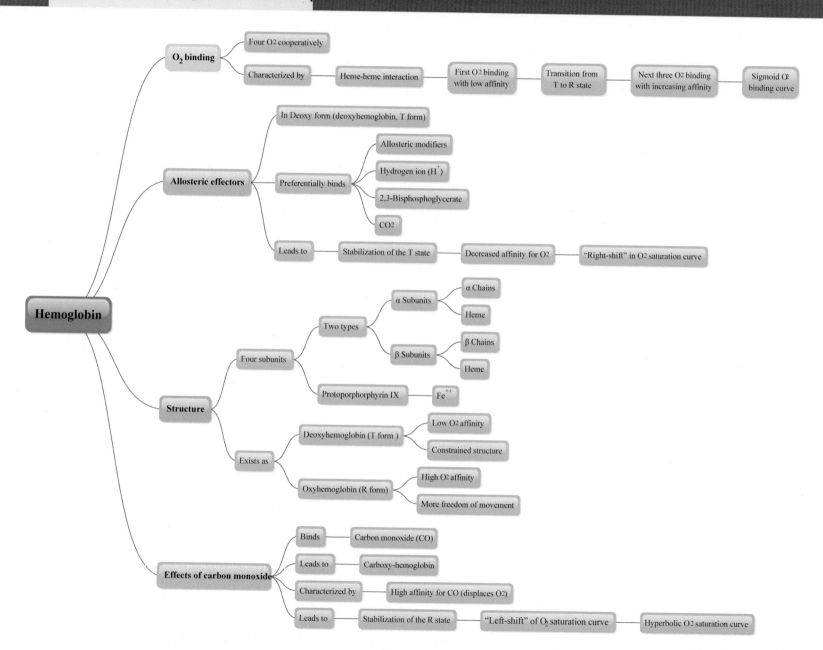

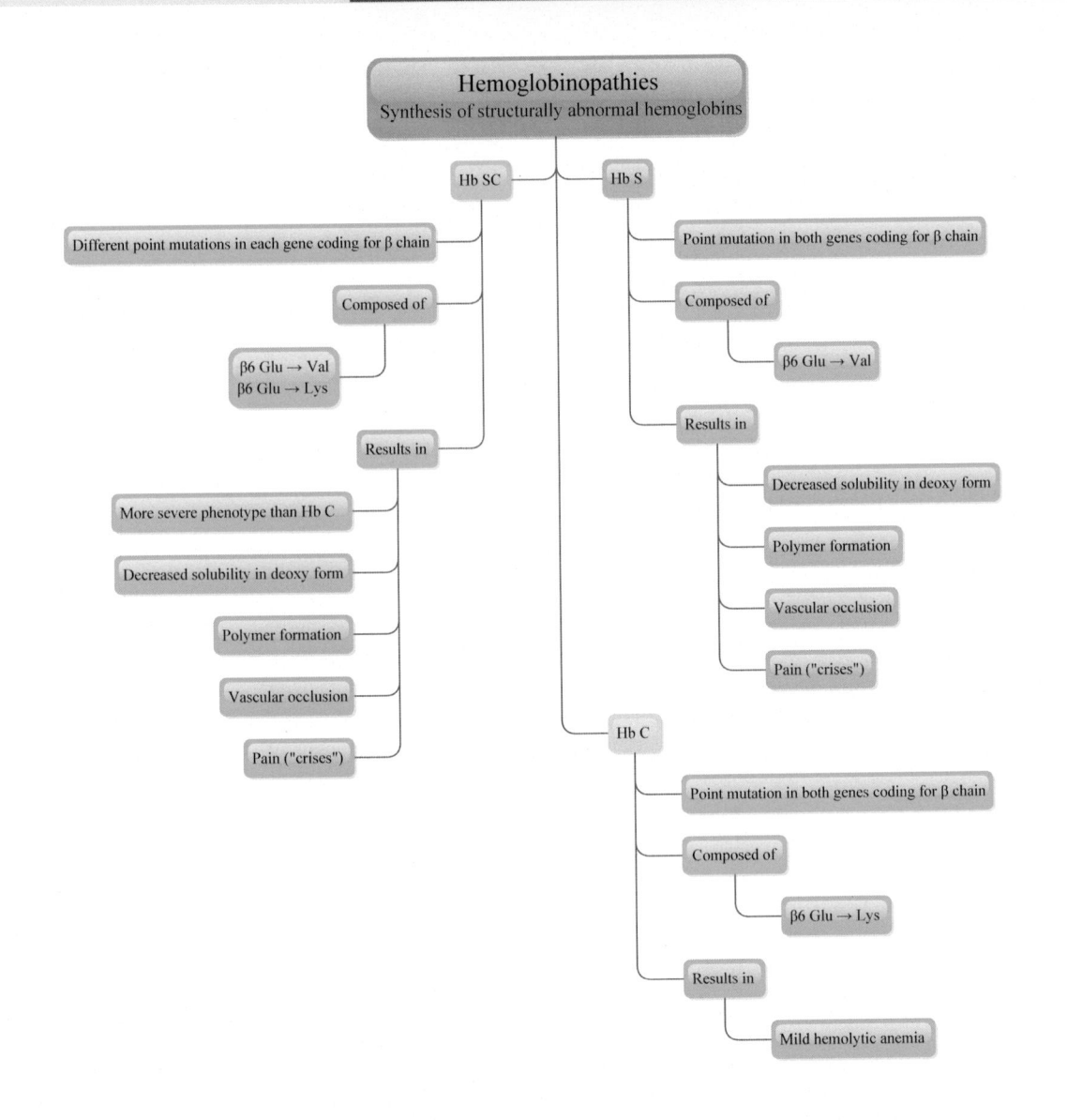

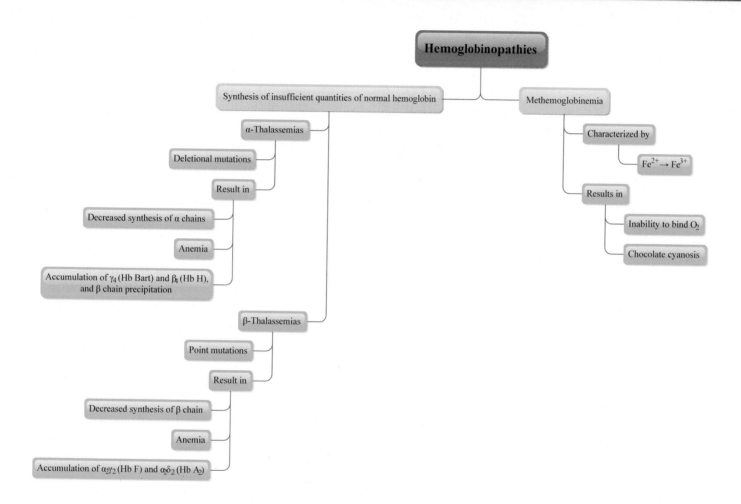

Globular proteins : E x e r c i s e s

Q 1: Circle the best correct answer:

1. Iron in the center of the heme that bond to the four nitrogen's of the porphyrin ring and two additional bond with:
a. One coordinated to the histidine residue , the other position is free .
b. One coordinated to the histidine residue , the other position is to bind oxygen.
c. Two positions is coordinated to the side chain of a histidine residue.
d. Two position is available to bind oxygen.

2. Myoglobin structure is:
a. each α-helix terminated by proline.
b. eight stretches of α-helix.
c. stabilized by hydrogen bonds and ionic bonds.
d. all of these

3. Hemoglobin stabilized by:
a. hydrogen bonds.
b. ionic bonds.
c. hydrophobic interaction
d. all of these

4. The function of distal histidine (E7) is:
a. helps stabilize the binding of oxygen to the ferrous iron.
b. helps stabilize the heme group.
c. helps stabilize the binding of CO_2 to the ferrous iron.
d. no function

5. Myoglobin can transfer:
a. Four molecule of oxygen
b. Two molecule of oxygen
c. One molecule of oxygen
d. one atom of oxygen

6. Hemoglobin A, the major hemoglobin in adults, is composed of:
a. Two α chains and two β chains, held together by noncovalent interactions.
b. Two α chains and two β chains, held together by covalent interactions.
c. Two α chains and two β chains, held together by disulfide bond interactions.
d. Two α chains separated from another two β chains.

7. In hemoglobin, α and β-subunits within each dimer $(\alpha\beta)_1$ and $(\alpha\beta)_2$ are held together by:
a. ionic bond
b. hydrogen bond.
c. hydrophobic interactions
d. all of these

8. Taut (T) form is:
a. The deoxy form of hemoglobin.
b. two αβ dimers interact through high No. of ionic bonds and hydrogen bonds
c. low oxygen affinity form of hemoglobin.
d. all of these.

9. Relax (R) form is:
a. The oxyhemogobin form.
b. high oxygen affinity form of hemoglobin.
c. rupture of some of the ionic bonds and hydrogen bonds between the αβ dimers
d. all of these

10. What is the different between T form and R form?
a. Oxygen binding to the R form, but T form is not.
b. Partial ruptures in ionic bonds and hydrogen bonds between the (αβ) dimers.
c. both a and b.
d. The T form is the high oxygen affinity form of hemoglobin.

11. Hemoglobin can bind with:
a. Four molecule of oxygen
b. Two molecule of oxygen
c. One molecule of oxygen
d. four atom of oxygen

Globular proteins : Exercises

Q 1: Circle the best correct answer:

12. Which of the following statements is true about Oxygen dissociation curve?
a. The myoglobin has a higher oxygen affinity at all pO_2 values than does hemoglobin.
b. The myoglobin has a lower oxygen affinity at all pO_2 values than does hemoglobin.
c. The myoglobin and hemoglobin has a equal oxygen affinity at all pO_2 values.
d. all of these

13. Sigmoidal oxygen dissociation curve is a property of
a. Hemoglobin
b. Carboxyhaemoglobin
c. Myoglobin
d. Methaemoglobin

14. The oxygen dissociation curve for myoglobin has a
a. hyperbolic shape
b. sigmoidal shape
c. allosteric effect
d. hemoglobin

15. As hemoglobin binds oxygen molecules, its affinity for oxygen increases, driving the binding of further oxygen molecules. Which term best describes this phenomenon?
a. Catalysis
b. Saturation
c. allosteric effect
d. isomerism

16. Which of the following statements about Bohr Effect is incorrect?
a. Shifting of oxyhemoglobin dissociation curve to the right
b. Shifting of oxyhemoglobin dissociation curve to the left
c. T(deoxy) form is stable
d. Increased pCO_2 and decreased pO_2

17. Mutations in two β-globin gene, at position six the glutamate converts to valine cause the:
a. Hb C disease
b. Hb S disease
c. β- Thalassemias
d. α- Thalassemias

18. Mutations in two β-globin gene, at position six the glutamate converts to lysine cause the:
a. Hb C disease
b. Hb S disease (sickle cell)
c. β- Thalassemias
d. α- Thalassemias

19. Which of the following statements about heterozygous is correct?
a. less susceptible to malaria because the RBCs has short life.
b. have one normal and one sickle cell gene in β-globin gene of hemoglobin.
c. do not show clinical symptoms and can have a normal life span.
d. all of these

20. When the synthesis of β-globin chains in chromosome No 11 is complete absent that can be cause:
a. minor β-thalassemia
b. major β-thalassemia
c. Hemoglobin SC disease
d. α-Thalassemia

21. When the synthesis of α-globin chains in chromosome No 16 is decreased or absent that can be cause:
a. minor β-thalassemia
b. major β-thalassemia
c. Hemoglobin SC disease
d. α-thalassemia

Globular proteins : E xe r c i s e s

Q 1: Circle the best correct answer:

22.The reason of the major β-thalasemia is:
a. absent on one β-globin gene
b. absent one α-globin gene
c. absent on two β-globin gene
d. absent on four α-globin gene

23. Hemoglobin SC disease migrates to the negative electrode in electrophoresis because:
a. mutant β-globin chains, in which glutamate at position six has been replaced with valine
b. decrease or absent on four α-globin gene
c. mutant β-globin chains, in which glutamate at position six has been replaced with lysine
d. All off these

24.When oxygen binds to a heme-containing protein, the two open coordination bonds of Fe^{2+} are occupied by:
a. One O atom and one amino acid atom
b. One O_2 molecule and one amino acid atom
c. One O_2 molecule and one heme atom
d. Two O_2 molecules

Q 2: Write short notes on:

a. The difference between (T form) and (R form)
b. Sickle cell anemia
c. allosteric effects
d. Bohr effect
e. Major β-thalasemia
f. Oxygen dissociation curve for myoglobin and hemoglobin
g. Myoglobin

OVERVIEW

Fibrous proteins, also called scleroproteins, are long filamentous proteinmolecules. Fibrous proteins form 'rod' or 'wire' - like shapes and are usually inert structural or storage proteins. They are generally water-insoluble in water.Collagen is a member of a family of naturally occurring proteins. It is one of the most abundant proteins present in mammals and it is responsible for performing a variety of important biological functions. It is most well-known for the structural role it plays in the body. It is present in large quantities in connective tissue and provides tendons and ligaments with tensile strength and skin with elasticity and bones strength. It often works in conjunction with other important proteins such as keratin and elastin.Collagen and elastin are examples of common, well-characterized fibrous proteins of the extracellular matrix that serve structural functions in the body. For example, collagen and elastin are found as components of skin, connective tissue, blood vessel walls, and sclera and cornea of the eye. Each fibrous protein exhibits special mechanical properties, resulting from its unique structure, which are obtained by combining specific amino acids into regular, secondary structural elements.

Chapter 4 : Fibrous protein

4.1.1.Structure of collagen

The collagen molecules themselves are made from 3 individual polypeptides or strings of amino acids. The strands wind around one another in an alpha-chain. The helix forms because of the regular amino acid sequence of the strands. The sequence is a repeating pattern of glycine-proline-X, where X can be hydroxyproline or hydroxylysine. A special amino acid sequence makes the tight collagen triple helix particularly stable. The glycine forms a tiny elbow packed inside the helix, and the proline and hydroxyproline smoothly bend the chain back around the helix by increase number of hydrogen bond between the triple alpha-chain.

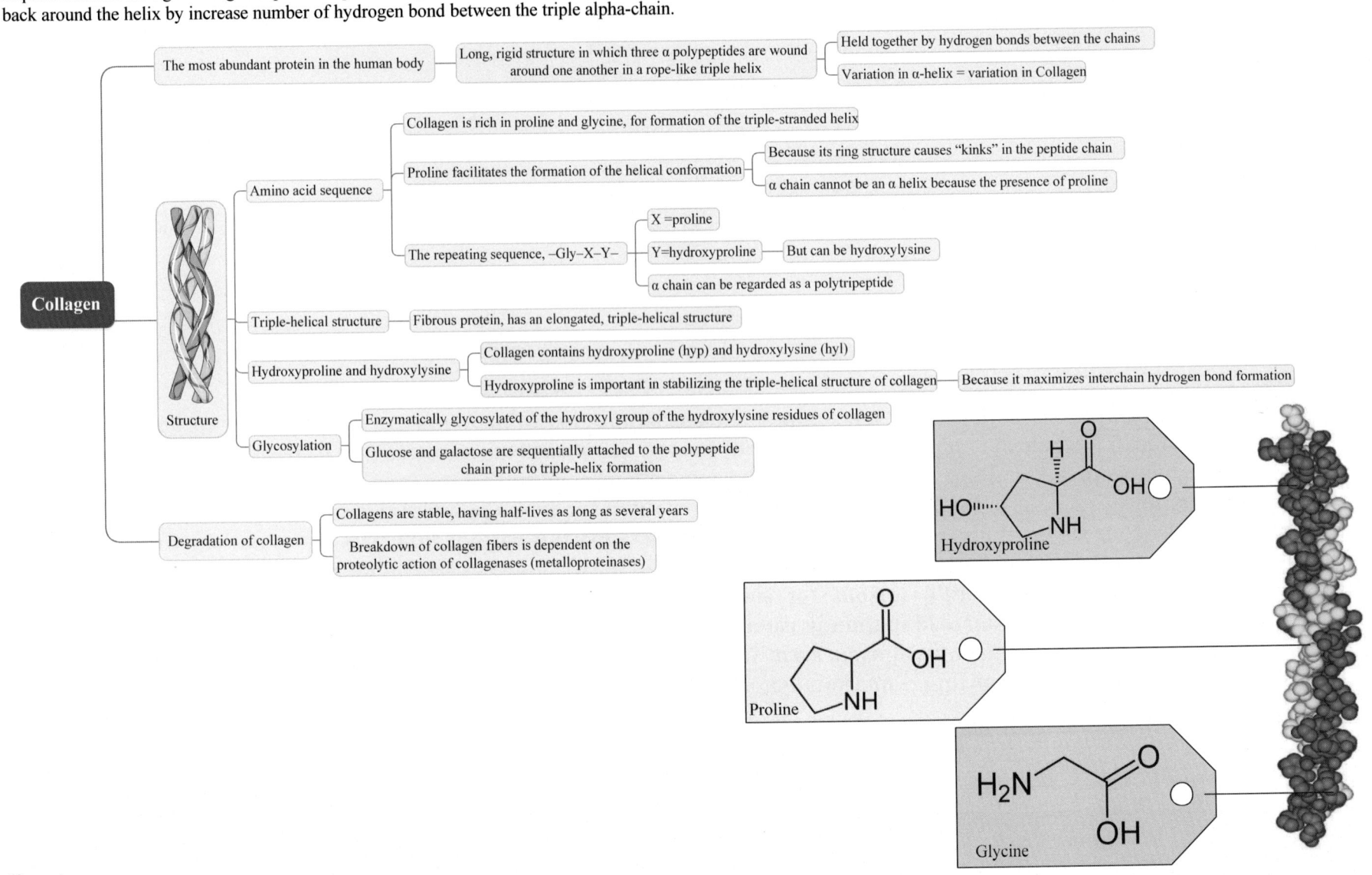

Chapter 4 : Fibrous protein

4.1.2.Types of collagen

Collagen occurs in many places throughout the body. Over 90% of the collagen in the human body, however, is type I. So far, more than 25 types of collagen have been identified and described. They can be divided into several groups according to the structure they form:

Types of collagen

Fibril-forming collagens: (Type I, II, III)

Network-forming collagens:(Types IV, VIII)

Fibril-associated collagens: (Types IX and XII)

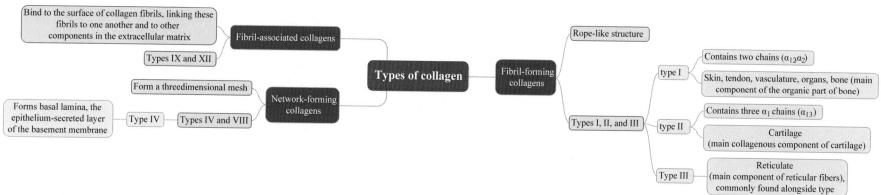

4.1.3.Collagen formation

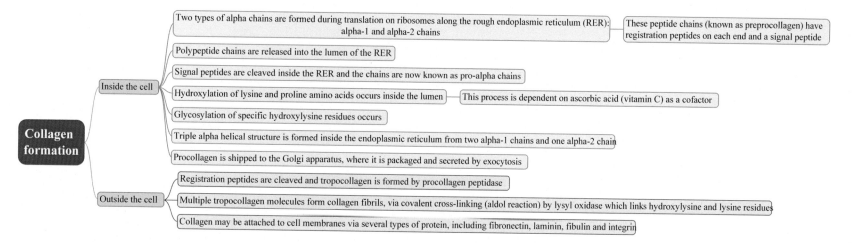

Chapter 4 : Fibrous protein

4.1.4. Collagenopathies

Ehlers-Danlos syndrome (EDS): are a group of genetic connective tissue disorders. Symptoms may include loose joints, stretchy skin, and abnormal scar formation. These can be noticed at birth or in early childhood. Complications may include aortic dissection, joint dislocations, scoliosis, chronic pain, or early osteoarthritis. Osteogenesis imperfecta (OI), also known as brittle bone disease, is a group of genetic disorders that mainly affect the bones. It results in bones that break easily. The severity may be mild to severe. The underlying mechanism is usually a problem with connective tissue due to a lack of type I collagen because the mutation cause replacement of glycine in (-Gly-X-Y-) with amino acid with bulky side chains. The resultant abnormal α-chains so prevent triple-helical conformation.

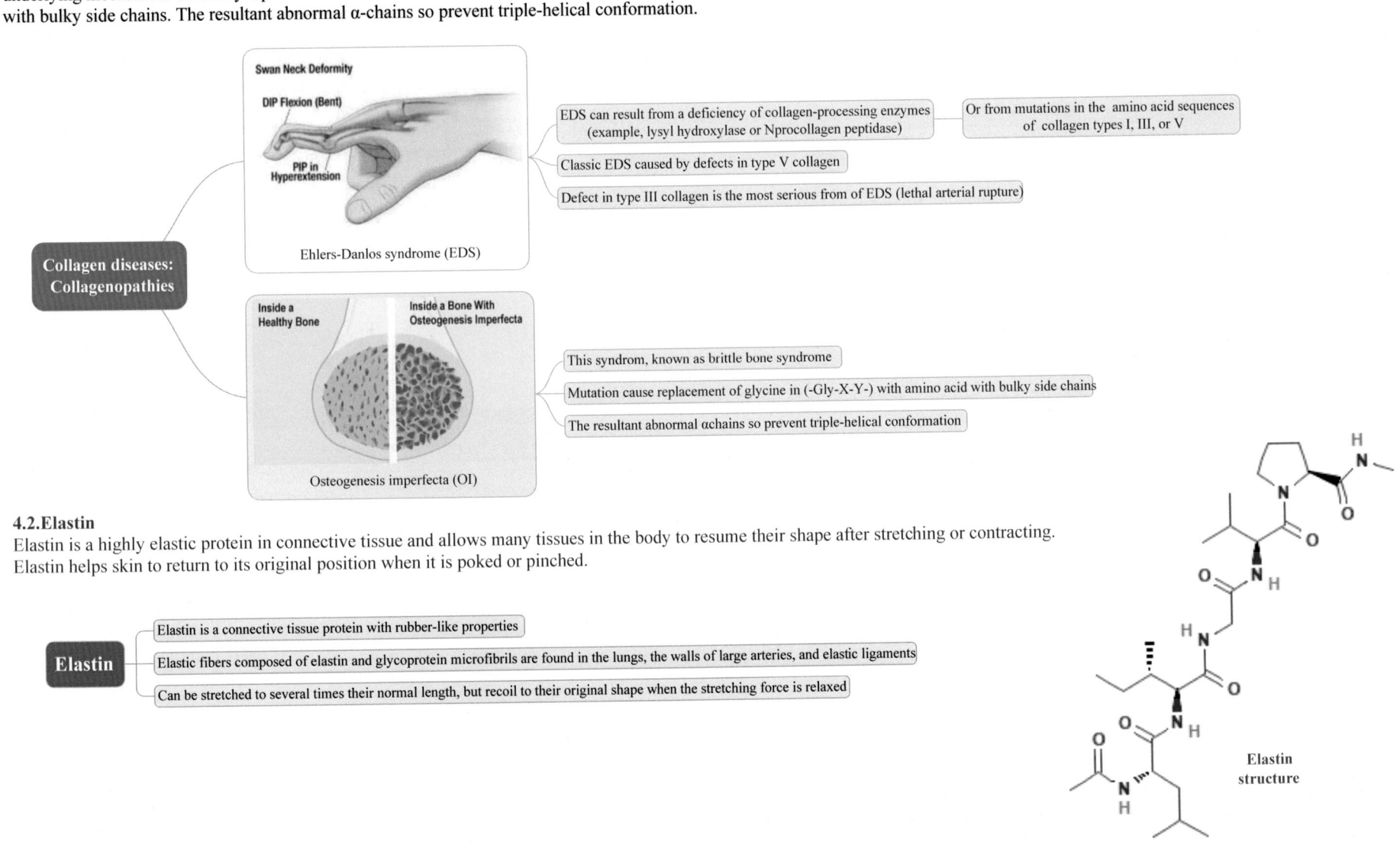

Swan Neck Deformity
DIP Flexion (Bent)
PIP in Hyperextension

Ehlers-Danlos syndrome (EDS)

Collagen diseases: Collagenopathies

EDS can result from a deficiency of collagen-processing enzymes (example, lysyl hydroxylase or Nprocollagen peptidase)

Or from mutations in the amino acid sequences of collagen types I, III, or V

Classic EDS caused by defects in type V collagen

Defect in type III collagen is the most serious from of EDS (lethal arterial rupture)

Inside a Healthy Bone

Inside a Bone With Osteogenesis Imperfecta

This syndrom, known as brittle bone syndrome

Mutation cause replacement of glycine in (-Gly-X-Y-) with amino acid with bulky side chains

The resultant abnormal αchains so prevent triple-helical conformation

Osteogenesis imperfecta (OI)

4.2.Elastin

Elastin is a highly elastic protein in connective tissue and allows many tissues in the body to resume their shape after stretching or contracting. Elastin helps skin to return to its original position when it is poked or pinched.

Elastin

Elastin is a connective tissue protein with rubber-like properties

Elastic fibers composed of elastin and glycoprotein microfibrils are found in the lungs, the walls of large arteries, and elastic ligaments

Can be stretched to several times their normal length, but recoil to their original shape when the stretching force is relaxed

Elastin structure

4.2.1. Structure of elastin

Elastin is a major protein component of tissues that require elasticity such as arteries, lungs, bladder, skin and elastic ligaments and cartilage. It is composed of soluble tropoelastin protein containing primarily, glycine and valine and modified alanine and proline residues. Tropoelastin is a ~65kDa protein that is highly cross-linked to form an insoluble complex. The most common interchain cross-link in elastins is the result of the conversion of the amine groups of lysine to reactive aldehydes by lysyl oxidase. This results in the spontaneous formation of desmosine cross-links.

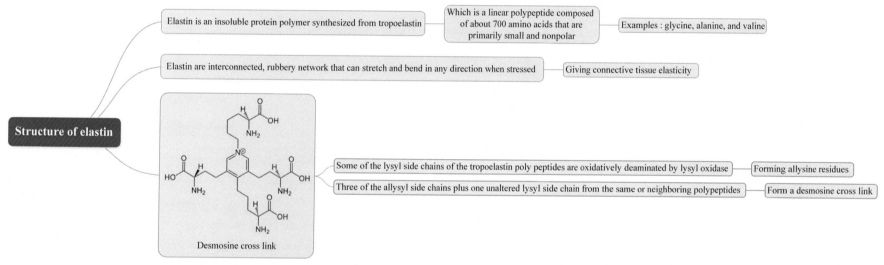

Alpha-1-antitrypsin or α1-antitrypsin (AAT) is a protein belonging to the serpin superfamily. It is encoded in humans by the SERPINA1 gene. A protease inhibitor, because it inhibits various proteases. it protects tissues from enzymes of inflammatory cells, especially neutrophil elastase. When the blood contains inadequate amounts of AAT or functionally defective AAT (such as in alpha-1 antitrypsin deficiency), neutrophil elastase is excessively free to break down elastin, degrading the elasticity of the lungs, which results in respiratory complications, such as emphysema and liver cirrhosis.

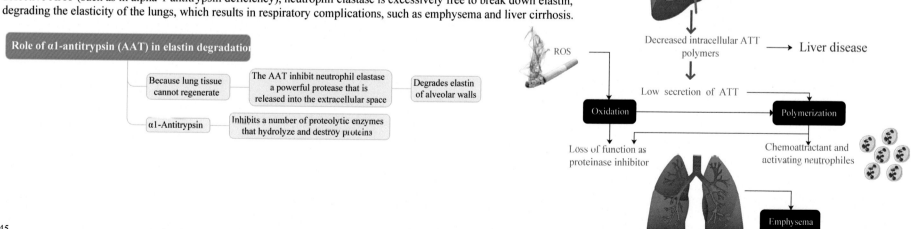

4.2.2.Emphysema

Emphysema is one type of chronic obstructive pulmonary disease (COPD). It means destruction of the lung. In emphysema, the breathing tubes are narrowed and the air sacs are damaged. These changes lead to shortness of breath with daily activities. The major cause of emphysema is smoking cigarettes.

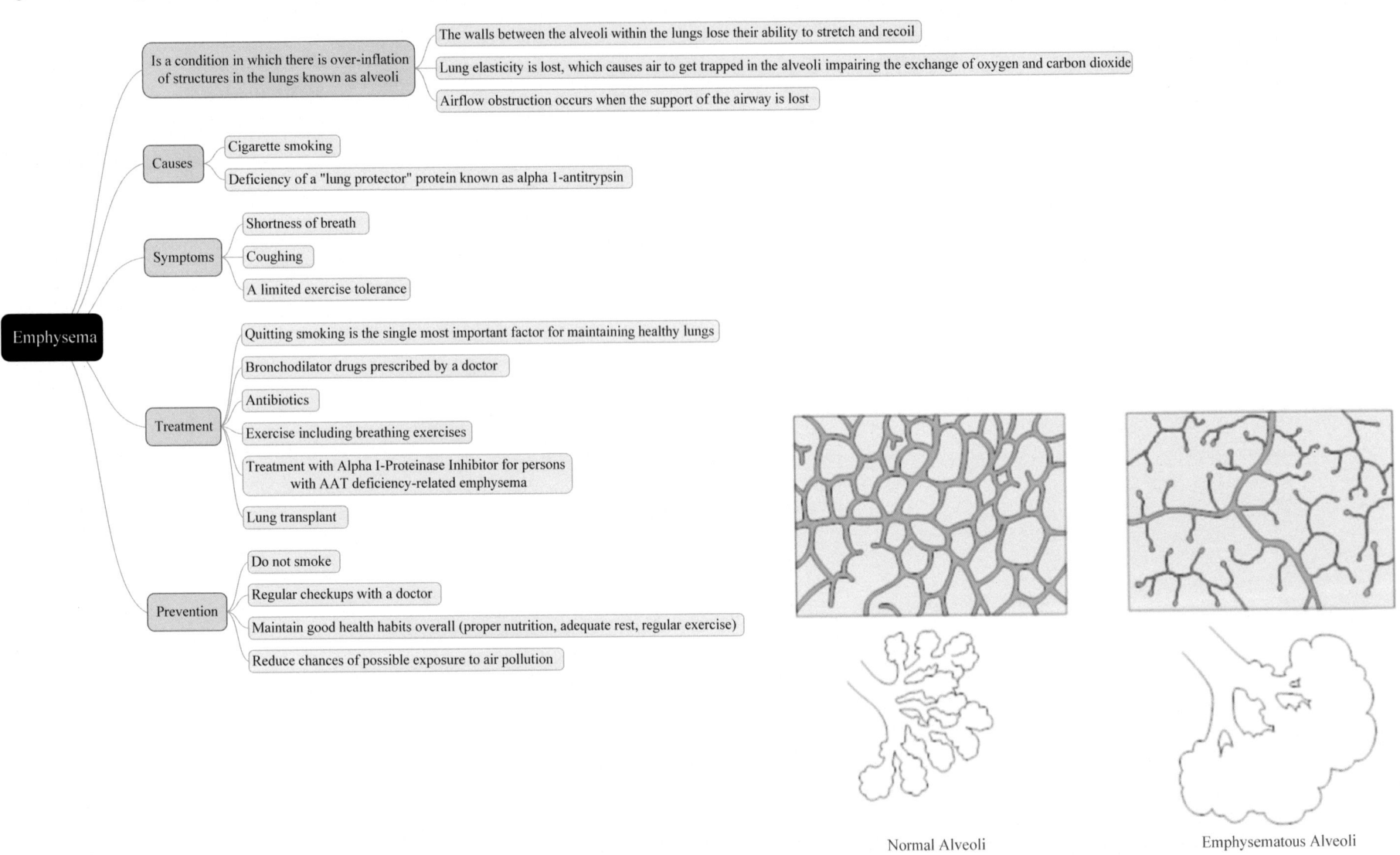

Normal Alveoli   Emphysematous Alveoli

4.3.Marfan syndrome (MFS)

Marfan syndrome (MFS) is a genetic disorder of the connective tissue. The degree to which people are affected varies. The most serious complications involve the heart and aorta, with an increased risk of mitral valve prolapse and aortic aneurysm. Other commonly affected areas include the lungs, eyes, bones and the covering of the spinal cord.

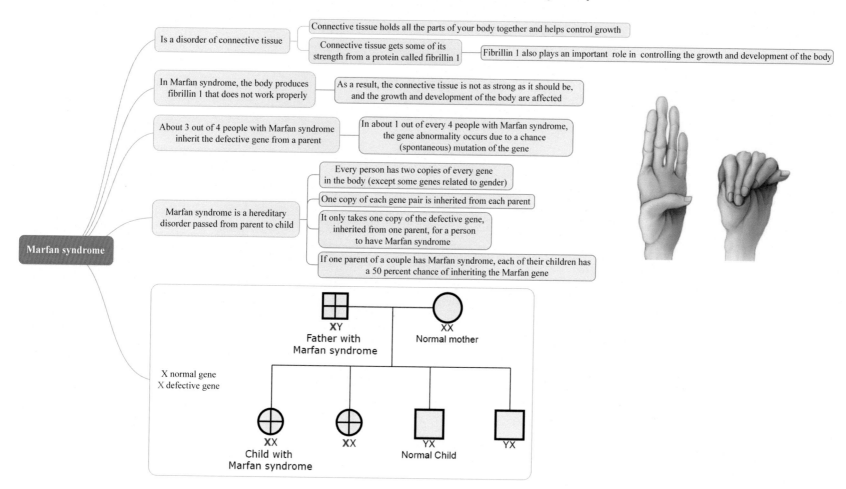

Marfan syndrome

Is a disorder of connective tissue
- Connective tissue holds all the parts of your body together and helps control growth
- Connective tissue gets some of its strength from a protein called fibrillin 1 — Fibrillin 1 also plays an important role in controlling the growth and development of the body

In Marfan syndrome, the body produces fibrillin 1 that does not work properly — As a result, the connective tissue is not as strong as it should be, and the growth and development of the body are affected

About 3 out of 4 people with Marfan syndrome inherit the defective gene from a parent — In about 1 out of every 4 people with Marfan syndrome, the gene abnormality occurs due to a chance (spontaneous) mutation of the gene

Marfan syndrome is a hereditary disorder passed from parent to child
- Every person has two copies of every gene in the body (except some genes related to gender)
- One copy of each gene pair is inherited from each parent
- It only takes one copy of the defective gene, inherited from one parent, for a person to have Marfan syndrome
- If one parent of a couple has Marfan syndrome, each of their children has a 50 percent chance of inheriting the Marfan gene

XY
Father with
Marfan syndrome

XX
Normal mother

X normal gene
X defective gene

XX
Child with
Marfan syndrome

XX

YX
Normal Child

YX

4.4.The Layers of Human Skin

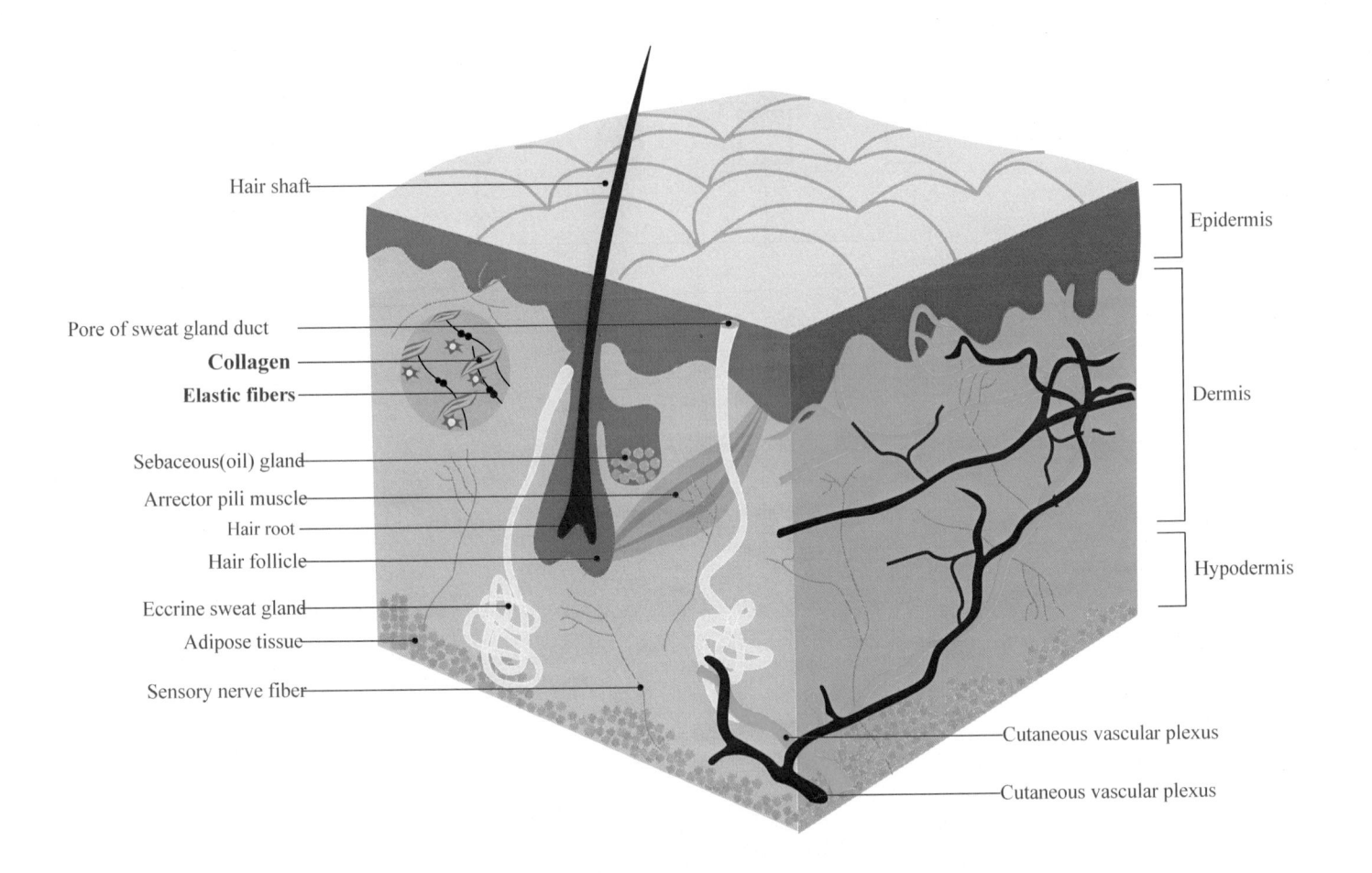

Hair shaft

Pore of sweat gland duct

Collagen

Elastic fibers

Sebaceous(oil) gland

Arrector pili muscle

Hair root

Hair follicle

Eccrine sweat gland

Adipose tissue

Sensory nerve fiber

Epidermis

Dermis

Hypodermis

Cutaneous vascular plexus

Cutaneous vascular plexus

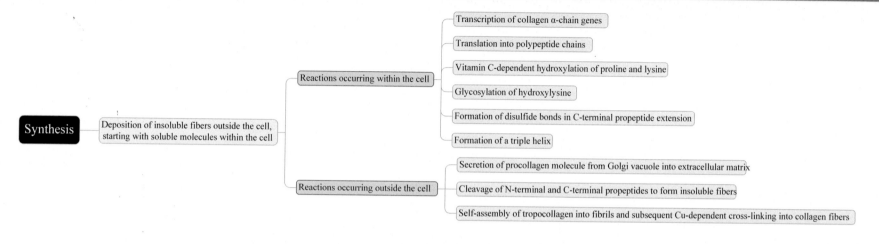

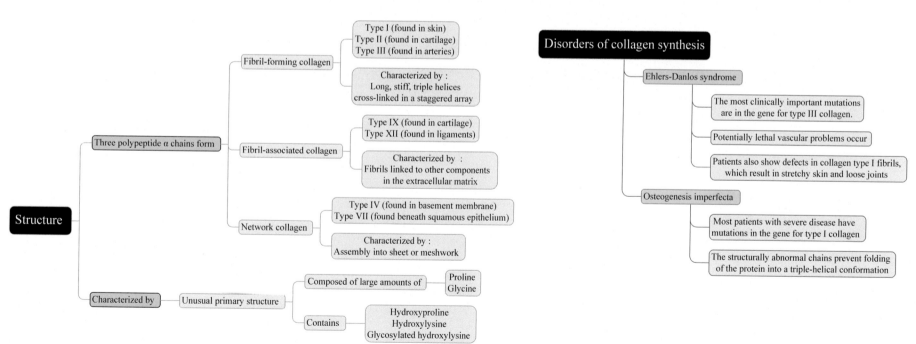

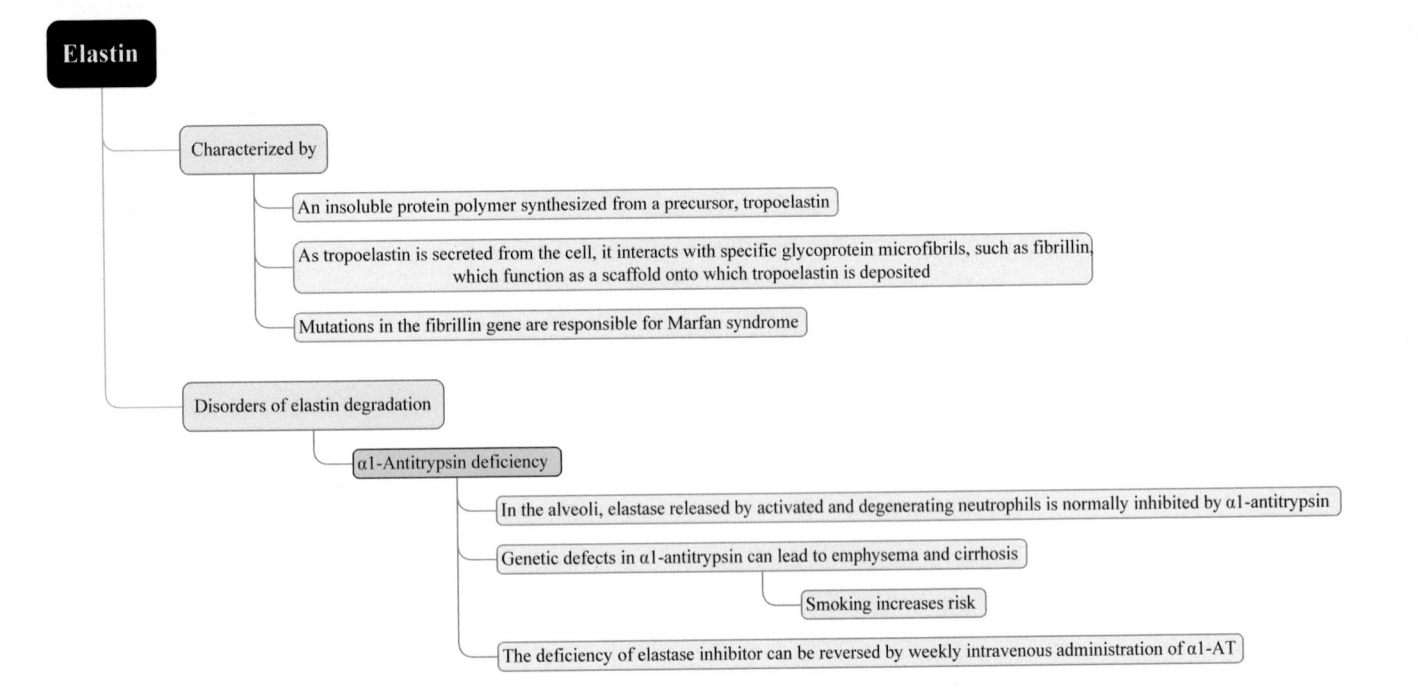

Elastin

Characterized by

- An insoluble protein polymer synthesized from a precursor, tropoelastin

- As tropoelastin is secreted from the cell, it interacts with specific glycoprotein microfibrils, such as fibrillin, which function as a scaffold onto which tropoelastin is deposited

- Mutations in the fibrillin gene are responsible for Marfan syndrome

Disorders of elastin degradation

- $\alpha 1$-Antitrypsin deficiency

  - In the alveoli, elastase released by activated and degenerating neutrophils is normally inhibited by $\alpha 1$-antitrypsin

  - Genetic defects in $\alpha 1$-antitrypsin can lead to emphysema and cirrhosis

    - Smoking increases risk

  - The deficiency of elastase inhibitor can be reversed by weekly intravenous administration of $\alpha 1$-AT

Fibrous protein : E x e r c i s e s

Q 1: Circle the best correct answer:

1.The most abundant protein in mammals is:
a.Hemoglobin
b.Myoglobin
c.Collagen
d.Elastin

2.The collagen structure regarded as:
a.Right handed triple helix
b.Folding & arrangement of domains in the polypeptide
c.Subunits of polypeptide
d.Folding & arrangement of domains in the polypeptide

3.Which of the following statements about collagen is correct?
a.Collagen is rope like structure
b.Collagen is a globular, intracellular protein
c.Collagen consist from small and nonpolar
d.Collagen is rubber-like structure

4.The most abundant proteins in cartilage is:
a.Collagen type II
b.Collagen type IX
c.Collagen type IV
d.Both a and b

5.Types I, II, and III structure are
a.The fibril-forming collagens (rope like structure).
b.The network-forming collagens, forming a three-dimensional mesh.
c.Bind to the surface of collagen fibrils.
d.Vascular endothelial &basement membrane.

6.Types IV and VII are:
a.Network-forming collagens, forming a three-dimensional mesh.
b.bind to the surface of collagen fibrils.
c.Fibril-forming collagens (rope like structure).
d.Skin, bone, tendon

7.Types IX and XII are:
a.Network-forming collagens, forming a three-dimensional mesh.
b.Fibril-forming collagens (rope like structure)
c.Fibril-associated collagens
d.All of these

8.The most abundant amino acid in collagen is:
a.Glycine and valine
b.Glycine and alanine
c.Glycine and proline
d.Proline and valine

9.Which of the following statements about collagen is correct?
a.Collagen is a globular, intracellular protein.
b.Hydroxyproline is stabilizing the structure of collagen because the hydrogen bond formation
c .Post-translational modification of collagen involves vitamin A.
d. The structure of collagen consists of a superhelix of three α helices twisted together.

10.Hydroxyproline is important in stabilizing the triple-helical structure of collagen because
a.It maximizes interchain ionic bond formation
b.It maximizes interchain, hydrophobic interaction.
c.It maximizes interchain hydrogen bond formation
d.It maximizes interchain by disulfide bond formation.

Fibrous protein : E x e r c i s e s

Q 1: Circle the best correct answer:

11.Hydroxylation and glycosylation in synthesis of collagen considered:

a.Translation

b.Transcription

c.Post translation or modification process

d.None of the above

12.In synthesis of collagen, cross link formation depends on:

a.Condensation of proline residue with hydroxylproline residue

b.Condensation of allysine residue with lysine residue

c.Condensation of amides group of amino acids with amine group of lysine

d.Condensation of glycine with proline

13.Stretch skin of classic Ehlers-Danlos syndrome (EDS) caused by:

a.Defect in collagen type V

b.Defect in Collagen type IX

c.Abnormal Collagen type V

d.All of these

14.The mutation of Osteogenesis imperfecta (OI) is replacement of glycine in (–Gly–X–Y–), where X =proline; Y=hydroxyproline or hydroxylysine with:

a.Serine

b.Isoleucine

c.Cysteine

d.Alanine

15.The elastine structure regarded as:

a.Tropoelastin that are primarily small and nonpolar amino acids.

b.Troponin that are primarily small and nonpolar amino acids.

c.Tropoelastin that are primarily small and polar amino acids.

d.tropoelastin that are primarily bulky side chain and polar amino acids.

16.Mutations in the fibrillin-1 protein are responsible for:

a.Marfan syndrome

b.Creutzfeldt-Jakob disease

c.Down syndrome

d.Alzheimer disease

17.............Prevent destruction of elastin by elastase in lungs.

a.Trypsin

b.Pepsin

c.α1-antitrypsin

d.Neutrophil elastase

18.Mutations in the gene for α_1- antitrypsin cause:

a.Emphysema

b.Sickle cell anemia

c.Liver cirrhosis

d.Both a and c

19.The protein present in connective tissue, skin, and cornea is

a.Keratin

b.Elastin

c.Myoglobin

d.Collagen

20.The number of helices present in a collagen molecule is

a.1

b.2

c.3

d.4

21.protein rich in glycine and proline is

a.Collagen

b.Keratin

c.Haemoglobin

d.Gelatin

22.The most abundant protein in bones is:

a.Collagen type I

b.Collagen type II

c.Collagen type III

d.Non-collagen proteins

Fibrous protein : E x e r c i s e s

Q 1: Circle the best correct answer:

23.Marfan's syndrome results from a mutation in the gene coding:
a.Collagen
b.Elastin
c.Fibrillin-1 protein
d.Keratin

24.Abnormal collagen structure is seen in all of the following except:
a.Marfan syndrome
b.Osteogenesis imperfecta
c.Ehlers-Danlos syndrome
d.both b and c

25.Self-assembly of tropocollagen into fibrils to form mature collagen fibers by:
a.Cross linking
b.Hydrogen bond
c.covalent bond
d.Disulfide bond

26.Which of the following statements is incorrect concerning Elastin?
a.Synthesized from tropoelastin, small non polar amino acids
b.Mutations in fibrillin gene are responsible for Marfins syndrome
c.Genetic defects in α-1antitrypsin can lead to emphysema
d.Its rich in hydroxyprolyine and hydroxylysine

Q 2. Write short note on:

a. Collagen
b. Elastin
c. Collagen diseases
d. Marfan syndrome

Q 3. What is the structure and function of collagen ?

Q 4. What is the structure and function of α_1 antitrypsin ?

Q 5. What is the structure and function of elastin ?

OVERVIEW

Enzymes are macromolecular biological catalysts. Enzymes accelerate chemical reactions. The molecules upon which enzymes may act are called substrates and the enzyme converts the substrates into different molecules known as products. Almost all metabolic processes in the cell need enzyme catalysis in order to occur at rates fast enough to sustain life. Metabolic pathways depend upon enzymes to catalyze individual steps. This chapter examines the nature of these catalytic molecules and their mechanism of action.

Chapter 5 : Enzymes

5.1.Nomenclature

The first is its short, recommended name, convenient for everyday use; example: pepsin, trypsin.

The second is the more complete systematic name, which is used when an enzyme must be identified without ambiguity, therefore the enzymes are classified into six different groups according to the reaction being catalyzed. The nomenclature was determined by the Enzyme Commission in 1961 (with the latest update having occurred in 1992), hence all enzymes are assigned an "EC" number. For a given enzyme for numerous subgroups, the suffix -ase is attached to a fairly complete description of the chemical reaction catalyzed, including the names of all the substrates. Systematic name EnzymesSubstrate - chemical reaction – ase

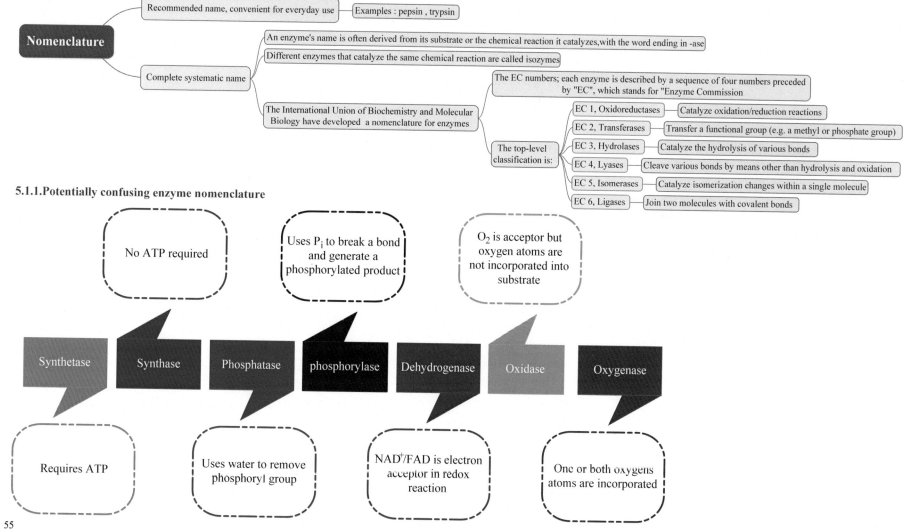

5.1.1.Potentially confusing enzyme nomenclature

5.2. Properties of Enzymes

Enzymes act on specific substances and catalyze specific reactions. This indicates that an enzyme has two types of specificity a substrate specificity and a reaction specificity.
An enzyme displays its catalytic activity by identifying and binding to its specific substrate therefor the enzymes has many properties.

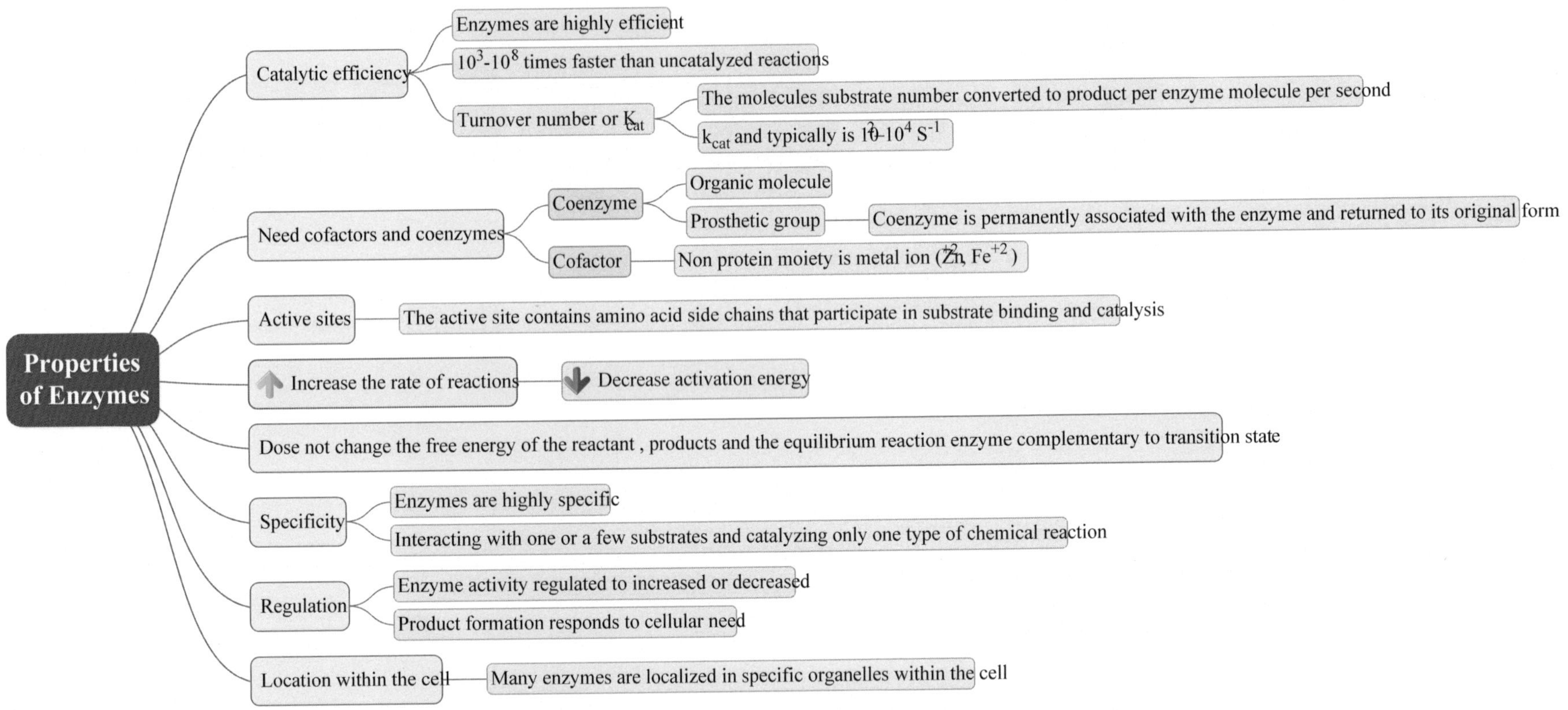

Properties of Enzymes

- Catalytic efficiency
  - Enzymes are highly efficient
  - 10^3-10^8 times faster than uncatalyzed reactions
  - Turnover number or K_{cat}
    - The molecules substrate number converted to product per enzyme molecule per second
    - k_{cat} and typically is 10-10^4 S^{-1}
- Need cofactors and coenzymes
  - Coenzyme
    - Organic molecule
    - Prosthetic group — Coenzyme is permanently associated with the enzyme and returned to its original form
  - Cofactor — Non protein moiety is metal ion (Zn^{+2}, Fe^{+2})
- Active sites — The active site contains amino acid side chains that participate in substrate binding and catalysis
- Increase the rate of reactions — Decrease activation energy
- Dose not change the free energy of the reactant , products and the equilibrium reaction enzyme complementary to transition state
- Specificity
  - Enzymes are highly specific
  - Interacting with one or a few substrates and catalyzing only one type of chemical reaction
- Regulation
  - Enzyme activity regulated to increased or decreased
  - Product formation responds to cellular need
- Location within the cell — Many enzymes are localized in specific organelles within the cell

5.3. Factor affecting reaction velocity

Enzymes lower the activation energy required to get the reaction started.There are several factors that affect the speed of an enzyme's action, such as the concentration of the enzyme, the concentration of the substrate, temperature, hydrogen ion concentration (pH)

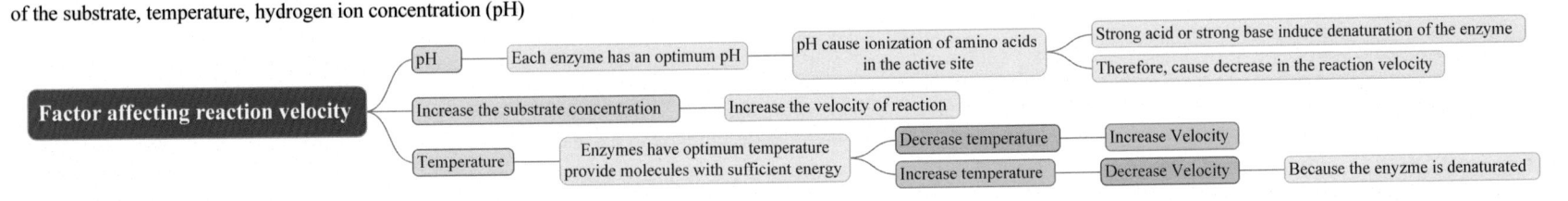

Factor affecting reaction velocity

- pH — Each enzyme has an optimum pH — pH cause ionization of amino acids in the active site
  - Strong acid or strong base induce denaturation of the enzyme
  - Therefore, cause decrease in the reaction velocity
- Increase the substrate concentration — Increase the velocity of reaction
- Temperature — Enzymes have optimum temperature provide molecules with sufficient energy
  - Decrease temperature — Increase Velocity
  - Increase temperature — Decrease Velocity — Because the enyzme is denaturated

5.4. Michaelis–Menten kinetics

V_{max} is equal to the product of the catalyst rate constant (k_{cat}) and the concentration of the enzyme. The Michaelis-Menten equation can then be rewritten as $V = K_{cat}[Enzyme][S] / (Km + [S])$. Kcat, and it measures the number of substrate molecules "turned over" converted to product per enzyme per second.

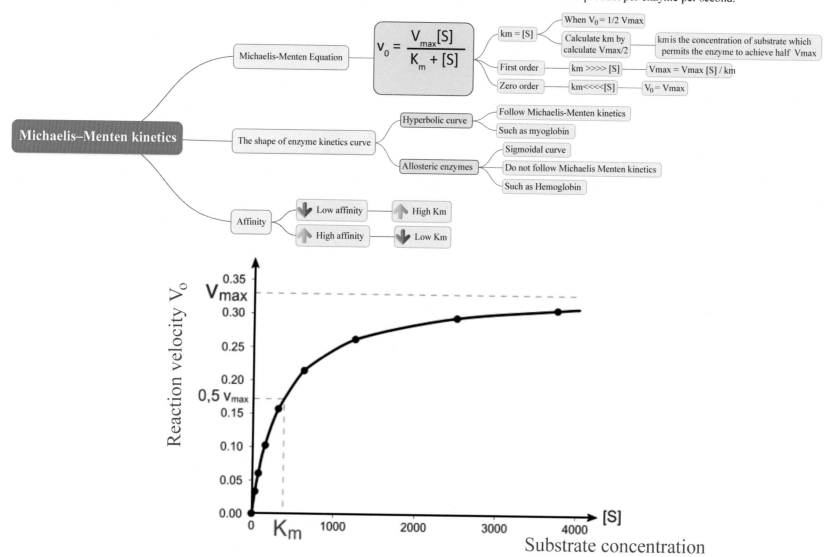

Substrate concentration

In biochemistry, the Lineweaver–Burk plot (or double reciprocal plot) is a graphical representation of the Lineweaver–Burk equation of enzyme kinetics, described by Hans Lineweaver and DeanBurk in 1934

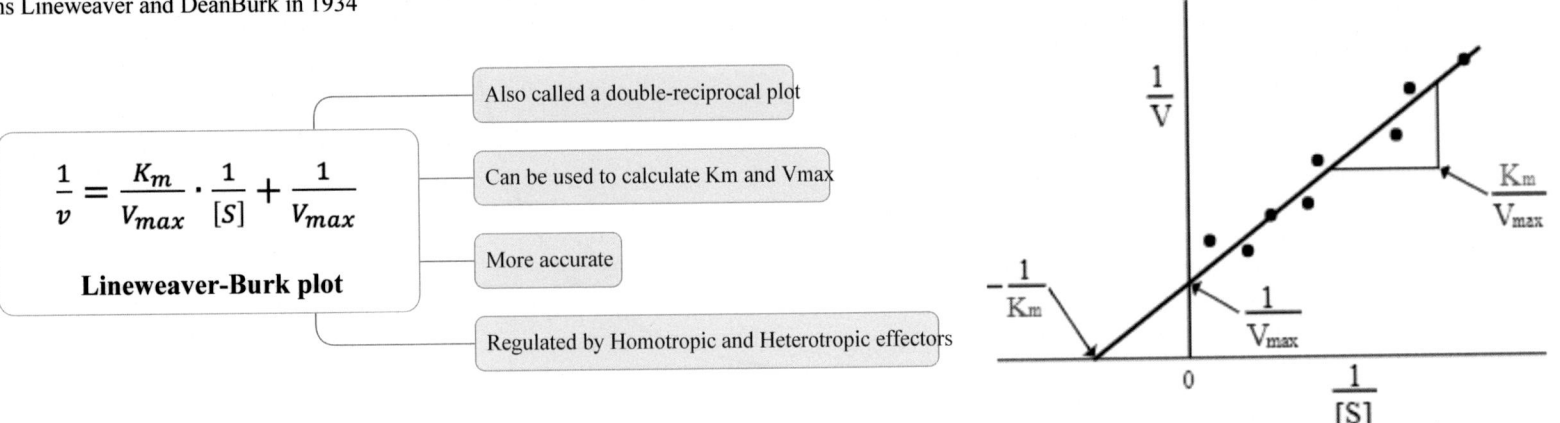

$$\frac{1}{v} = \frac{K_m}{V_{max}} \cdot \frac{1}{[S]} + \frac{1}{V_{max}}$$

Lineweaver-Burk plot

Also called a double-reciprocal plot

Can be used to calculate Km and Vmax

More accurate

Regulated by Homotropic and Heterotropic effectors

5.5.Enzyme inhibitors

Enzyme inhibitors are substances which alter the catalytic action of the enzyme and consequently slow down, or in some cases, stop catalysis. There are two types of inhibitor, irreversible inhibitors bind to enzymes through covalent bonds and reversible inhibitors attach to enzymes with non-covalent interactions such as hydrogen bonds, hydrophobic interactions and ionic bonds. reversible inhibitors generally do not undergo chemical reactions when bound to the enzyme and can be easily removed.

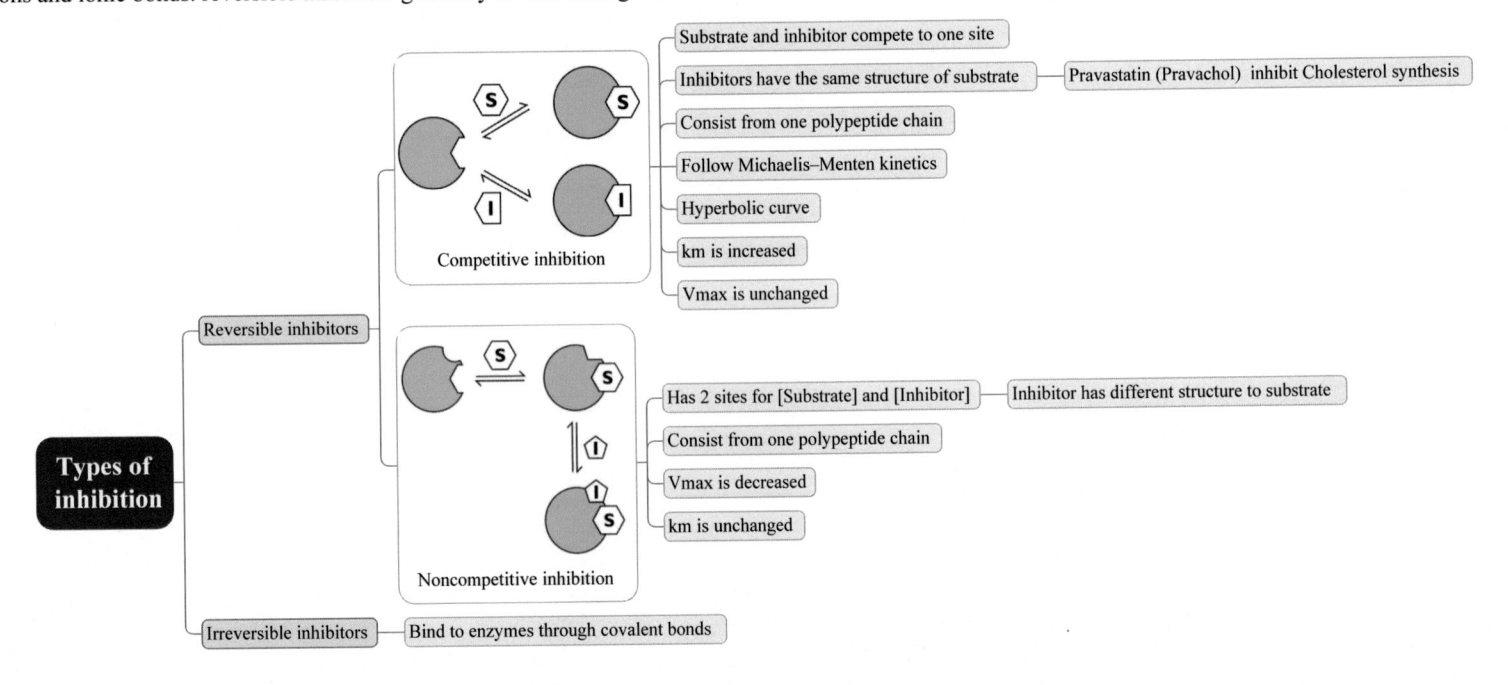

Substrate and inhibitor compete to one site

Inhibitors have the same structure of substrate — Pravastatin (Pravachol) inhibit Cholesterol synthesis

Consist from one polypeptide chain

Follow Michaelis–Menten kinetics

Hyperbolic curve

km is increased

Vmax is unchanged

Competitive inhibition

Has 2 sites for [Substrate] and [Inhibitor] — Inhibitor has different structure to substrate

Consist from one polypeptide chain

Vmax is decreased

km is unchanged

Noncompetitive inhibition

Types of inhibition

Reversible inhibitors

Irreversible inhibitors — Bind to enzymes through covalent bonds

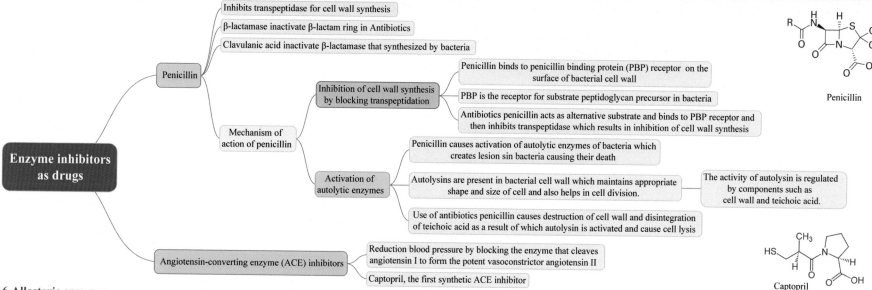

Enzyme inhibitors as drugs

Penicillin
- Inhibits transpeptidase for cell wall synthesis
- β-lactamase inactivate β-lactam ring in Antibiotics
- Clavulanic acid inactivate β-lactamase that synthesized by bacteria

Mechanism of action of penicillin
- Inhibition of cell wall synthesis by blocking transpeptidation
  - Penicillin binds to penicillin binding protein (PBP) receptor on the surface of bacterial cell wall
  - PBP is the receptor for substrate peptidoglycan precursor in bacteria
  - Antibiotics penicillin acts as alternative substrate and binds to PBP receptor and then inhibits transpeptidase which results in inhibition of cell wall synthesis
- Activation of autolytic enzymes
  - Penicillin causes activation of autolytic enzymes of bacteria which creates lesion sin bacteria causing their death
  - Autolysins are present in bacterial cell wall which maintains appropriate shape and size of cell and also helps in cell division.
    - The activity of autolysin is regulated by components such as cell wall and teichoic acid.
  - Use of antibiotics penicillin causes destruction of cell wall and disintegration of teichoic acid as a result of which autolysin is activated and cause cell lysis

Angiotensin-converting enzyme (ACE) inhibitors
- Reduction blood pressure by blocking the enzyme that cleaves angiotensin I to form the potent vasoconstrictor angiotensin II
- Captopril, the first synthetic ACE inhibitor

Penicillin

Captopril

5.6. Allosteric enzymes

Allosteric enzymes are enzymes that change their conformational ensemble upon binding of an effector, which results in an apparent change in binding affinity at a different ligand binding site. The site to which the effector binds is termed the allosteric site.

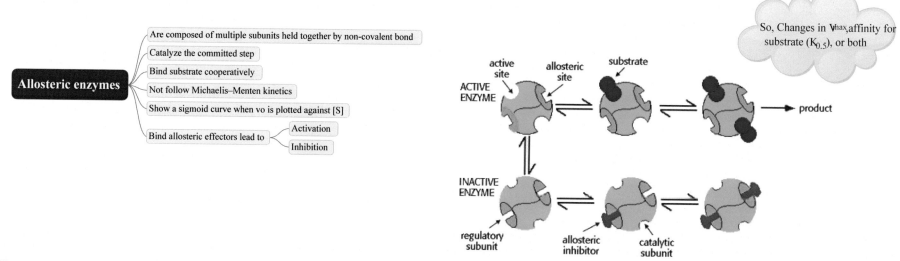

Allosteric enzymes
- Are composed of multiple subunits held together by non-covalent bond
- Catalyze the committed step
- Bind substrate cooperatively
- Not follow Michaelis–Menten kinetics
- Show a sigmoid curve when vo is plotted against [S]
- Bind allosteric effectors lead to
  - Activation
  - Inhibition

So, Changes in Vmax, affinity for substrate (K0.5), or both

5.7. Regulation of Enzyme Activity

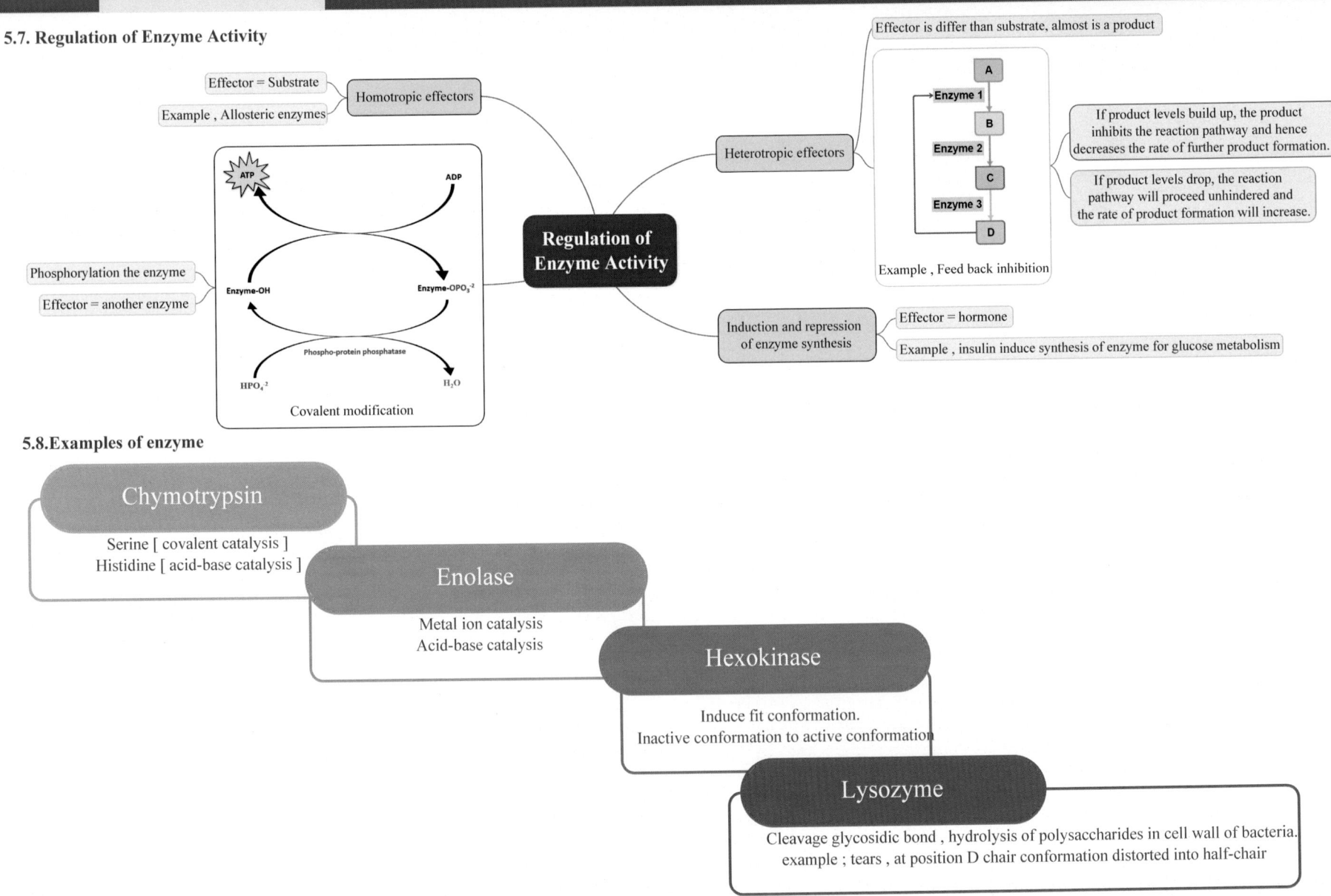

Effector = Substrate

Example , Allosteric enzymes

Homotropic effectors

Effector is differ than substrate, almost is a product

Heterotropic effectors

A

Enzyme 1

B

Enzyme 2

C

Enzyme 3

D

If product levels build up, the product inhibits the reaction pathway and hence decreases the rate of further product formation.

If product levels drop, the reaction pathway will proceed unhindered and the rate of product formation will increase.

Example , Feed back inhibition

Regulation of Enzyme Activity

ATP

ADP

Phosphorylation the enzyme

Effector = another enzyme

Enzyme-OH

Enzyme-OPO$_3^{-2}$

Phospho-protein phosphatase

HPO$_4^{-2}$

H$_2$O

Covalent modification

Induction and repression of enzyme synthesis

Effector = hormone

Example , insulin induce synthesis of enzyme for glucose metabolism

5.8. Examples of enzyme

Chymotrypsin

Serine [covalent catalysis]
Histidine [acid-base catalysis]

Enolase

Metal ion catalysis
Acid-base catalysis

Hexokinase

Induce fit conformation.
Inactive conformation to active conformation

Lysozyme

Cleavage glycosidic bond , hydrolysis of polysaccharides in cell wall of bacteria.
example ; tears , at position D chair conformation distorted into half-chair

5.9.Serine proteases (or serine endopeptidases)

Are enzymes that cleave peptide bonds in proteins, in which serine serves as the nucleophilic amino acid at the (enzyme's) active site.They are found ubiquitously in both eukaryotes and prokaryotes. Serine proteases are the related enzymes, trypsin, chymotrypsin, and elastase.

5.10.Therapeutic Application of enzymes

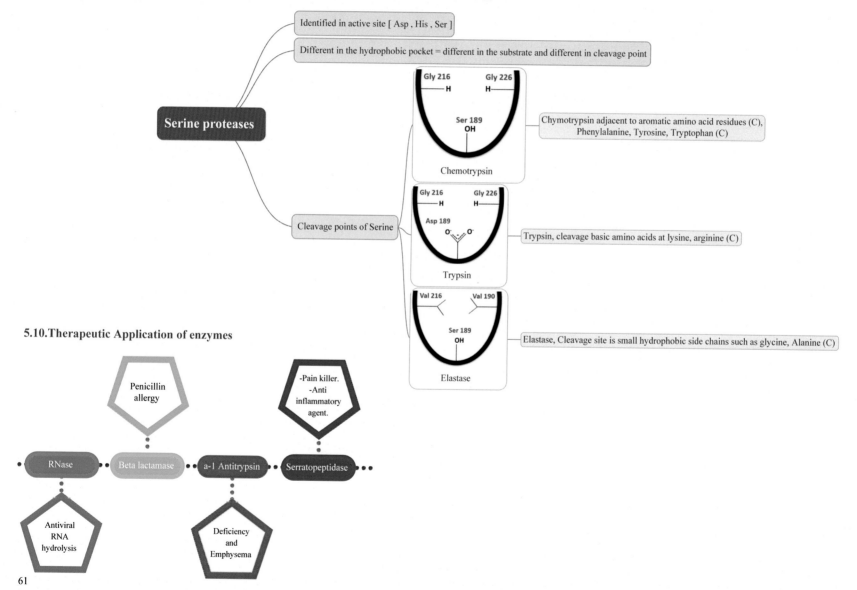

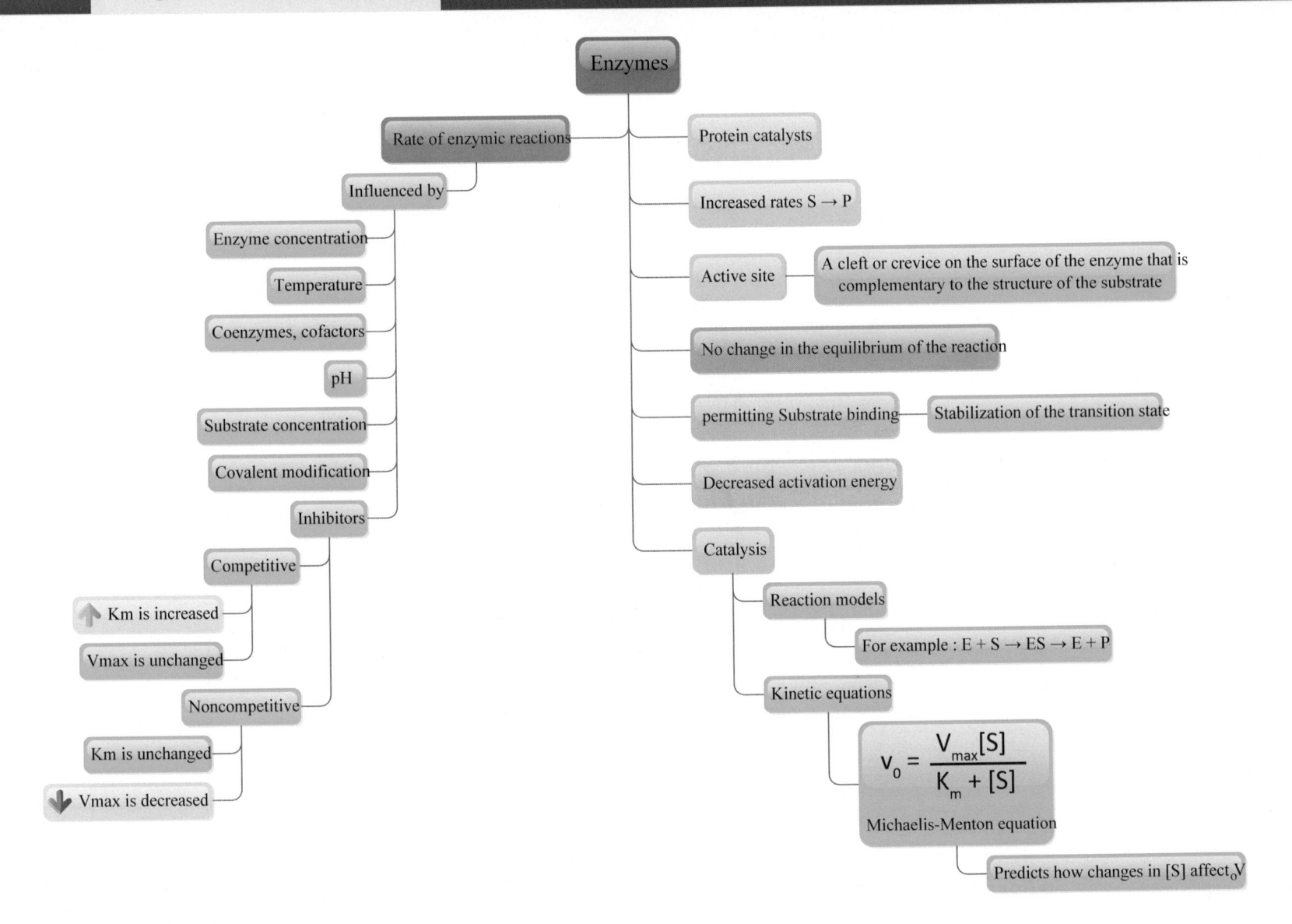

Enzymes : Exercises

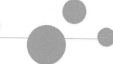

Q 1: Circle the best correct answer:

1.When Km <<<<< [S], therefore V_o = ...:
a.V_o=Vmax[S]/km
b.V_o = 1/2 Vmax
c.V_o=Vmax
d.V_o=Vmax/5

2.The false statement about Allosteric enzymes is:
a.Regulation by homotropic effectors and heterotropic effectors
b.Allosteric enzymes follow Michaelis-Menten Equation
c.These enzymes are usually composed of multiple subunits
d.Allosteric enzymes give sigmoidal curve

3.The function of Phosphatase enzymes is:
a.Phosphorylation
b.Removal of phosphate group
c.Oxidoreductase
d.Ligases

4.The substrate and chemical reaction for pyruvate decarboxylase are..............
a.Pyruvate & add carboxylase group respectively
b.Lactate & add carboxylase respectively
c.Pyruvate & remove of carboxylase group respectively
d.Urea & remove amino group respectively

5.Which of the following statements is false about enzymes?
a.Need cofactor or coenzyme
b.Interacting with one or a few substrates
c.Catalyzing many types of chemical reaction
d.Localized in specific organelles within the cell

6. Which of the following statements about covalent modification is true?
a.Heterotropic effectors; some enzymes are regulated by their own product
b.Induction or repression the enzyme synthesis, example insulin
c.Homotropic effectors; some enzymes are regulated by their ownsubstrate
d.Phosphorylation the enzyme by another enzyme

7.Which of the following statements about Allosteric enzymes is false?
a.Regulation by Homotropic effectors and Heterotropic effectors
b.Don't follow Michaelis-Menten Equation
c.These enzymes are usually composed of multiple subunits
d.Allosteric enzymes give hyperbolic curve

8.When Km = [S], therefore V_o=....................:
a.V_o = Vmax [S]/km
b.V_o = 1/2Vmax
c.V_o = Vmax
d.V_o = Vmax/5

9.What is the main function of enzymes in biological systems?
a.Catalysis of a reaction.
b.Altering the equilibrium of a reaction.
c.Energy transport
d.Protein synthesis

10.The cofactor is:
a.Organic molecules that is required by some enzymes
b.Inorganic ions that is required by some enzymes
c.None of the above
d.Both a and b

11.The optimum pH varies for different enzymes because:
a.Temperature increases the rate of reaction
b.High pH leads to activate the enzyme
c.pH provide molecules with sufficient energy
d.pH effects on the ionization (protonated or deprotonated) of the active site

12.Which one of the following is not among the six internationally accepted classes of enzymes?
a.Hydrolases
b.Polymerases
c.Ligases
d.Oxidoreductases

13.Which of the following statements is regarding the active site of an enzyme?
a.An active site contains amino acids that participate in substrate binding and catalysis
b.An active site is normally hydrophilic in nature
c.An active site is rigid and does not change shape
d.An active site at the center of globular proteins

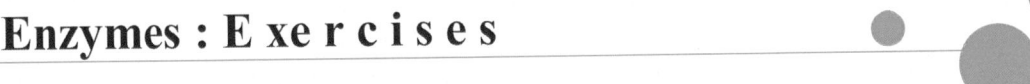

Q 1: Circle the best correct answer:

14.Which of the following statements is true?

a.Enzymes are not specific, interaction with many substrates

b.Enzymes are highly specific, interacting with a few substrates and catalyzing only one chemical reaction

c.Enzymes catalyzing many types of chemical reactions

d.Enzymes are proteins that decrease the velocity of the reaction

15.Steady-state assumption is:

a.Temperature increases the rate of reaction.

b.The rate of synthesis is more than the rate of degradation d. Inhibitor concentration.

c.The rate of synthesis is equal to its rate of degradation

d.High pH leads to denaturation of the enzyme

16.The optimum pH varies for different enzymes because:

a.Temperature increases the rate of reaction

b.High pH leads to denaturation of the enzyme

c.pH provide molecules with sufficient energy

d.pH effects on the ionization of the active site

17.The enzymes are sensitive to

a.Changes in pH

b.Changes in temperature

c.Both a and b

d.None of these

18.At high temperature the rate of enzyme action decreases because the high temperature.

a.Changes the pH of the system

b.Alters the active site of the enzyme up to denaturation

c.Neutralize acids and bases in the system

d.Increases the concentration of enzymes

19.The Michaelis-Menten constant, Km is.

a.Numerically equal to ½ Vmax

b.Independent temperature and pH

c.Numerically equal to the substrate concentration that gives half-maximum velocity

d.Dependent on the substrate concentration

20.At First order, When [S] <<<Km, V_0 equal to:

a.V_0 = Vmax

b.V_0 = 1/2 Vmax

c.V_0 = Vmax [S] / Km

d.V_0 = 2 Vmax

21.In competitive inhibition, an inhibitor:

a.Binds at several different sites on an enzyme

b.Binds covalently to the enzyme

c.Binds reversibly at the active site

d.Lowers the characteristic Vmax of the enzyme

22.A competitive inhibitor of an enzyme-catalyzed reaction:

a.Increases KM and unchanged Vmax

b.Decrease Vmax and unchanged Km

c.Decrease Vmax and decrease Km

d.Increase Km and decrease Vmax

23.A noncompetitive inhibitor of an enzyme-catalyzed reaction:

a.Increases KM and increases Vmax

b.Decrease Vmax and unchanged Km

c.Decrease Vmax and decrease Km

d.Increase Vmax and unchanged Km

24.A competitive inhibitor of an enzyme is usually:

a.A highly reactive compound

b.A metal ion such as Hg^{2+} or Pb^{2+}

c.Structurally similar to the substrate

d.Binds reversibly at different site on the enzyme

25.Which of the following statements is false about the Allosteric enzymes?

a.Usually catalyze several different reactions within a metabolic pathway

b.Usually have more than one polypeptide chain

c.Usually have only one active site

d.Usually do not follow Michaelis-Menten kinetics

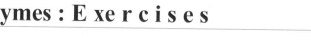

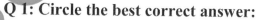

Q 1: Circle the best correct answer:

26. A small molecule that decreases the activity of an enzyme by binding to a site other than the catalytic site is termed a:
a.Allosteric inhibitor.
b.Alternative inhibitor.
c.Competitive inhibitor.
d.Transition-state analog.

27.As haemoglobin binds oxygen molecules, its affinity for oxygen increases, driving the binding of further oxygen molecules. Which term best describes this phenomenon?
a.Catalysis.
b.Allostery.
c.Saturation.
d.Isomerism.

28.The enzymes involved in Feedback inhibition called:
a.Allosteric enzyme
b.Holoenzyme
c.Apoenzyme
d.Coenzyme

29.Homotropic effector is:
a.Substrate itself serves as an effector
b.Product serves as an effector
c.Another enzyme serves as an effector
d.Hormone serves as an effector

30.Heterotropic effectors:
a.Substrate itself serves as an effector.
b.The effector different from the substrate.
c.Another enzyme serves as an effector.
d.Hormone serves as an effector.

31.The active site for enzymes regulated by covalent modification:
a.Substrate itself serves as an effector
b.The effector different from the substrate
c.Another enzyme serves as an effector
d.Hormone serves as an effector

32.Km value is too small that is mean:
a.Low affinity of the enzyme for substrate
b.High affinity of the enzyme for substrate
c.The affinity of the enzyme for substrate unchanged
d.None of these

33.Which of the following statements concerning enzyme regulation is incorrect?
a.Heterotropic effectors; some enzymes are regulated by their own product.
b.Allosteric effectors always increase $K_{0.5}$
c.Induction or repression the enzyme synthesis, example insulin.
d.Homotropic effectors; some enzymes are regulated by their own substrate.
e.Covalent modification (phosphorylation the enzyme)

34.Reaction with no inhibitor has Vmax=500, Km=2; so the Vmax with present competitive inhibitor equal:
a.250
b.500
c.2
d.1

35.Reaction with no inhibitor has Vmax=500, Km=2; so the Km with present noncompetitive inhibitor equal:
a.250
b.500
c.2
d.1

36.Which of the following chemical reactions catalyzed by urease?
a.Oxidoreductases
b.Lyases
c.Hydrolases
d.Ligases

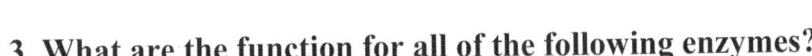

Q 1: Circle the best correct answer:

37.Which of the following statements is false about the Properties of enzymes?
a.Enzymes has few substrate
b.Enzymes need cofactor or coenzyme
c.Enzymes are localized in specific organelles
d.Enzymes has 2 or more type of chemical reaction

38.Trypsin is specific for cleavage of:
a.Glycosidic bond
b.Peptide bonds adjacent to aromatic amino acid residues.
c.Peptide bonds adjacent to basic amino acid residues
d.Hydrogen and ionic bonds.

39.The cleavage point of serine proteases is different due to:
a.Different specific hydrophobic pocket in the enzyme.
b.Identical in the active site (serine, histidine, and aspartate).
c.Change conformations of the individual proteins.
d.Acid base catalysis

40.Chymotrypsin is specific for cleavage of:
a.Glyosidic bond
b.Peptide bonds adjacent to aromatic amino acid residues.
c.Peptide bonds adjacent to basic amino acid residues
d.Hydrogen and ionic bonds.

Q 2. Write short note on:

1.Decrease velocity rate of reaction with high temperature.
2.Decrease the velocity of reaction when increase pH or decrease pH comparing with optimum pH for the enzymes .
3.Describe the regulation of allosteric enzyme.
4.Affinity of enzyme to substrate is decrease in competitive inhibitor.
5.The relation between the Km and the affinity.
6.Turnover number.
7.The cleavage point of serine proteases is different
8.Structure of hydrophobic pocket for (Chymotrypsin, Trypsin, and elastase)

Q 3. What are the function for all of the following enzymes?

1.Chymotrypsin
2.Trypsin
3.Serratopeptidase

Q 4. Describe the types of regulation enzymes.

Q 5. What are the effects of temperature and pH on enzymes?

Q 6. What are the properties of enzymes?

Q 7. Write short note about enzyme specificity.

Enzymes : E x e r c i s e s

Q 8. Comparing between the competitive inhibitor and non-competitive inhibitor for all of the following:

	COMPETITIVE INHIBITOR	NON-COMPETITIVE INHIBITOR
number of site on the enzyme		
structure of inhibitor is similar or different with substrate		
Km		
Vmax		

Q 9. The rate of an enzymatic reaction is measured with three similar but different substrates.
From the experiments, the Km and Kcat values were determined for each substrate.

	Km	Kcat	Km Kcat Kcat/Km (M^{-1}S^{-1})
Substrate A	1	$5*10^3$	$5*10^3$
Substrate B	0.1	$5*10^{-2}$	$5*10^{-2}$
Substrate C	100	$5*10^4$	$5*10^2$

Based on this data, answer all the following questions:
1. With which compound the enzyme has the highest affinity? Explain your answer.
2. With which compound the enzyme has maximum Velocity? Explain your answer.
3. With which compound the enzyme has highest catalytic efficiency? Explain your answer

Q 10. After study all of the following figures, answer all the questions.

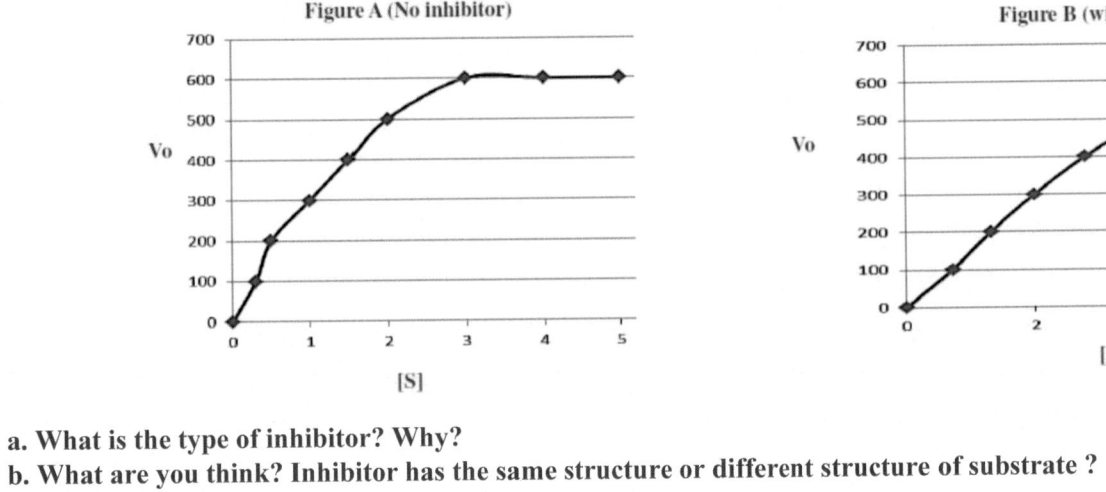

a.

Vmax =

....

Km =

....

b.

What is the type of
inhibitor?
why?

c.

What is the type of inhibitor?
Why?

Q 11: A biochemist obtains the following data for two charts for an enzyme without inhibitor and with inhibitor that is known to follow Michaelis-Menten kinetics

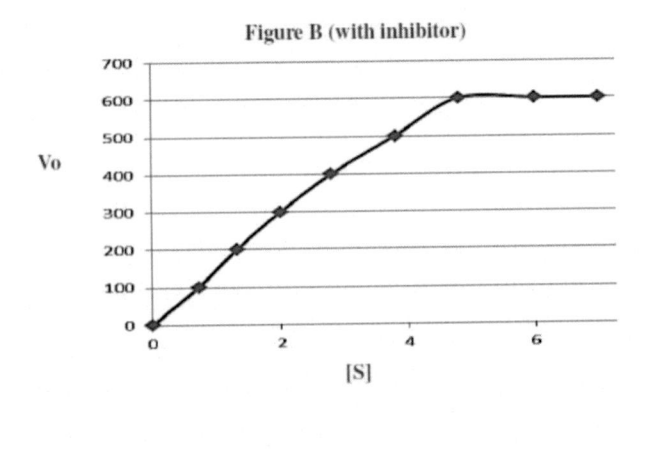

a. What is the type of inhibitor? Why?

b. What are you think? Inhibitor has the same structure or different structure of substrate ?

Q 12. After study the following figures, Answer the questions. If you know are given the concentration for two types of inhibitor.

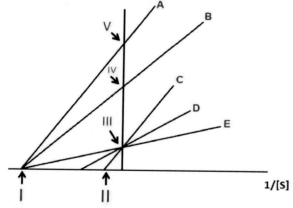

1. Which represents competitive inhibitor with concentration 30 mM?
a) A b) B c) C d) D e) E

2. Which represents competitive inhibitor with concentration 20 mM?
a) A b) B c) C d) D e) E

3. How can we calculate Km for non-competitive inhibitor with concentration 10 mM ?
a) I b) II c) III d) IV e) V

4. Which represent enzyme alone (without Non- competitive inhibitor)?
a) A b) B c) C d) D e) E

5. How can we calculate Vmax for competitive inhibitor with concentration 30 mM ?
a) I b) II c) III d) IV e) V

OVERVIEW

Bioenergetics describes the transfer and utilization of energy in biologic systems. It makes use of a few basic ideas from the field of thermo - dynamics, particularly the concept of free energy. Changes in free energy (ΔG) provide a measure of the energetic feasibility of a chemical reaction and can, therefore, allow prediction of whether a reaction or process can take place. Bioenergetics concerns only the initial and final energy states of reaction components, not the mechanism or how much time is needed for the chemical change to take place. In short, bio - energetics predicts if a process is possible, whereas kinetics measures how fast the reaction occurs.

Chapter 6 : Bioenergetics and Oxidative Phosphorylation

6.1.Bioenergetics

Is a field in biochemistry and cell biology that concerns energy flow through living systems. This is an active area of biological research that includes the study of the transformation of energy in living organisms and the study of thousands of different cellular processes such as cellular respiration and the many other metabolic and enzymatic processes that lead to production and utilization of energy in forms such as adenosine triphosphate (ATP) molecules. That is, the goal of bioenergetics is to describe how living organisms acquire and transform energy in order to perform biological work.The study of metabolic pathways is thus essential to bioenergetics.

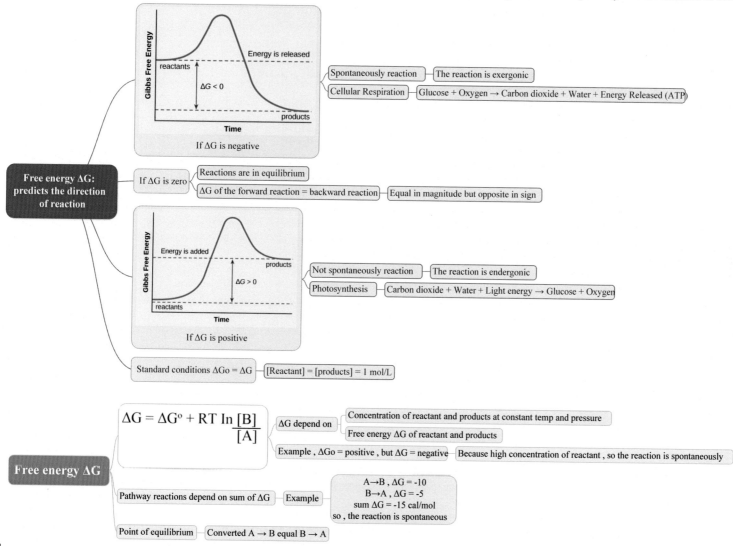

Free energy ΔG: predicts the direction of reaction

If ΔG is negative
- Spontaneously reaction — The reaction is exergonic
- Cellular Respiration — Glucose + Oxygen → Carbon dioxide + Water + Energy Released (ATP)

If ΔG is zero
- Reactions are in equilibrium
- ΔG of the forward reaction = backward reaction — Equal in magnitude but opposite in sign

If ΔG is positive
- Not spontaneously reaction — The reaction is endergonic
- Photosynthesis — Carbon dioxide + Water + Light energy → Glucose + Oxygen

Standard conditions ΔGo = ΔG — [Reactant] = [products] = 1 mol/L

Free energy ΔG

$$\Delta G = \Delta G^o + RT \ln \frac{[B]}{[A]}$$

ΔG depend on
- Concentration of reactant and products at constant temp and pressure
- Free energy ΔG of reactant and products

Example , ΔGo = positive , but ΔG = negative — Because high concentration of reactant , so the reaction is spontaneously

Pathway reactions depend on sum of ΔG — Example
- A→B , ΔG = -10
- B→A , ΔG = -5
- sum ΔG = -15 cal/mol
- so , the reaction is spontaneous

Point of equilibrium — Converted A → B equal B → A

6.2. Photosynthesis

Is a process used by plants and other organisms to convert light energy into chemical energy that can later be released to fuel the organisms activities. This chemical energy is stored in carbohydrate molecules, such as sugars, which are synthesized from carbon dioxide and water hence the name photosynthesis.

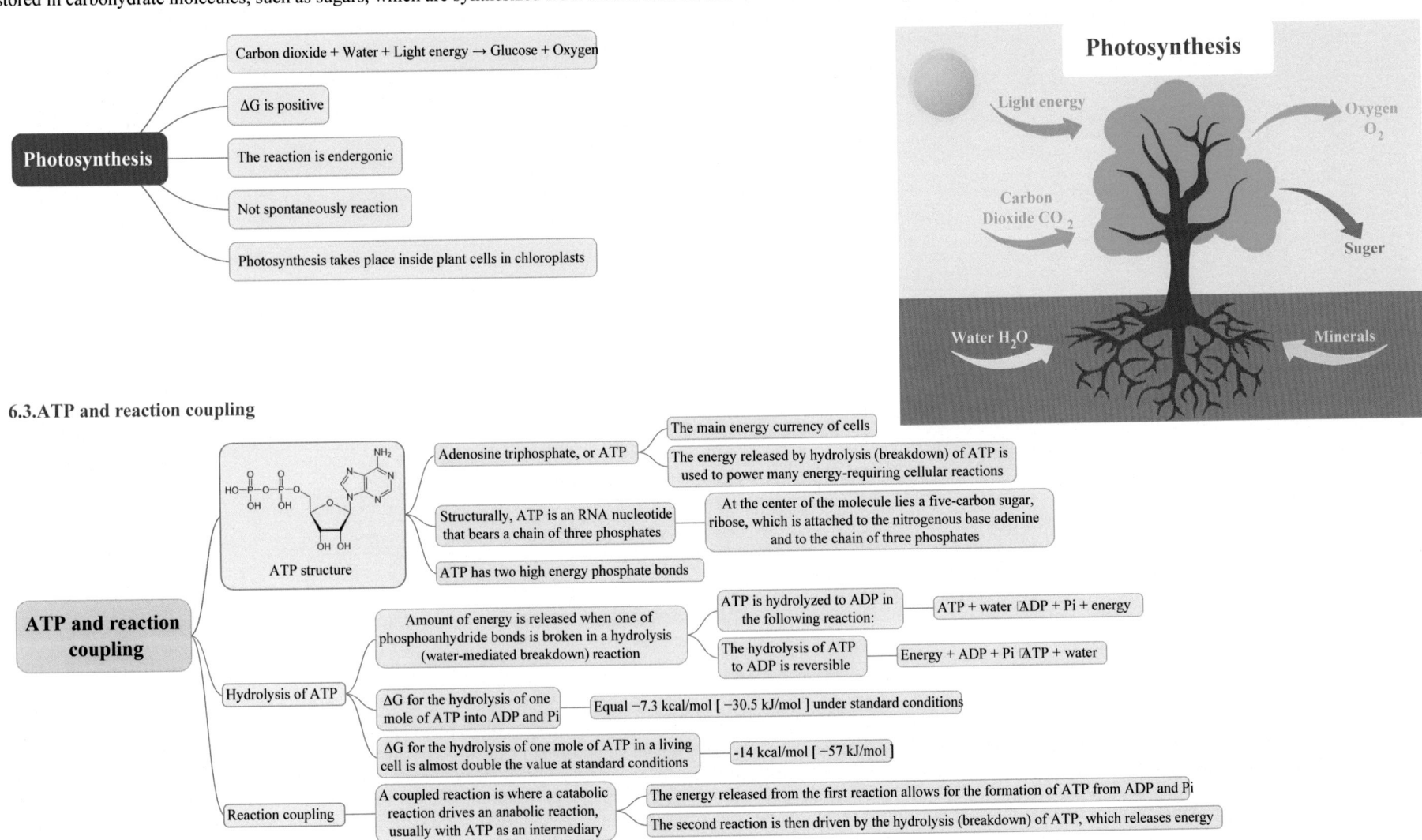

6.3. ATP and reaction coupling

Photosynthesis
- Carbon dioxide + Water + Light energy → Glucose + Oxygen
- ΔG is positive
- The reaction is endergonic
- Not spontaneously reaction
- Photosynthesis takes place inside plant cells in chloroplasts

ATP and reaction coupling

ATP structure
- Adenosine triphosphate, or ATP
  - The main energy currency of cells
  - The energy released by hydrolysis (breakdown) of ATP is used to power many energy-requiring cellular reactions
- Structurally, ATP is an RNA nucleotide that bears a chain of three phosphates
  - At the center of the molecule lies a five-carbon sugar, ribose, which is attached to the nitrogenous base adenine and to the chain of three phosphates
- ATP has two high energy phosphate bonds

Hydrolysis of ATP
- Amount of energy is released when one of phosphoanhydride bonds is broken in a hydrolysis (water-mediated breakdown) reaction
  - ATP is hydrolyzed to ADP in the following reaction: — ATP + water ⟶ ADP + Pi + energy
  - The hydrolysis of ATP to ADP is reversible — Energy + ADP + Pi ⟶ ATP + water
- ΔG for the hydrolysis of one mole of ATP into ADP and Pi — Equal −7.3 kcal/mol [−30.5 kJ/mol] under standard conditions
- ΔG for the hydrolysis of one mole of ATP in a living cell is almost double the value at standard conditions — -14 kcal/mol [−57 kJ/mol]

Reaction coupling
- A coupled reaction is where a catabolic reaction drives an anabolic reaction, usually with ATP as an intermediary
  - The energy released from the first reaction allows for the formation of ATP from ADP and Pi
  - The second reaction is then driven by the hydrolysis (breakdown) of ATP, which releases energy

6.4.Cyclic photophosphorylation

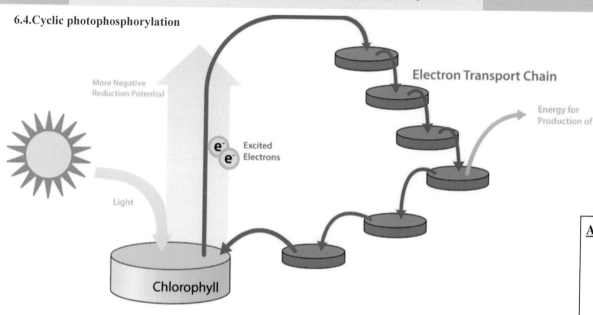

A coupled reaction is where a catabolic reaction drives an anabolic reaction, usually with ATP as an intermediary.

<u>An ATP molecule</u>

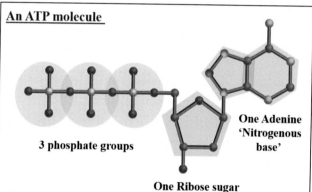

3 phosphate groups

One Adenine 'Nitrogenous base'

One Ribose sugar

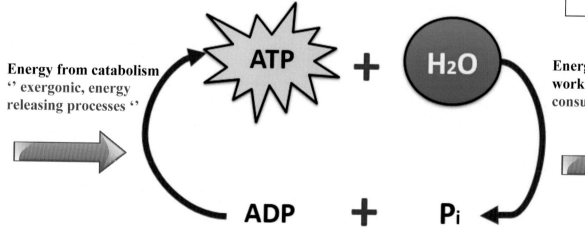

Energy from catabolism '' exergonic, energy releasing processes ''

Energy from cellular work '' endergonic, energy consuming processes ''

ATP + H₂O

ADP + Pᵢ

6.5. Structure of mitochondrion

The mitochondrion (plural mitochondria) is a double-membrane-bound organelle found in most eukaryoticorganisms. Some cells in some multicellular organisms may, however, lack them (for example, mature mammalian red blood cells). In addition, Mitochondria are rod-shaped organelles that can be considered the power generators of the cell, converting oxygen and nutrients into adenosine triphosphate (ATP). ATP is the chemical energy "currency" of the cell that powers the cell's metabolic activities.

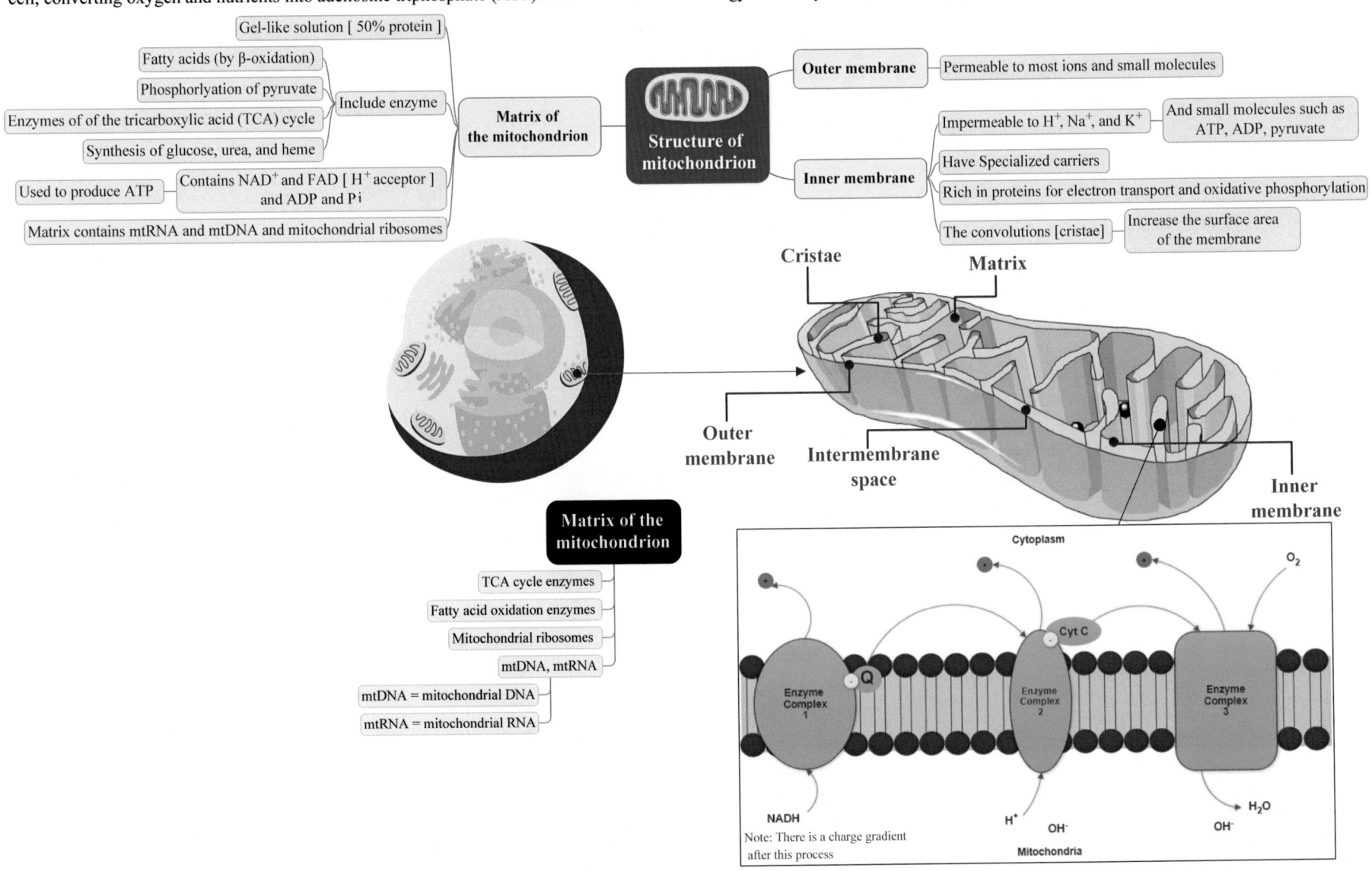

Gel-like solution [50% protein]

Fatty acids (by β-oxidation)

Phosphorlyation of pyruvate

Enzymes of of the tricarboxylic acid (TCA) cycle

Synthesis of glucose, urea, and heme

Include enzyme

Used to produce ATP

Contains NAD^+ and FAD [H^+ acceptor] and ADP and Pi

Matrix contains mtRNA and mtDNA and mitochondrial ribosomes

Matrix of the mitochondrion

Structure of mitochondrion

Outer membrane — Permeable to most ions and small molecules

Inner membrane

Impermeable to H^+, Na^+, and K^+ — And small molecules such as ATP, ADP, pyruvate

Have Specialized carriers

Rich in proteins for electron transport and oxidative phosphorylation

The convolutions [cristae] — Increase the surface area of the membrane

Cristae   Matrix

Outer membrane   Intermembrane space   Inner membrane

Matrix of the mitochondrion

TCA cycle enzymes

Fatty acid oxidation enzymes

Mitochondrial ribosomes

mtDNA, mtRNA

mtDNA = mitochondrial DNA

mtRNA = mitochondrial RNA

Cytoplasm

O_2

Cyt C

Enzyme Complex 1

Q

Enzyme Complex 2

Enzyme Complex 3

NADH

H^+ OH^-

OH^-

H_2O

Note: There is a charge gradient after this process

Mitochondria

6.6.The electron transport chain

Electron Transport Chain is a series of protein complexes (called Complexes I, II, III, and IV) found in the inner mitochondrial membrane whose main goal is to shuttle electrons to oxygen and couples this electron transfer with the transfer of protons (H+ ions) across a membrane. This creates an electrochemical proton gradient that that can be used to synthesized ATP molecules, a molecule that stores energy chemically in the form of highly strained bonds.

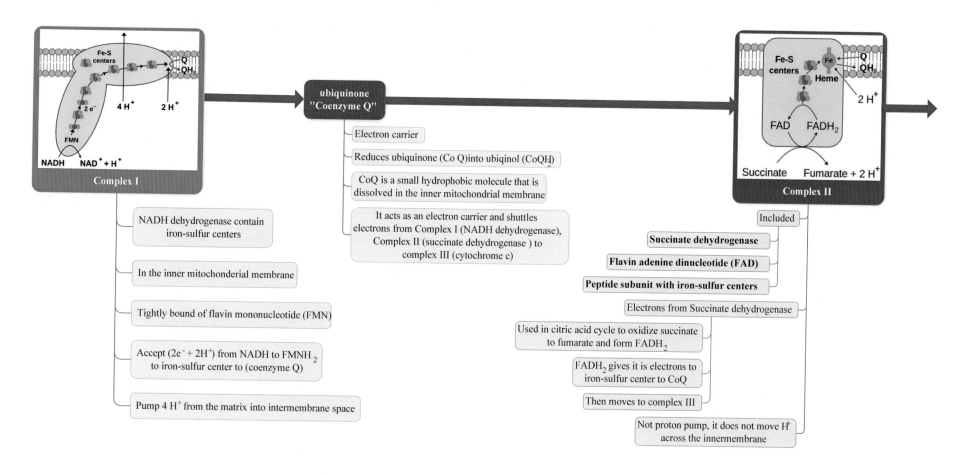

Complex I

- NADH dehydrogenase contain iron-sulfur centers
- In the inner mitochonderial membrane
- Tightly bound of flavin mononucleotide (FMN)
- Accept $(2e^- + 2H^+)$ from NADH to FMNH$_2$ to iron-sulfur center to (coenzyme Q)
- Pump 4 H$^+$ from the matrix into intermembrane space

ubiquinone "Coenzyme Q"

- Electron carrier
- Reduces ubiquinone (Co Q)into ubiqinol (CoQH$_2$)
- CoQ is a small hydrophobic molecule that is dissolved in the inner mitochondrial membrane
- It acts as an electron carrier and shuttles electrons from Complex I (NADH dehydrogenase), Complex II (succinate dehydrogenase) to complex III (cytochrome c)

Complex II

Included
- **Succinate dehydrogenase**
- **Flavin adenine dinucleotide (FAD)**
- **Peptide subunit with iron-sulfur centers**

- Electrons from Succinate dehydrogenase
- Used in citric acid cycle to oxidize succinate to fumarate and form FADH$_2$
- FADH$_2$ gives it is electrons to iron-sulfur center to CoQ
- Then moves to complex III
- Not proton pump, it does not move H$^+$ across the innermembrane

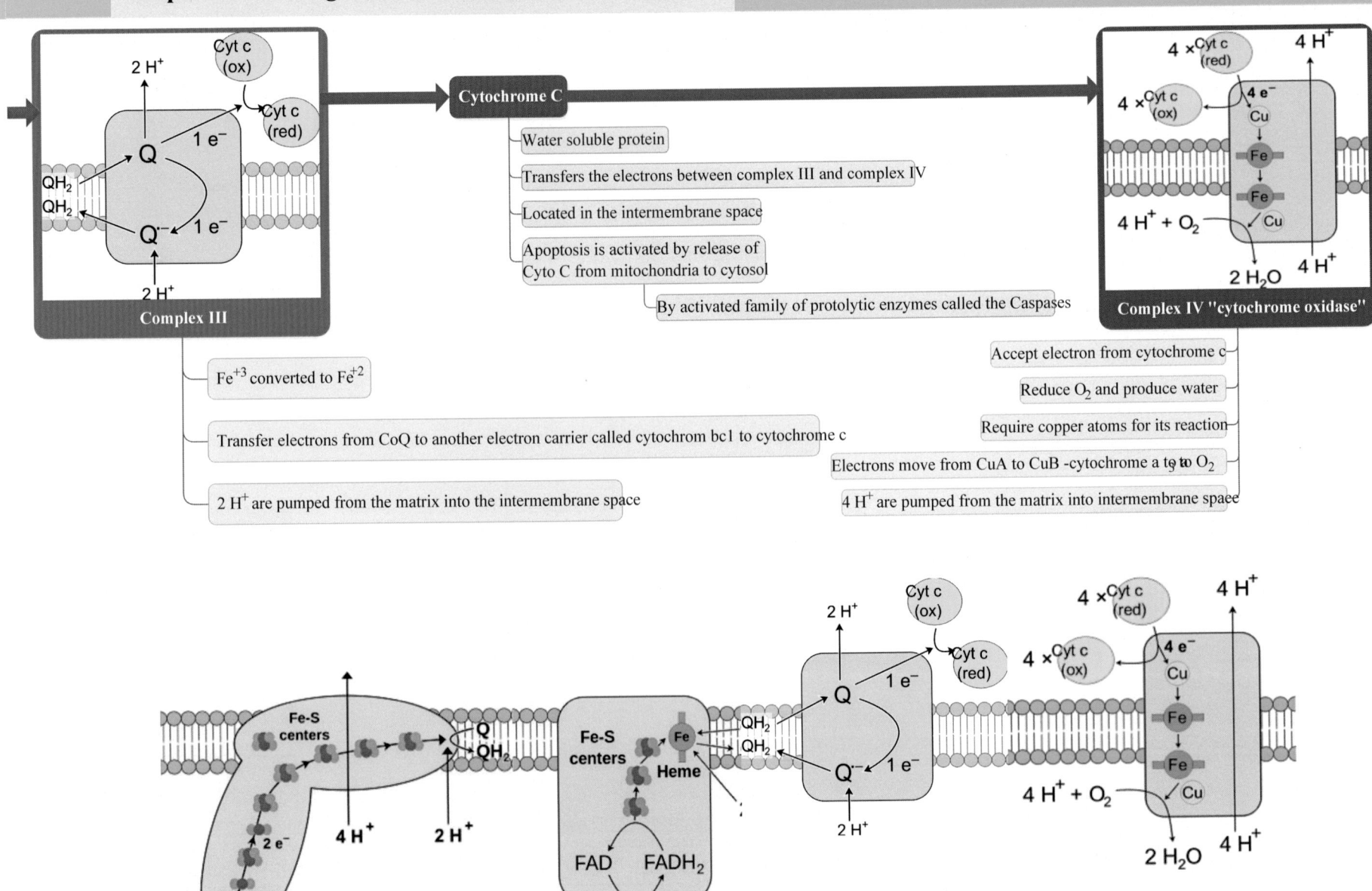

Complex III

Cytochrome C

- Water soluble protein
- Transfers the electrons between complex III and complex IV
- Located in the intermembrane space
- Apoptosis is activated by release of Cyto C from mitochondria to cytosol
- By activated family of protolytic enzymes called the Caspases

Complex IV "cytochrome oxidase"

- Fe^{+3} converted to Fe^{+2}
- Transfer electrons from CoQ to another electron carrier called cytochrom bc1 to cytochrome c
- 2 H^+ are pumped from the matrix into the intermembrane space

- Accept electron from cytochrome c
- Reduce O_2 and produce water
- Require copper atoms for its reaction
- Electrons move from CuA to CuB -cytochrome a to O_2
- 4 H^+ are pumped from the matrix into intermembrane space

Chapter 6 : Bioenergetics and Oxidative Phosphorylation

Chemiosmotic hypothesis OR (Mitchell hypothesis) explains how the free energy generated by the transport of electrons by the electron transport chain is used to produce ATP from ADP + Pi. ATP-ADP transport OR ADP/ATP translocases, are transporter proteins that enable the exchange of cytosolic adenosine diphosphate (ADP) and mitochondrial adenosine triphosphate (ATP) across the inner mitochondrial membrane. Free ADP is transported from the cytoplasm to the mitochondrial matrix, while ATP produced from oxidative phosphorylation is transported from the mitochondrial matrix to the cytoplasm, thus providing the cells with its main energy currency.

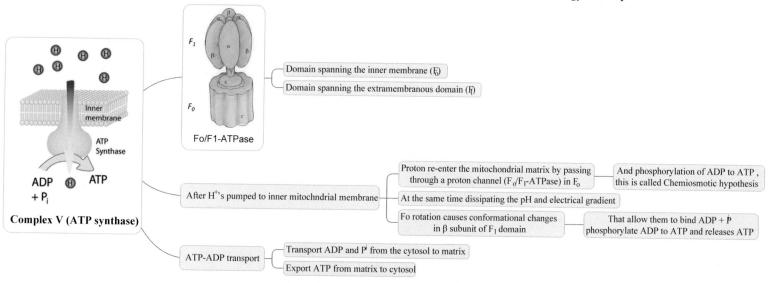

Fo/F1-ATPase

- Domain spanning the inner membrane (F_o)
- Domain spanning the extramembranous domain (F_1)

Complex V (ATP synthase)

After H$^+$'s pumped to inner mitochndrial membrane
- Proton re-enter the mitochondrial matrix by passing through a proton channel (F$_o$/F$_1$-ATPase) in F$_o$ — And phosphorylation of ADP to ATP , this is called Chemiosmotic hypothesis
- At the same time dissipating the pH and electrical gradient
- Fo rotation causes conformational changes in β subunit of F$_1$ domain — That allow them to bind ADP + P^i phosphorylate ADP to ATP and releases ATP

ATP-ADP transport
- Transport ADP and P^i from the cytosol to matrix
- Export ATP from matrix to cytosol

Non-shivering thermogenesis occurs in brown adipose tissue (brown fat) that is present in almost all eutherians (swine being the only exception currently known). Brown adipose tissue has a unique uncoupling protein (thermogenin, also known as uncoupling protein 1) that allows the uncoupling of protons moving down their mitochondrial gradient from the synthesis of ATP, thus allowing the energy to be dissipated as heat.

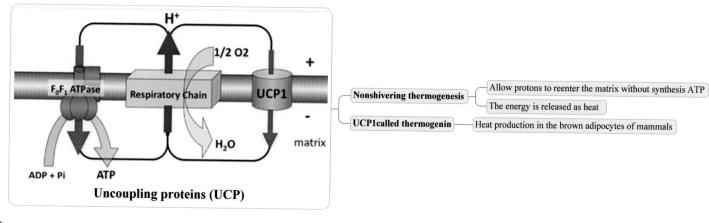

Uncoupling proteins (UCP)

Nonshivering thermogenesis
- Allow protons to reenter the matrix without synthesis ATP
- The energy is released as heat

UCP1called thermogenin
- Heat production in the brown adipocytes of mammals

NADH transported from cytosol into mitochondrial matrix by

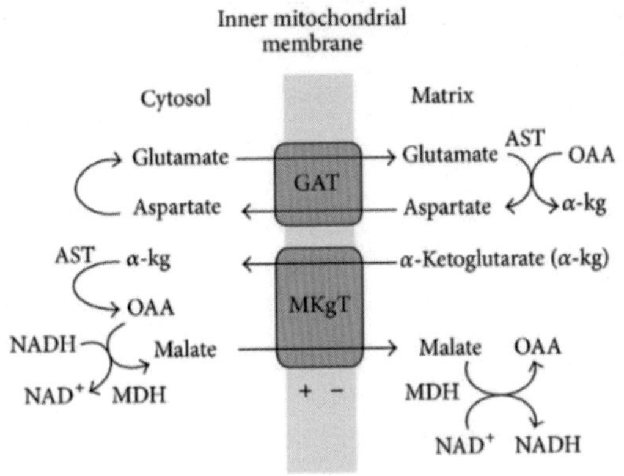

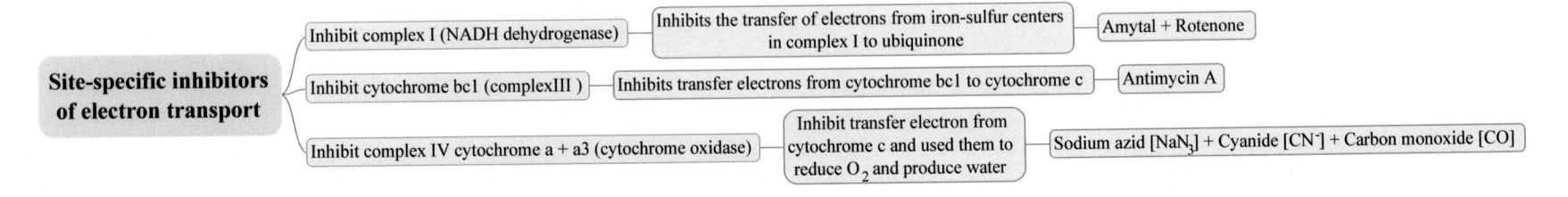

Malate-Aspartate shuttle

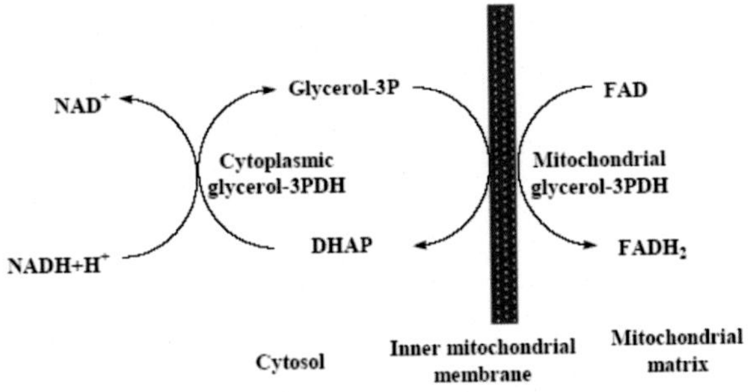

Glycerol 3-Phosphate Shuttle

Produced **3 ATPs**

Due to NADH oxidation in Complex I

Produced **2 ATPs**

Due to FADH$_2$ reduction in Complex IV

6.7. Site-specific inhibitors of electron transport
Inhibition of electron transport inhibits ATP synthesis because these processes are tightly coupled

Site-specific inhibitors of electron transport

Inhibit complex I (NADH dehydrogenase) — Inhibits the transfer of electrons from iron-sulfur centers in complex I to ubiquinone — Amytal + Rotenone

Inhibit cytochrome bc1 (complexIII) — Inhibits transfer electrons from cytochrome bc1 to cytochrome c — Antimycin A

Inhibit complex IV cytochrome a + a3 (cytochrome oxidase) — Inhibit transfer electron from cytochrome c and used them to reduce O$_2$ and produce water — Sodium azid [NaN$_3$] + Cyanide [CN$^-$] + Carbon monoxide [CO]

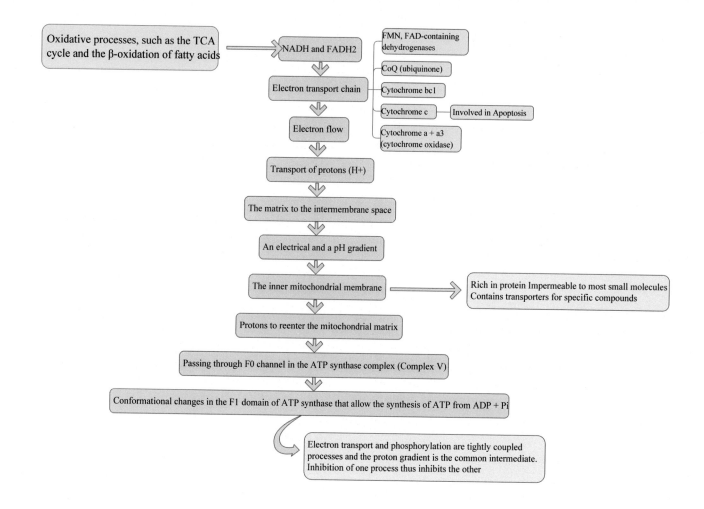

Oxidative processes, such as the TCA cycle and the β-oxidation of fatty acids

NADH and FADH2

FMN, FAD-containing dehydrogenases

CoQ (ubiquinone)

Cytochrome bc1

Cytochrome c — Involved in Apoptosis

Cytochrome a + a3 (cytochrome oxidase)

Electron transport chain

Electron flow

Transport of protons (H+)

The matrix to the intermembrane space

An electrical and a pH gradient

The inner mitochondrial membrane → Rich in protein Impermeable to most small molecules Contains transporters for specific compounds

Protons to reenter the mitochondrial matrix

Passing through F0 channel in the ATP synthase complex (Complex V)

Conformational changes in the F1 domain of ATP synthase that allow the synthesis of ATP from ADP + Pi

Electron transport and phosphorylation are tightly coupled processes and the proton gradient is the common intermediate. Inhibition of one process thus inhibits the other

Oxidative Phosphorylation : Exercises

Q 1: Circle the best correct answer:

1. The number of ATP produced in the oxidation of 1 molecule of NADH is...... and oxidation of $FADH_2$ is...... in oxidative phosphorylation is :
a. 3, 2
b. 2, 3
c. 3, 3
d. 2, 2

2. The location of electron transport chain is:
a. Cytoplasm
b. Endoplasmic reticulum
c. Mitochondria
d. Nucleus

3. The complex that act as NADH dehydrogenase is :
a. Complex I
b. Complex II
c. Complex III
d. Complex IV

4. The complex that act as succinate dehydrogenase is:
a. Complex I
b. Complex II
c. Complex III
d. Complex IV

5. Which of the following statement is false about CoQ?
a. It is accept electrons from complex I and complex II
b. It is a small hydrophobic molecule that is dissolved in the inner mitochondrial membrane.
c. Called ubiquinone
d. Reduce O_2 and produce water

6. Which of the following statement is false about Complex IV?
a. It is called cytochrome oxidase
b. It is pump proton
c. It is called cytochrome reductase
d. Reduce O_2 and produce water

7. Which of the following protein complexes is not proton pump?
a. Complex I
b. Complex II
c. Complex III
c. Complex IV

8. Sodium azide inhibit ETC at...............
a. Complex I
b. Complex II
c. Complex III
d. Complex IV

9. Which of the following statement about uncoupling protein is true?:
a. Proton re-enter the matrix without energy captured as ATP
b. Energy released as heat (called nonshivering thermogenesis)
c. uncoupling protein produced heat in brown adipocytes of mammals
d. all of these

10. The true statement about complex V (ATP synthase):
a. also called Fo/F1-ATPase
b. Consist from the inner membrane (F_o) and extra membranous domain (F_1)
c. Allow phosphorylated ADP and release ATP
d. All of these

11. NADH is oxidized in complex..................therefore, the total number of proton pumped during oxidation NADH is...............
a. Complex II, 6 H^+
b. Complex I, 10H^+
c. Complex III, 2H^+
d. Complex IV, 4H^+

12. The toxicity of amytal due to inhibit:
a. Complex I
b. Complex II
c. Complex III
d. Complex IV

Q 1: Circle the best correct answer:

13. The number of ATP that is produced from both Glycerol -3- phosphate shuttle is........and Malate-Aspartate shuttle is.........
a. 2ATP,3ATP
b.3ATP,2ATP
c.1ATP,2ATP
d.3ATP,6ATP

14. The true statement about ATP-ADP transport is:
a. Found in inner mitochondrial membrane
b. Imports one molecule of ADP from the cytosol into mitochondria
c. Exporting one ATP from the matrix back into the cytosol
d. All of these

15. The true statement about cytochrome C is:
a. Located in the intermembrane space
b. Water soluble protein
c. Transfer electrons between complex III and complex IV
d. All of these

Q 2: Write short notes on:

1. The chemiosmotic theory of oxidative phosphorylation.
2. The nonshivering thermogenesis.
3. Describe Glycerol 3-Phosphate Shuttle and Malate-Aspartate shuttle.
4. Explain, NADH transported from cytosol into mitochondrial matrix by Glycerol 3-Phosphate Shuttle produced 2 ATP.
5. Explain, $FADH_2$ produced 2ATP by oxidative phosphorylation.
6. Explain, If NADH transported from cytosol into mitochondrial matrix by Malate-Aspartate shuttle produce 3ATP.

OVERVIEW

Carbohydrates are the most abundant organic molecules in nature. Carbohydrates are found in a wide array of both healthy and unhealthy foods, bread, beans, milk, popcorn, potatoes, cookies, spaghetti, soft drinks, corn, and cherry pie. They also come in a variety of forms. The most common and abundant forms are sugars, fibers, and starches. Carbohydrates provide the body with glucose, which is converted to energy used to support bodily functions and physical activity, and serving as cell membrane components that mediate some forms of intercellular communication. Carbohydrates also serve as a structural component of many organisms, including the cell walls of bacteria, the exoskeleton of many insects, and the fibrous cellulose of plants. The empiric formula for many of the simpler carbo - hydrates is $(CH_2O)_n$. This formula holds true for monosaccharaides .Some exceptions exist.

Chapter 7 : Introduction to Carbohydrates

Carbohydrates, together with lipids, proteins and nucleic acids, are one of the four major classes of biologically essential organic molecules found in all living organism

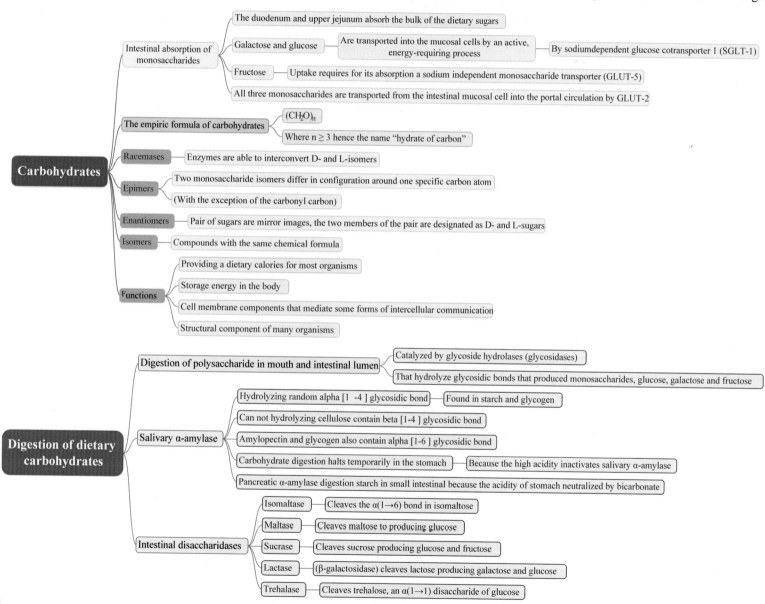

Carbohydrates

- **Intestinal absorption of monosaccharides**
  - The duodenum and upper jejunum absorb the bulk of the dietary sugars
  - Galactose and glucose — Are transported into the mucosal cells by an active, energy-requiring process — By sodiumdependent glucose cotransporter 1 (SGLT-1)
  - Fructose — Uptake requires for its absorption a sodium independent monosaccharide transporter (GLUT-5)
  - All three monosaccharides are transported from the intestinal mucosal cell into the portal circulation by GLUT-2
- **The empiric formula of carbohydrates**
  - $(CH_2O)_n$
  - Where $n \geq 3$ hence the name "hydrate of carbon"
- **Racemases** — Enzymes are able to interconvert D- and L-isomers
- **Epimers**
  - Two monosaccharide isomers differ in configuration around one specific carbon atom
  - (With the exception of the carbonyl carbon)
- **Enantiomers** — Pair of sugars are mirror images, the two members of the pair are designated as D- and L-sugars
- **Isomers** — Compounds with the same chemical formula
- **Functions**
  - Providing a dietary calories for most organisms
  - Storage energy in the body
  - Cell membrane components that mediate some forms of intercellular communication
  - Structural component of many organisms

Digestion of dietary carbohydrates

- **Digestion of polysaccharide in mouth and intestinal lumen**
  - Catalyzed by glycoside hydrolases (glycosidases)
  - That hydrolyze glycosidic bonds that produced monosaccharides, glucose, galactose and fructose
- **Salivary α-amylase**
  - Hydrolyzing random alpha [1 -4] glycosidic bond — Found in starch and glycogen
  - Can not hydrolyzing cellulose contain beta [1-4] glycosidic bond
  - Amylopectin and glycogen also contain alpha [1-6] glycosidic bond
  - Carbohydrate digestion halts temporarily in the stomach — Because the high acidity inactivates salivary α-amylase
  - Pancreatic α-amylase digestion starch in small intestinal because the acidity of stomach neutralized by bicarbonate
- **Intestinal disaccharidases**
  - Isomaltase — Cleaves the $\alpha(1{\rightarrow}6)$ bond in isomaltose
  - Maltase — Cleaves maltose to producing glucose
  - Sucrase — Cleaves sucrose producing glucose and fructose
  - Lactase — (β-galactosidase) cleaves lactose producing galactose and glucose
  - Trehalase — Cleaves trehalose, an $\alpha(1{\rightarrow}1)$ disaccharide of glucose

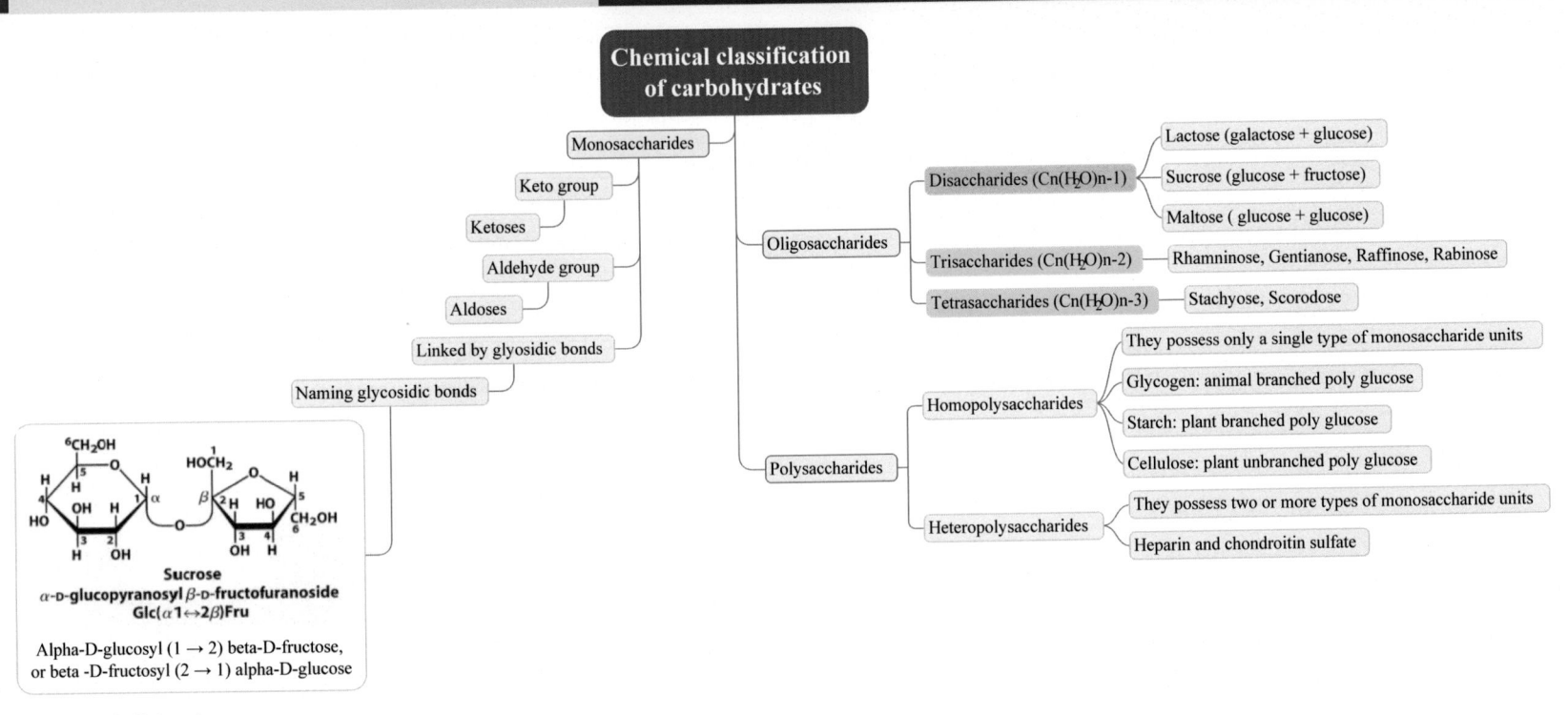

7.1. Digestive enzyme deficiencies

If carbohydrate degradation is deficient (heredity, intestinal disease, malnutrition, or drugs that injure the mucosa of the small intestine), undigested carbohydrate will pass into the large intestine, where it can cause:

1. osmotic diarrhea.
2. Bacterial fermentation of the compounds produces large volumes of CO_2 and H_2 gas, causing abdominal cramps, diarrhea, and flatulence.
3. Lactose intolerance, caused by a lack of lactase or age dependent loss of lactase due to mutation in chromosome 2 that control the gene of lactase and also Sucrase-isomaltase complex deficiency results in an intolerance of ingested sucrose.

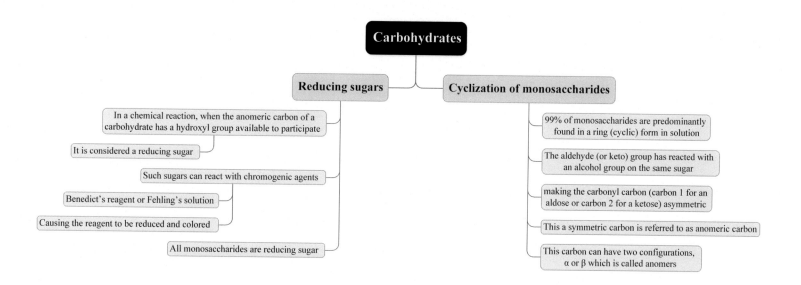

Carbohydrates

Reducing sugars

- In a chemical reaction, when the anomeric carbon of a carbohydrate has a hydroxyl group available to participate
- It is considered a reducing sugar
- Such sugars can react with chromogenic agents
- Benedict's reagent or Fehling's solution
- Causing the reagent to be reduced and colored
- All monosaccharides are reducing sugar

Cyclization of monosaccharides

- 99% of monosaccharides are predominantly found in a ring (cyclic) form in solution
- The aldehyde (or keto) group has reacted with an alcohol group on the same sugar
- making the carbonyl carbon (carbon 1 for an aldose or carbon 2 for a ketose) asymmetric
- This a symmetric carbon is referred to as anomeric carbon
- This carbon can have two configurations, α or β which is called anomers

OVERVIEW

Metabolic pathway. In biochemistry, a metabolic pathway is a linked series of chemical reactions occurring within a cell. The reactants, products, and intermediates of an enzymatic reaction are known as metabolites, which are modified by a sequence of chemical reactions catalyzed by enzymes. Most pathways can be classified as either catabolic (degradative) or anabolic (synthetic). Catabolic reactions break down complex molecules, such as proteins, polysaccharides, and lipids, to a few simple molecules, for example, CO_2, NH_3 (ammonia), and water. Anabolic pathways form complex end products from simple precursors, for example, the synthesis of the polysaccharide, glycogen, from glucose.

Chapter 8 : Glycolysis

8.1. Sodium-monosaccharide cotransporter system.

The secondary active transport of glucose in the kidney is Na^+ linked; therefore an Na^+ gradient must be established. This is achieved through the action of the Na^+/K^+ pump, the energy for which is provided through the hydrolysis of ATP. Three Na+ ions are extruded from the cell in exchange for two K^+ ions entering through the intramembranous enzyme Na^+/K^+-ATPase; this leaves a relative deficiency of Na^+ in the intracellular compartment. Na^+ ions diffuse down their concentration gradient into the columnar epithelia, co-transporting glucose. Once inside the epithelial cells, glucose reenters the bloodstream through facilitated diffusion through GLUT-2 transporters

8.2. Sodium-independent facilitated diffusion transport

Glucose transporters are a wide group of membrane proteins that facilitate the transport of glucose across the plasma membrane. Because glucose is a vital source of energy for all life, these transporters are present in all phyla. The GLUT family are a protein family that is found in most mammalian cells.

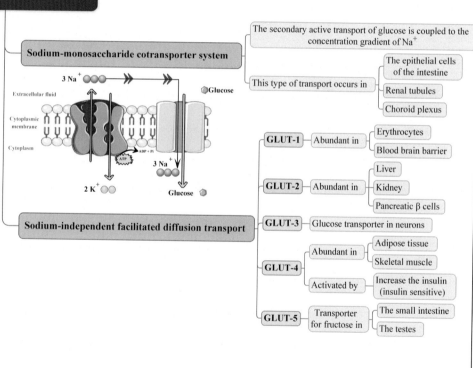

Schematic representation of the facilitated transport of glucose through a cell membrane. [Note: GLUT proteins contain 12 trans-membrane helices.]

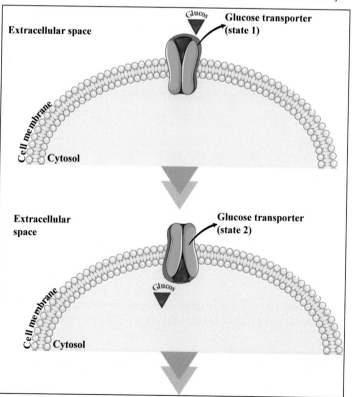

8.3.Glycolysis

Glycolysis (occurs in cytosol) is the metabolic pathway that converts glucose , into pyruvate, The free energy released in this process is used to form the high-energy molecules ATP (adenosine triphosphate) and NADH (reduced nicotinamide adenine dinucleotide). Glycolysis is a sequence of ten enzyme-catalyzed reactions. Most monosaccharides, such as fructose and galactose, can be converted to one of these intermediates. The intermediates may also be directly useful. For example, the intermediate dihydroxyacetone phosphate (DHAP) is a source of the glycerol that combines with fatty acids to form fat. The overall reaction of glycolysis which occurs in the cytoplasm is represented simply as:

$C_6H_{12}O_6$ + 2 NAD$^+$ + 2 ADP + 2 P$_i$ → 2 pyruvic acid, (CH$_3$(C=O)COOH + 2 ATP + 2 NADH + 2 H

Glycolysis occurs in two stages

Energy investment phase [from step 1 to 5] — Phosphorylated forms of intermediates by consuming 2 ATP

Energy generation phase [from step 6 to 10] — Generated 4 ATP and 2 NADH

8.3.1.The first step: Phosphorylation of glucose "To trapped within the cell"

the first step of glycolysis is phosphorylation by hexokinase and glucokinase of glucose to glucose-6-phosphate (G6P) trapped within the cells. magnesium (Mg) is also involved to help shield the negative charges from the phosphate groups on the ATP molecule.

Glucose ($C_6H_{12}O_6$) + ATP + Hexokinase → Glucose 6-Phosphate ($C_6H_{11}O_6P_1$) + ADP

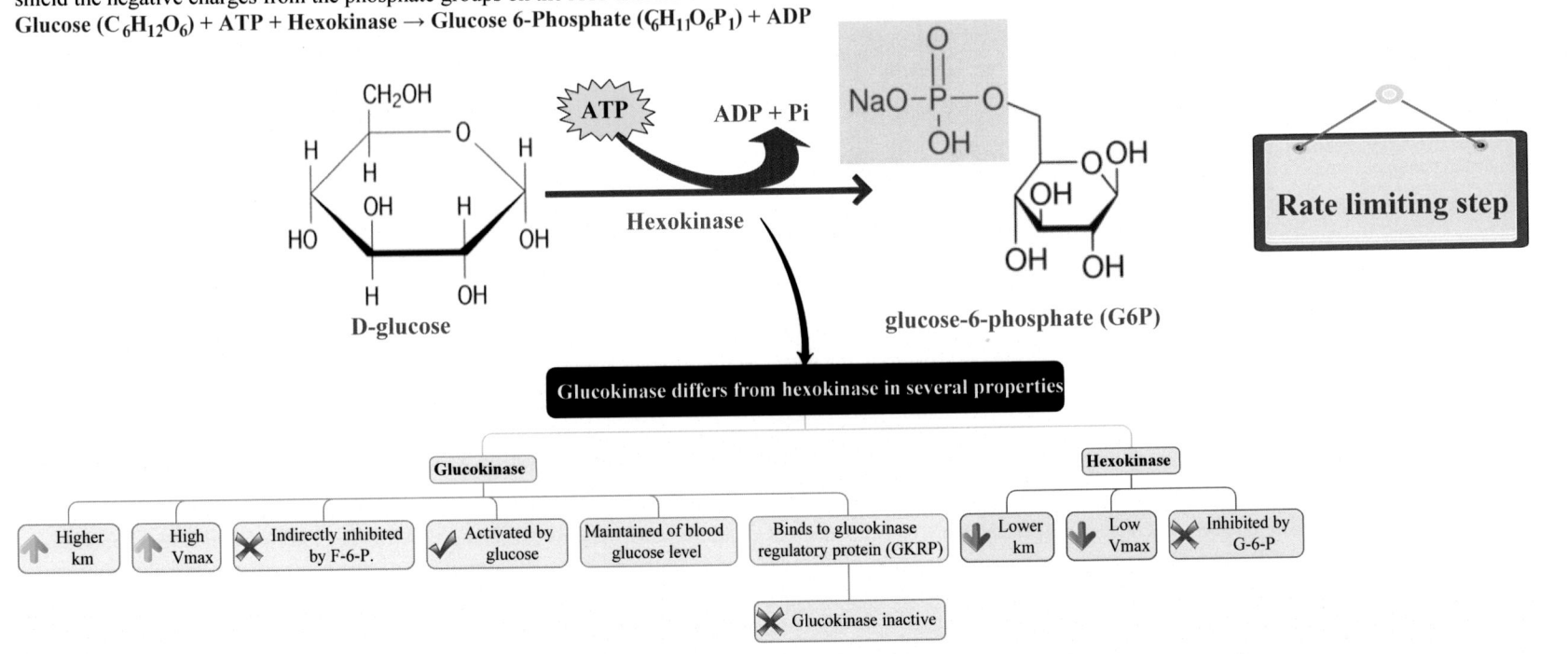

D-glucose

glucose-6-phosphate (G6P)

Rate limiting step

Glucokinase differs from hexokinase in several properties

Glucokinase
- ↑ Higher km
- ↑ High Vmax
- ✖ Indirectly inhibited by F-6-P.
- ✔ Activated by glucose
- Maintained of blood glucose level
- Binds to glucokinase regulatory protein (GKRP)
  - ✖ Glucokinase inactive

Hexokinase
- ↓ Lower km
- ↓ Low Vmax
- ✖ Inhibited by G-6-P

8.3.2.The second step: Isomerization of glucose 6-phosphate

The second reaction of glycolysis is the rearrangement of glucose 6-phosphate (G6P) into fructose 6-phosphate (F6P) by glucose phosphate isomerase

Glucose 6-Phosphate ($C_6H_{11}O_6P_1$) + Phosphoglucoisomerase (Enzyme) → Fructose 6-Phosphate ($C_6H_{11}O_6P_1$)

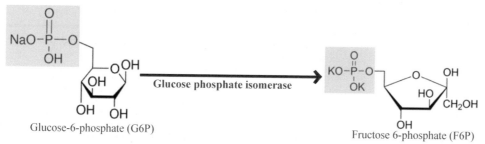

Glucose-6-phosphate (G6P)   Fructose 6-phosphate (F6P)

8.3.3.The third step: Phosphorylation of fructose 6-phosphate

Fructose-6-phosphate is converted to Fructose- 1,6-bisphosphate (FBP) by irreversible phosphorylation reaction catalyzed by phospho- fructokinase-1 (PFK-1) is important control point and the rate-limiting and committed step of glycolysis. A second molecule of ATP provides the phosphate group that is added on to the F6P molecule. A magnesium atom is involved to help shield negative charges.

Fructose 6-Phosphate ($C_6H_{11}O_6P_1$) + phosphofructokinase (Enzyme) + ATP → Fructose 1, 6-diphosphate ($C_6H_{10}O_6P_2$)

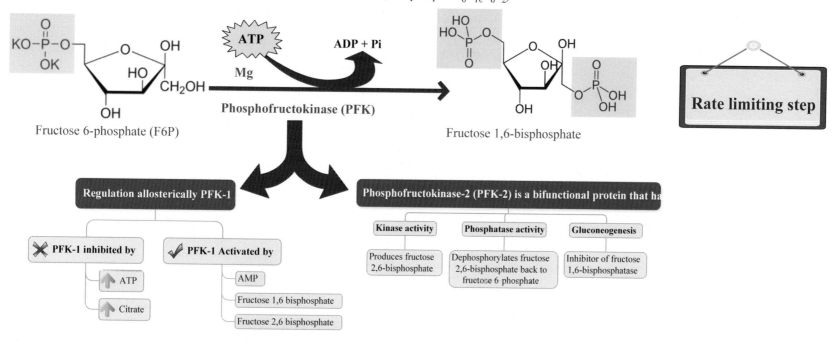

8.3.4.The 4th Step: litting of Fructose 1, 6-Diphosphate

The enzyme aldolase, which catalyzes the cleavage of FBP to yield two 3-carbon molecules. One of these molecules is called glyceraldehyde-3-phosphate (GAP) and the other is called dihydroxyacetone phosphate (DHAP).

Fructose 1, 6-diphosphate ($C_6H_{10}O_6P_2$) + Aldolase (Enzyme) → Glyceraldehyde Phosphate ($C_3H_5O_3P_1$) + Dihydroxyacetone phosphate ($C_3H_5O_3P_1$)

Fructose 1,6-bisphosphate

Aldolase

Dihydroxyacetone phosphate (DHAP)   Triose phosphate isomerase   Glyceraldehyde 3-phosphate (GAP)

8.3.5.The 5th step:Interconversion of the Two Sugars

The enzyme Triose phosphate isomerase interconverts the molecules dihydroxyacetone phosphate (DHAP) and glyceraldehyde 3-phosphate (GAP). Glyceraldehyde phospso it can continue in glycolysis.

Dihydroxyacetone phosphate ($C_3H_5O_3P_1$) + Triose Phosphate → Glyceraldehyde phosphate ($C_3H_5O_3P_1$)

8.3.6.The 6th step:Oxidation of glyceraldehyde 3-phosphate

The oxidation aldehyde group of glyceraldehyde 3-phosphate to a carboxyl group which attached to Pi to form
 1,3-bisphosphoglycerate by glyceraldehyde 3-phosphate dehydrogenase is the first oxidation-reduction reaction of glycolysis so produced NADH.

Triose phosphate dehydrogenase (Enzyme) + 2 NA$_i^+$ + 2 H$^-$ → 2NADH (Reduced Nicotinamide Adenine Dinucleotide) + 2 $\overset{+}{H}$

Triose phosphate dehydrogenase + 2 Glyceraldehyde phosphate ($C_3H_5O_3P_1$) + 2P (from cytoplasm) → 2 molecules of 1,3-diphoshoglyceric acid ($C_3H_4O_4P_2$)

Oxidation-reduction reaction

Glyceraldehyde 3-phosphate (GAP)

NAD$^+$ NADH

Glyceraldehyde-3-phosphate dehydrogenase (GAPDH)

1,3-bisphosphoglycerate

Mutase

In Red Blood Cells

No ATP production

2,3-bisphosphoglycerate

Phosphatase

2-phosphoglycerate

8.3.7. The 7th step: Synthesis of 3-phosphoglycerate producing ATP

Phosphoglycerate kinase transfers a phosphate group from 1,3-bisphosphoglycerate to ADP to form ATP and 3-phosphoglycerate.

2 molecules of 1,3-diphoshoglyceric acid ($C_3H_4O_4P_2$) + 2ADP + phosphoglycerokinase → 2 molecules of 3-Phosphoglyceric acid ($C_3H_5O_4P_1$) + 2ATP (Adenosine Triphosphate)

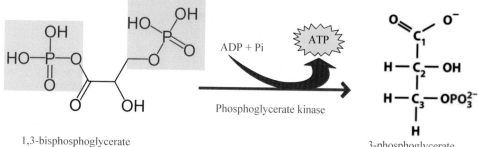

1,3-bisphosphoglycerate

ADP + Pi

ATP

Phosphoglycerate kinase

3-phosphoglycerate

substrate-level phosphorylation
Synthesize 2 ATP from 2 ADP

8.3.8. The 8th step: Relocation of Phosphorus Atom

The shift of the phosphate group from carbon 3 to carbon 2 of phosphoglycerate by phosphoglycerate mutase is freely reversible.

2 molecules of 3-Phosphoglyceric acid ($C_3H_5O_4P_1$) + phosphoglyceromutase (enzyme) → 2 molecules of 2-Phosphoglyceric acid ($C_3H_5O_4P_1$)

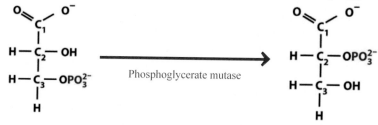

3-phosphoglycerate

Phosphoglycerate mutase

2-phosphoglycerate

8.3.9. The 9th step: Removal of Water

Dehydration of 2-phosphoglycerate by enolase to form phosphoenolpyruvate (PEP). The reaction is reversible

2 molecules of 2-Phosphoglyceric acid ($C_3H_5O_4P_1$) + Enolase (Enzyme) → 2 molecules of phosphoenolpyruvic acid (PEP) ($C_3H_3O_3P_1$) + 2 H_2O

2-phosphoglycerate

Enolase

phosphoenolpyruvic acid
(PEP)

+

H_2O

Water

8.3.10.The 10th step: Creation of Pyruvic Acid and ATP

The final step of glycolysis converts phosphoenolpyruvate into pyruvate with the help of the enzyme pyruvate kinase. As the enzyme's name suggests, this reaction involves the transfer of a phosphate group. The phosphate group attached to the 2' carbon of the PEP is transferred to a molecule of ADP, yielding ATP. Again, since there are two molecules of PEP, here we actually generate 2 ATP molecules. (substrate level phosphorylation).

2 molecules of phosphoenolpyruvic acid (PEP) ($C_3H_3O_3P_1$) + 2ADP + Pyruvate kinase (Enzyme) → 2ATP + 2 molecules of pyruvic acid.

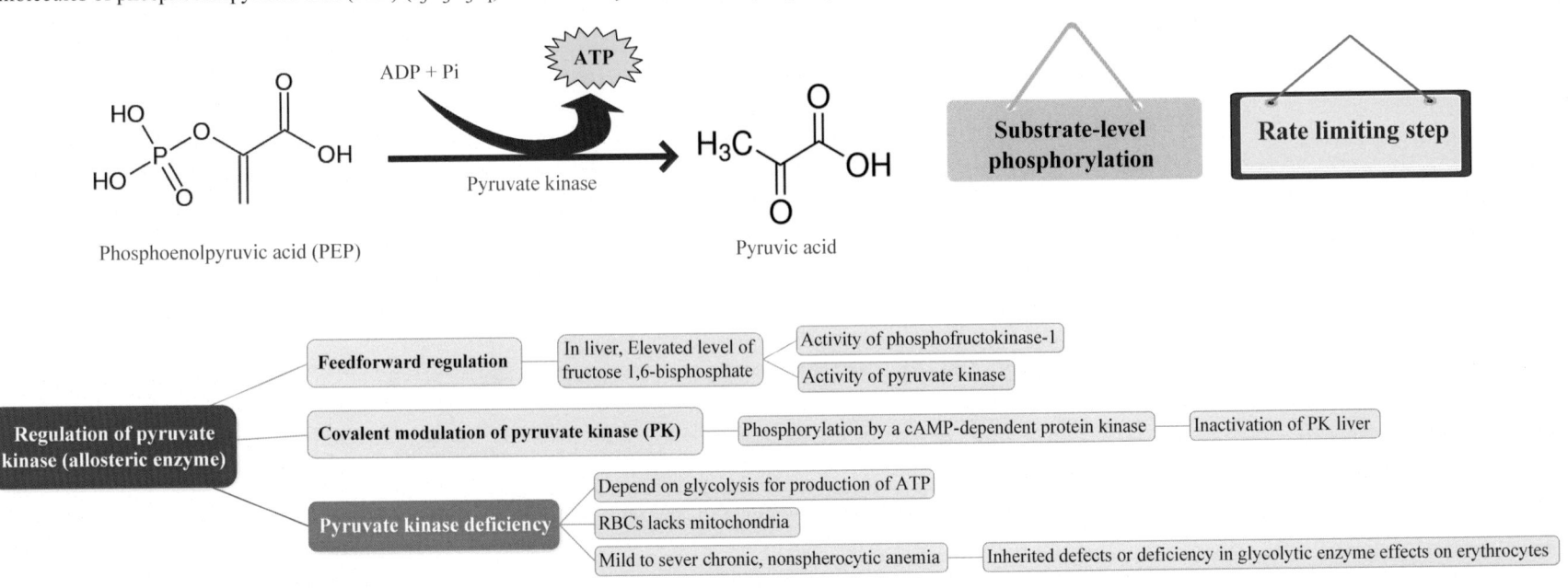

8.4.Fates of Pyruvate

In the absence of oxygen (anaerobic conditions) pyruvate undergoes fermentation either lactic acid fermentation or alcohol fermentation. In this fermentation reaction NO ATP molecules is generated, however reduced NAD^+ is generated from fermentation. The NAD^+ regenerated is used in the glycolysis process to make ATP. Therefore these cells only get energy (2 ATP) from glycolysis and not from the TCA cycle. Example of such cell are red blood cells. In the presence of oxygen (aerobic condition) pyruvate is converted to acetyl-CoA by the enzyme pyruvate dehydrogenase complex which enters the TCA The other fate of pyruvate is carboxylated to oxaloacetate (a TCA cycle intermediate) by pyruvate carboxylase.

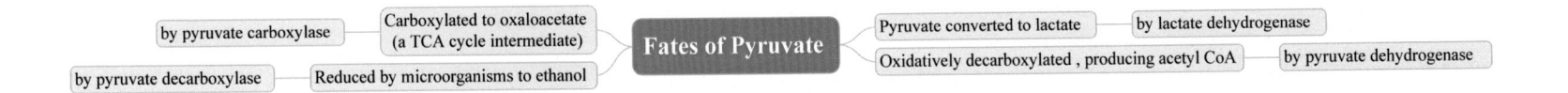

Glycolysis regulated steps

Hexokinase
- Inhibited by glucose -6-phosphate (G-6-P)
- Activated by glucose

Glucokinase
- Activated by glucose
- Inhibited by fructose-6-phosphate (F-6-P)

Phosphofructokinase-1 (PFK-1)
- Activated by
  - Fructose 2,6-bisphosphate
  - AMP
  - Fructose 1,6-bisphosphate
- Inhibited by
  - ATP
  - Citrate

**Activated by insulin
Inhibited by glucagon**

Pyruvate kinase (PK)
- activated by
  - Fructose 1,6-bisphosphate
- Covalent modulation

Pyruvate kinase (PK)

- Mutation in gene for PK
  - Altered primary structure of enzyme
  - Altered folding
  - Pyruvate kinase deficiency disease
  - causing hemolytic anemia

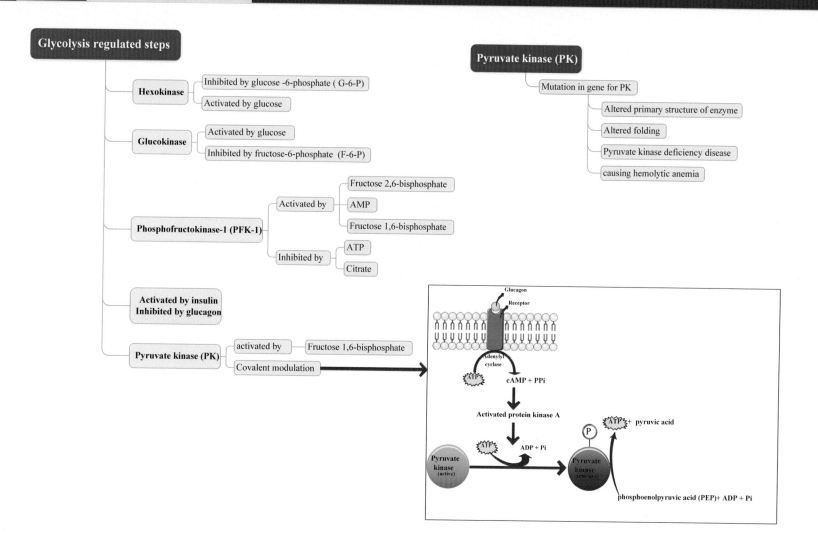

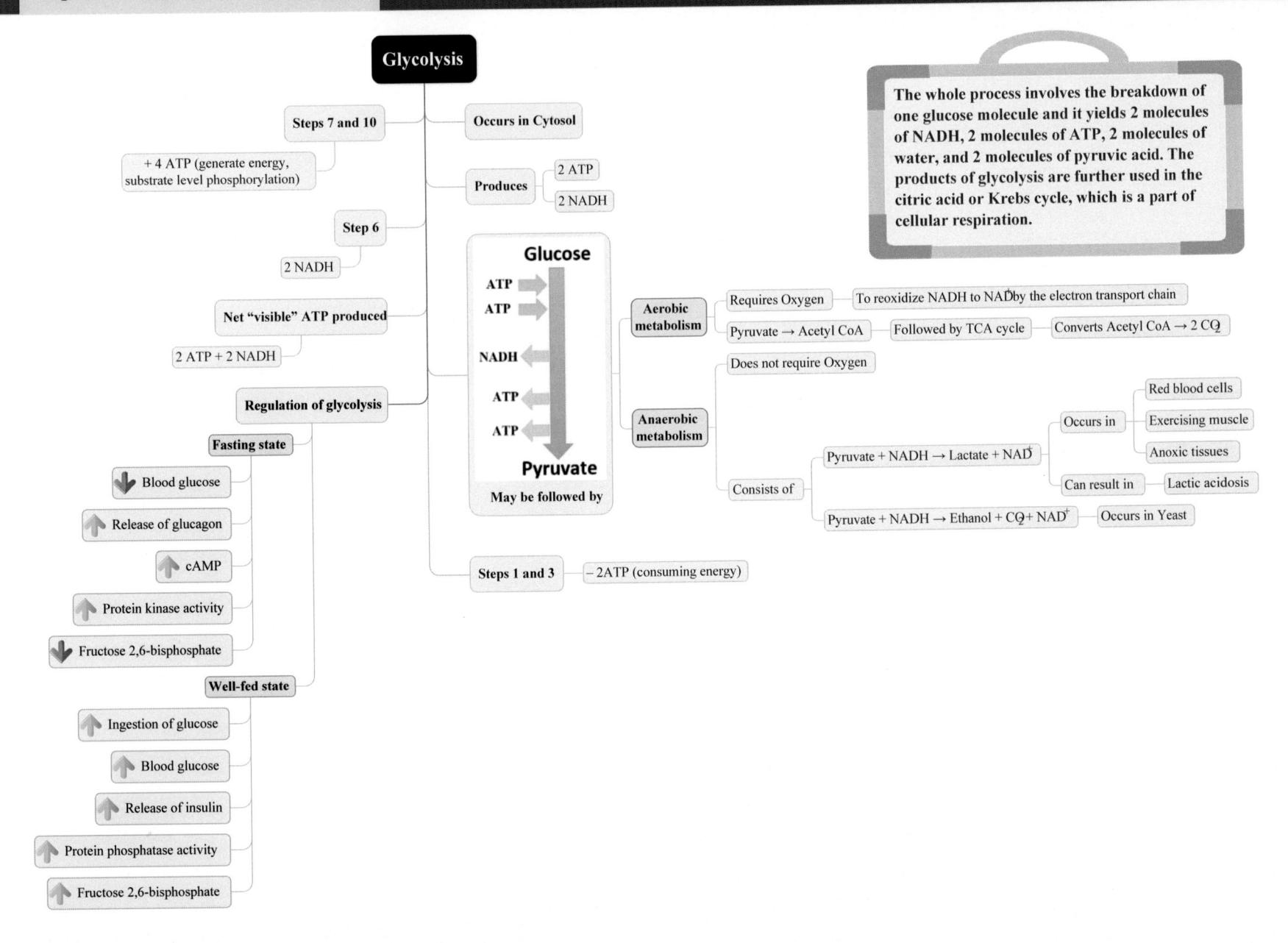

Glycolysis

Steps 7 and 10

+ 4 ATP (generate energy, substrate level phosphorylation)

Step 6

2 NADH

Net "visible" ATP produced

2 ATP + 2 NADH

Regulation of glycolysis

Fasting state

Blood glucose

Release of glucagon

cAMP

Protein kinase activity

Fructose 2,6-bisphosphate

Well-fed state

Ingestion of glucose

Blood glucose

Release of insulin

Protein phosphatase activity

Fructose 2,6-bisphosphate

Occurs in Cytosol

Produces

2 ATP

2 NADH

Glucose

ATP

ATP

NADH

ATP

ATP

Pyruvate

May be followed by

Steps 1 and 3 — 2ATP (consuming energy)

Aerobic metabolism

Requires Oxygen — To reoxidize NADH to NAD$^+$ by the electron transport chain

Pyruvate → Acetyl CoA — Followed by TCA cycle — Converts Acetyl CoA → 2 CO_2

Anaerobic metabolism

Does not require Oxygen

Consists of

Pyruvate + NADH → Lactate + NAD$^+$

Occurs in

Red blood cells

Exercising muscle

Anoxic tissues

Can result in — Lactic acidosis

Pyruvate + NADH → Ethanol + CO_2 + NAD$^+$ — Occurs in Yeast

The whole process involves the breakdown of one glucose molecule and it yields 2 molecules of NADH, 2 molecules of ATP, 2 molecules of water, and 2 molecules of pyruvic acid. The products of glycolysis are further used in the citric acid or Krebs cycle, which is a part of cellular respiration.

OVERVIEW

The citric acid cycle is a key metabolic pathway that connects carbohydrate, fat, and protein metabolism. The reactions of the cycle are carried out by eight enzymes that completely oxidize acetate (a two carbon molecule), in the form of acetyl-CoA, into two molecules each of carbon dioxide and water.This oxidation provides energy for the production of the majority of ATP in most animals, including humans. The cycle occurs totally in the mitochondria and is, therefore, in close proximity to the reactions of electron transport, which oxidize the reduced coenzymes produced by the cycle. The TCA cycle is an aerobic pathway, because O_2 is required as the final electron acceptor. Most of the body's catabolic pathways converge on the TCA cycle. Reactions such as the catabolism of some amino acids generate intermediates of the cycle and are called anaplerotic reactions. The citric acid cycle also supplies intermediates for a number of important synthetic reactions. For example, the cycle functions in the formation of glucose from the carbon skeletons of some amino acids, and it provides building blocks for the synthesis of some amino acids and heme.Therefore, this cycle should not be viewed as a closed circle, but instead as a traffic circle with compounds entering and leaving as required.

9.1.Pyruvate dehydrogenase complex (PDC)

Is a complex of three enzymes that converts pyruvate into acetyl-CoA by a process called pyruvate decarboxylation. Acetyl-CoA may then be used in the citric acid cycle to carry out cellular respiration, and this complex links the glycolysis metabolic pathway to the citric acid cycle. Pyruvate decarboxylation is also known as the "pyruvate dehydrogenase reaction" because it also involves the oxidation of pyruvate.

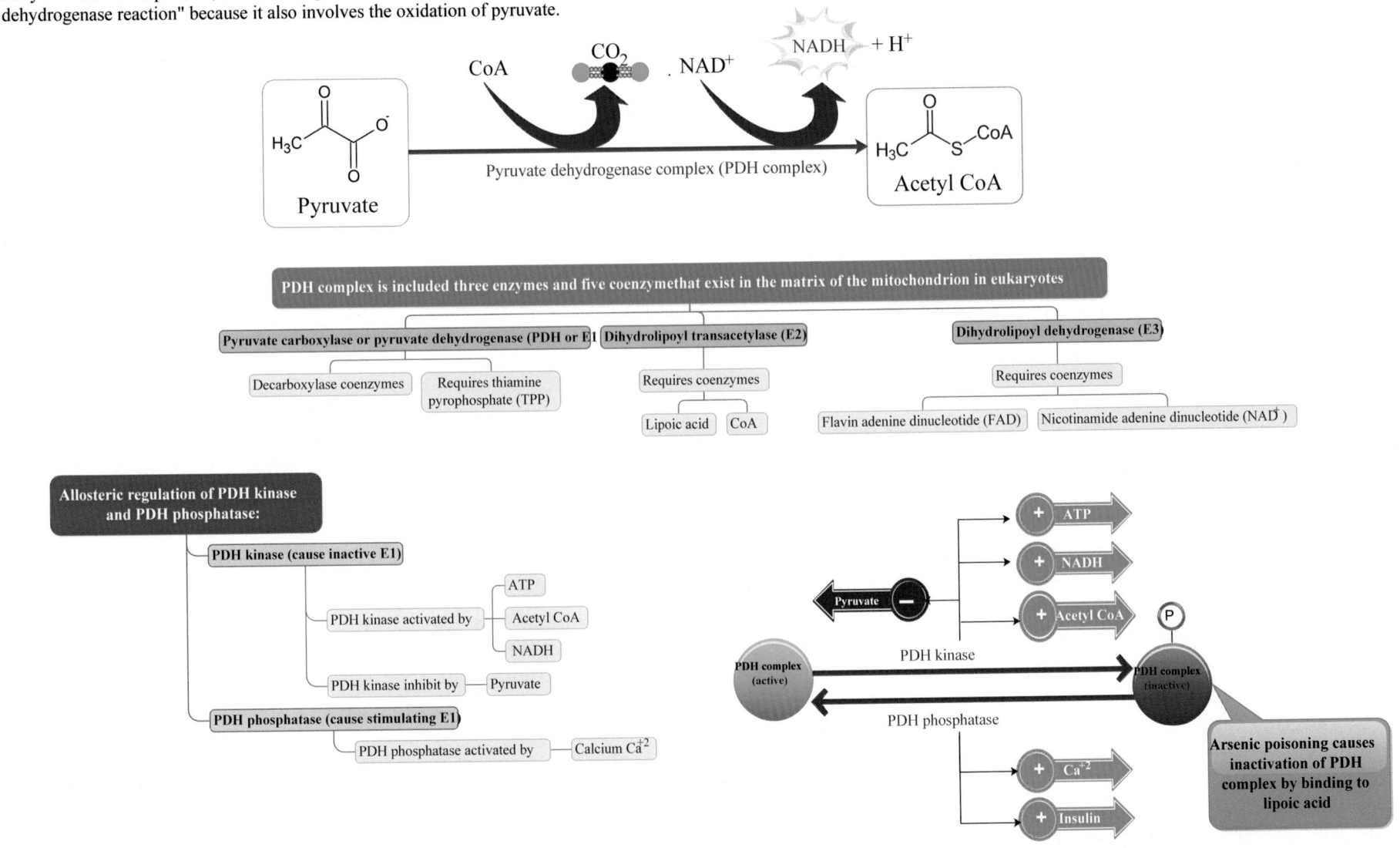

These are five steps of the process :

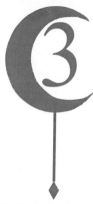

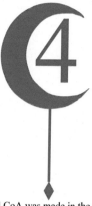

Pyruvate is decarboxylated by pyruvate dehydrogenase with help from TPP

The reactive carbon (between the N and the S of the five membered ring) of the TPP is oxidized and transferred as the acetyl group to lipoamide (which is the prosthetic group of the dihydrolipoyl transacetylase). This forms hydroxyethyl-TPP. An H^+ ion is required for the intermediate to give off CO_2

E_2(dihydrolipoyl transacetylase with cofactor lipoamide)oxidizes hydroxyethyl- to acetyl- and then transfers acetyl- to CoA, forming acetyl-CoA.

Acetyl CoA was made in the previous step. However, the process is incomplete. The $E_2$is still attached to the acetyl CoA molecule. So, E $_3$ (dihydrolipoyl dehydrogenase) oxidizes the thiol groups of the dihydrolipoamide back to lipoamide.

As a side reaction, NAD $^+$becomes reduced to NADH

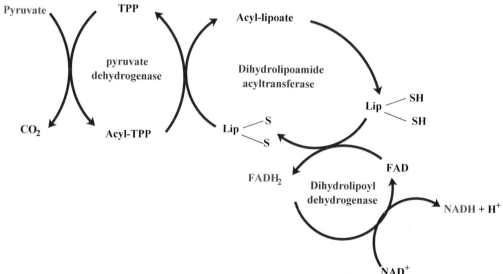

9.2.The citric acid cycle

Or TCA cycle (tricarboxylic acid cycle) or the Krebs cycle is a series of chemical reactions used by all aerobic organisms to release stored energy through the oxidation of acetyl-CoA derived from carbohydrates, fats, and proteins, into adenosine triphosphate (ATP) and carbon dioxide. In addition, the cycle provides precursors of certain amino acids, as well as the reducing agent NADH, that are used in numerous other reactions. Its central importance to many biochemical pathways suggests that it was one of the earliest established components of cellular metabolism and may have originated abiogenically. Even though it is branded as a 'cycle', it is not necessary for metabolites to follow only one specific route; at least three segments of the citric acid cycle have been recognized.

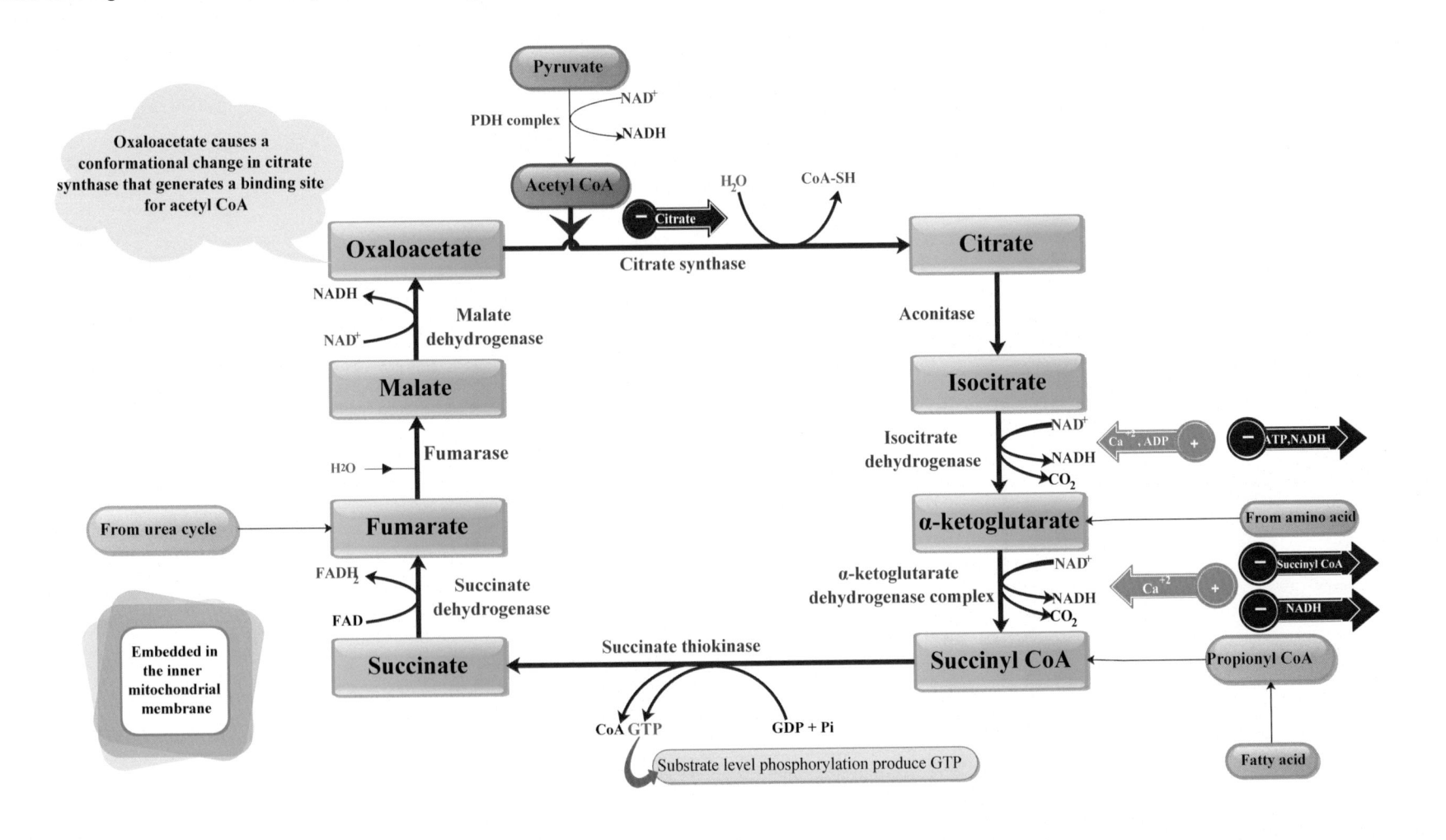

Chapter 9 : Tricarboxylic Acid Cycle and Pyruvate Dehydrogenase Complex

The cycle consumes acetyl-CoA and water, reduces NAD and FAD to NADH and $FADH_2$ and produces carbon dioxide as a waste byproduct. The overall yield of energy-containing compounds from the TCA cycle is three NADH, one $FADH_2$ and one GTP. The NADH generated by the citric acid cycle is fed into the oxidative phosphorylation (electron transport) pathway. The net result of these two closely linked pathways is the oxidation of nutrients to produce usable chemical energy in the form of ATP.

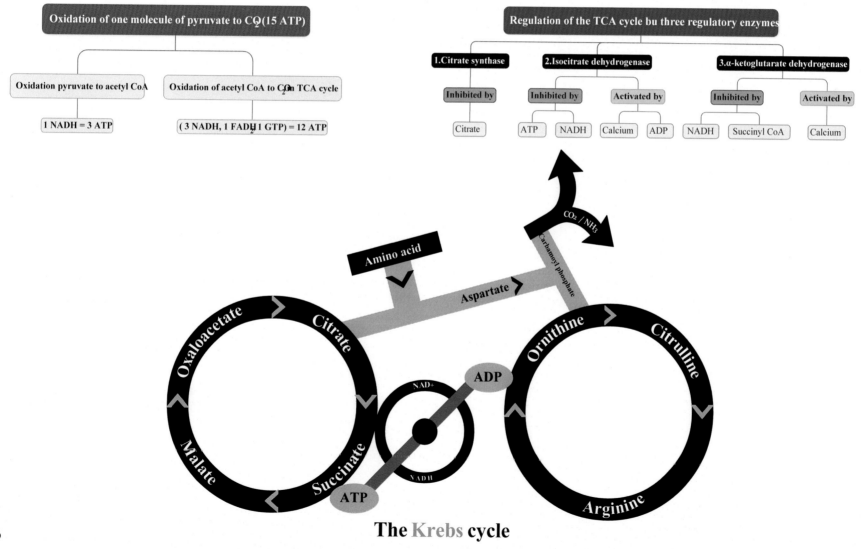

Oxidation of one molecule of pyruvate to CO_2 (15 ATP)

- Oxidation pyruvate to acetyl CoA
  - 1 NADH = 3 ATP
- Oxidation of acetyl CoA to CO_2 in TCA cycle
  - (3 NADH, 1 $FADH_2$ 1 GTP) = 12 ATP

Regulation of the TCA cycle bu three regulatory enzymes

- **1. Citrate synthase**
  - Inhibited by
    - Citrate
- **2. Isocitrate dehydrogenase**
  - Inhibited by
    - ATP
    - NADH
  - Activated by
    - Calcium
    - ADP
- **3. α-ketoglutarate dehydrogenase**
  - Inhibited by
    - NADH
    - Succinyl CoA
  - Activated by
    - Calcium

The Krebs cycle

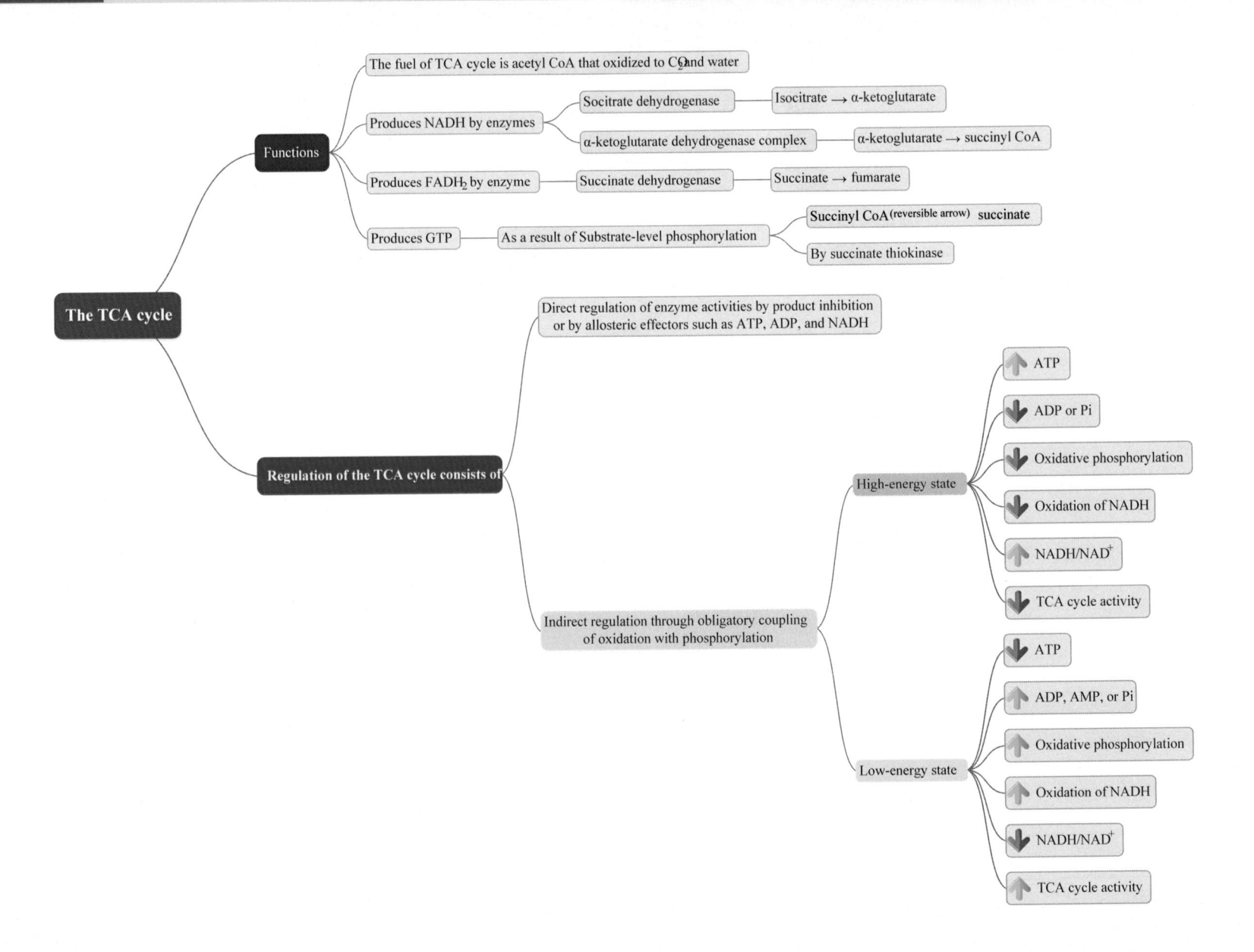

The TCA cycle

Functions

- The fuel of TCA cycle is acetyl CoA that oxidized to CO_2 and water
- Produces NADH by enzymes
  - Socitrate dehydrogenase — Isocitrate $\longrightarrow$ α-ketoglutarate
  - α-ketoglutarate dehydrogenase complex — α-ketoglutarate $\longrightarrow$ succinyl CoA
- Produces $FADH_2$ by enzyme — Succinate dehydrogenase — Succinate $\longrightarrow$ fumarate
- Produces GTP — As a result of Substrate-level phosphorylation
  - Succinyl CoA (reversible arrow) succinate
  - By succinate thiokinase

Regulation of the TCA cycle consists of

- Direct regulation of enzyme activities by product inhibition or by allosteric effectors such as ATP, ADP, and NADH
- Indirect regulation through obligatory coupling of oxidation with phosphorylation
  - High-energy state
    - ⬆ ATP
    - ⬇ ADP or Pi
    - ⬇ Oxidative phosphorylation
    - ⬇ Oxidation of NADH
    - ⬆ $NADH/NAD^+$
    - ⬇ TCA cycle activity
  - Low-energy state
    - ⬇ ATP
    - ⬆ ADP, AMP, or Pi
    - ⬆ Oxidative phosphorylation
    - ⬆ Oxidation of NADH
    - ⬇ $NADH/NAD^+$
    - ⬆ TCA cycle activity

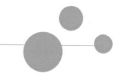

Q 1: Circle the best correct answer:

1. The reaction succinyl CoA to succinate by succinate thiokinase generate:
a. CDP
b. ADP
c. GTP
d. $NADP^+$

2. Which of the following enzymes are NOT reduced NAD^+ in TCA cycle to NADH?
a. Acotinas
b. α-ketoglutarate dehydrogenase
c. Isocitrate dehydrogenase
d. Malate dehydrogenase

3. Oxidative degradation of acetyl CoA in the TCA cycle gives a net yield of all the following <u>EXEPT</u>:
a. $FADH_2$
b. 3 NADH
c. 2 ATP
d. 2 CO_2

4. The first step of the TCA cycle is:
a. Conversion of pyruvate to acetyl-CoA
b. Condensation of acetyl-CoA with oxaloacetate
c. Conversion of citrate to isocitrate
d. Formation of alpha-ketoglutarate catalyzed by isocitrate dehydrogenase

5. In TCA cycle, GDP is phosphorylated to GTP by:
a. Succinate dehydrogenase
b. Aconitase
c. Succinate thiokinase
d. Fumarse

6. All of the following compounds are intermediates of TCA cycle except:
a. Maleate
b. Pyruvate
c. Oxaloacetate
d. Fumarate

7. The enzyme that NOT regulated in TCA cycle is:
a. Citrate synthase
b. α-ketoglutarate dehydrogenase
c. Malate dehydrogenase
d. Isocitrate dehydrogenase

8. $FADH_2$ is formed in TCA cycle in the reaction catalyzed by:
a. Isocitrate dehydrogenase
b. Malate dehydrogenase
c. Succinate thiokinase
d. Succinate dehydrogenase

9. GTP is formed in citric acid cycle in the reaction catalyzed by:
a. Isocitrate dehydrogenase
b. malate dehydrogenase
c. Succinate thiokinase
d. Succinate dehydrogenase

10. The fuel of the citric acid cycle is
a. Acetyl-CoA
b. Fumarate
c. Malate
d. Oxaloacetate

11. Citrate is converted to isocitrate by aconitase which contains:
a. Ca^{++}
b. Fe^{++}
c. Zn^{++}
d. Mg^{++}

12. Which of the following reactions is a substrate level reaction in TCA cycle?
a. Converting Citrate to isocitrate
b. Converting succinyl Co-A to succinate
c. Converting fumarate to malate
d. Converting isocitrate to α-ketoglutarate

TCA Cycle : Exercises

Q 1: Circle the best correct answer:

13.The second step in TCA cycle is:
a. Converting of Citrate to isocitrate
b. Condensation of oxaloacetate with acetyl-CoA
c. Converting of pyruvate to acetyl CoA
d. Converting of isocitrate to alpha-ketoglutarate

14.The integrator between the TCA cycle and urea cycle is:
a. Fumarate
b. Malate
c. Pyruvate
d. Citrate

Q 2: Write short notes on:

1.Explain:
The importance and regulation of TCA cycle.

2.What are the sources of oxaloacetate and acetyl CoA?

3.Describe:
The regulations and energetics of TCA cycle.

OVERVIEW

Gluconeogenesis is one of several main mechanisms used by humans and many other animals to maintain blood glucose levels, avoiding low levels (hypoglycemia). Other means include the degradation of glycogen (glycogenolysis) and fatty acid catabolism. Some tissues, such as the brain, red blood cells, kidney medulla, lens and cornea of the eye, testes, and exercising muscle, require a continuous supply of glucose as a metabolic fuel. Liver glycogen, an essential postprandial source of glucose, can meet these needs for only 10–18 hours in the absence of dietary intake of carbohydrate . During a prolonged fast, however, hepatic glycogen stores are depleted, and glucose is formed from precursors such as lactate, pyruvate, glycerol, and α-ketoacids. The formation of glucose does not occur by a simple reversal of glycolysis, because the overall equilibrium of glycolysis strongly favors pyruvate formation. Instead, glucose is synthesized by a special pathway, gluconeogenesis, that requires both mitochondrial and cytosolic enzymes. During an overnight fast, approximately 90% of gluconeogenesis occurs in the liver, with the kidneys providing 10% of the newly synthesized glucose molecules. However, during prolonged fasting, the kidneys become major glucoseproducing organs, contributing an estimated 40% of the total glucose production.

10.1.Gluconeogenesis

Is a metabolic pathway that results in the generation of glucose from non-carbohydrate carbon substrates such as lactate, breakdown of lipids (such as triglycerides), they include glycerol, and glucogenic amino acids. Glucose is the only energy source used by the brain (with the exception of ketone bodies during times of fasting), testes, erythrocytes, and kidney medulla. In mammals this process occurs in the liver and kidneys.

$$2 \text{ pyruvate} + 2 \text{ NADH} + 4 \text{ ATP} + 2\text{GTP} + 6 H_2O + 2 H^+ \rightarrow \text{Glucose} + 2 \text{ NAD}^+ + 4 \text{ ADP} + 2 \text{ GDP} + 6 \text{ Pi}$$

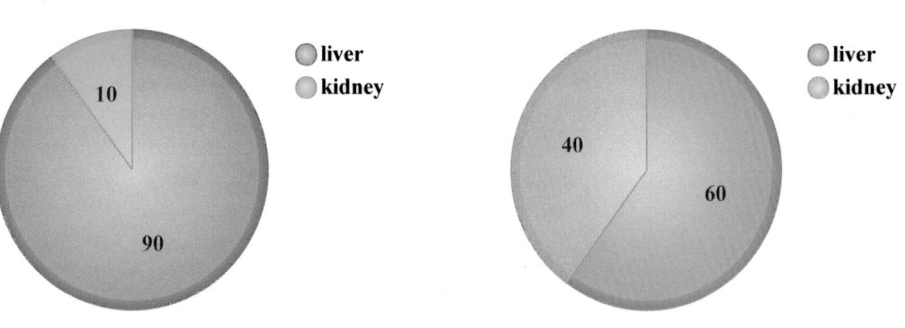

Gluconeogenesis occurs during overnight fast

○ liver
○ kidney

10
90

Gluconeogenesis occurs during prolonged fast

○ liver
○ kidney

40
60

The need for energy is important to sustain life. Organisms have evolved ways of producing substrates required for the catabolic reactions necessary to sustain life when desired substrates are unavailable. The main source of energy for eukaryotes is glucose. When glucose is unavailable, organisms are capable of metabolizing glucose from other non-carbohydrate precursors. The process that coverts pyruvate into glucose is called gluconeogenesis. Another way organisms derive glucose is from energy stores like glycogen and starch.

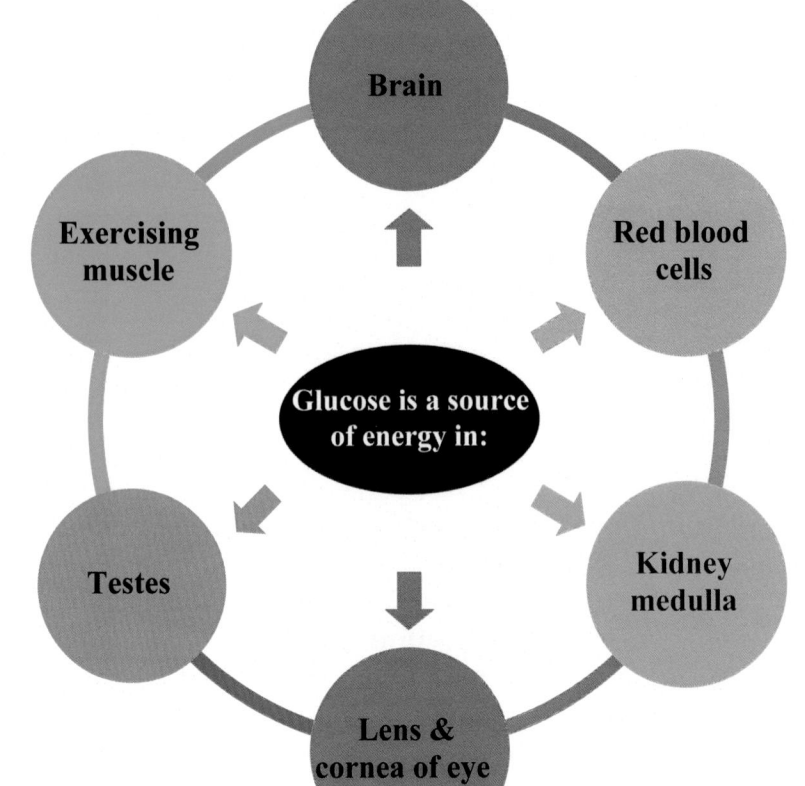

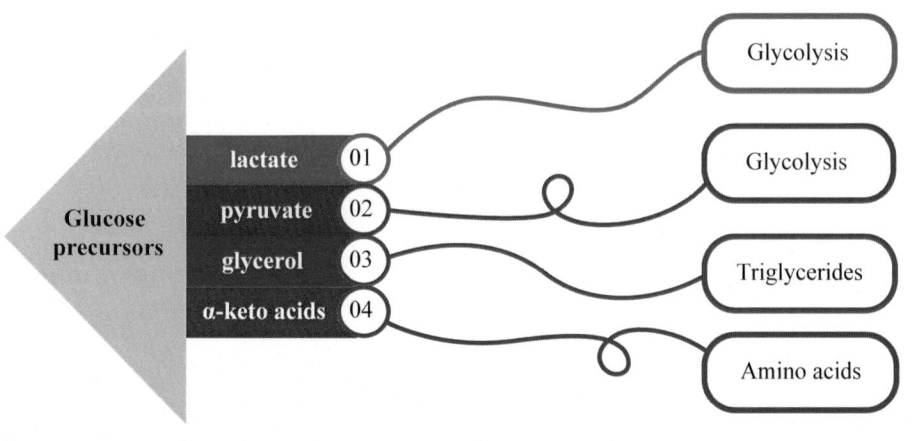

Glucose precursors

lactate	01
pyruvate	02
glycerol	03
α-keto acids	04

Glycolysis

Glycolysis

Triglycerides

Amino acids

Muscular activity requires ATP, which is provided by the breakdown of glycogen in the skeletal muscles. The breakdown of glycogen, a process known as glycogenolysis, releases glucose in the form of glucose-1-phosphate (G-1-P). The G-1-P is converted to G-6-P by the enzyme phosphoglucomutase. G-6-P is readily fed into glycolysis. When oxygen supply is insufficient, typically during intense muscular activity, energy must be released through anaerobic metabolism. Lactic acid fermentation converts pyruvate to lactate by lactate dehydrogenase. This lactate produced by anaerobic glycolysis in the muscles moves to the liver and is converted to glucose, which then returns to the muscles and is metabolized back to lactate which called cori cycle.

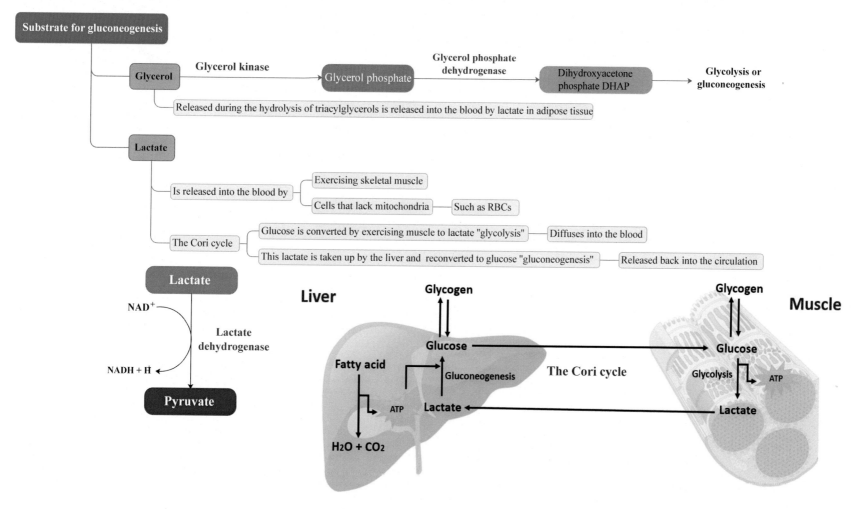

Gluconeogenesis is much like glycolysis only the process occurs in reverse. However, there are exceptions. In glycolysis there are three highly exergonic steps (steps 1,3,10). These are also regulatory steps which include the enzymes hexokinase, phosphofructokinase, and pyruvate kinase. Biological reactions can occur in both the forward and reverse direction. If the reaction occurs in the reverse direction the energy normally released in that reaction is now required. If gluconeogenesis were to simply occur in reverse the reaction would require too much energy to be profitable to that particular organism. In order to overcome this problem, nature has evolved three other enzymes to replace the glycolysis enzymes hexokinase, phosphofructokinase, and pyruvate kinase when going through the process of gluconeogenesis:

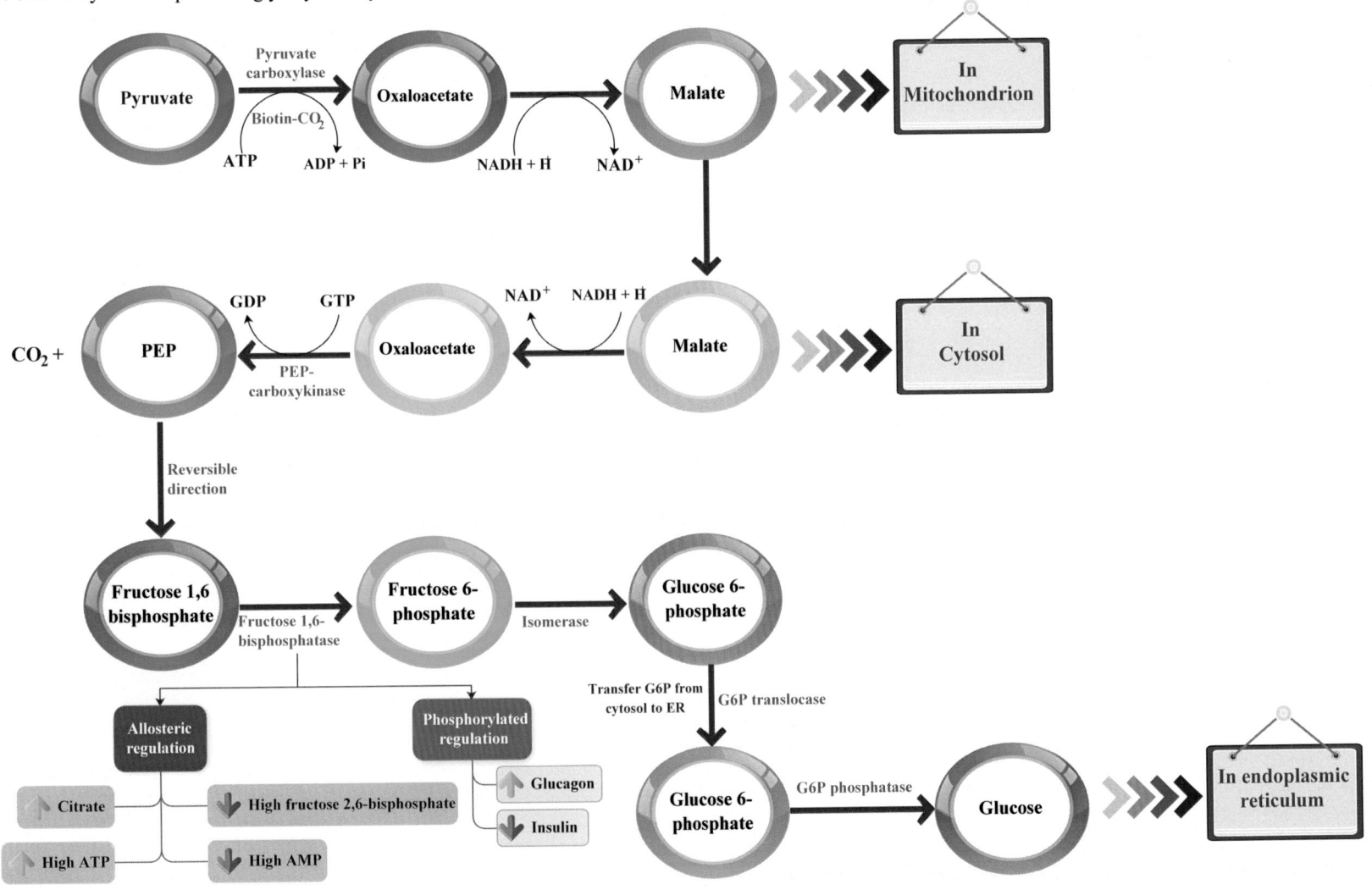

10.2.Regulation of gluconeogenesis

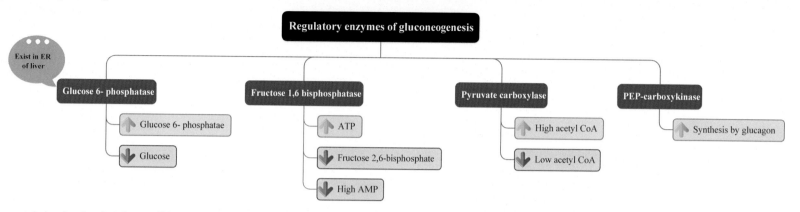

Gluconeogenesis is stimulated under conditions of fasting and starvation under the effect of glucagon and catecholamines. The regulation is mainly brought by induction/repression, covalent modifications. The key enzymes of regulation are Pyruvate carboxylase, PEP Carboxykinase, Fructose 1,6-bisphosphatase, and glucose 6-phosphatase which are stimulated if there need for glucose production. These effects are reversed in the fed state in the presence of insulin where the glycolytic enzymes are stimulated to promote glucose utilization and enzymes of gluconeogenesis are inhibited. Thus glycolysis and gluconeogenesis do not occur at the same time, they are reciprocally regulated.

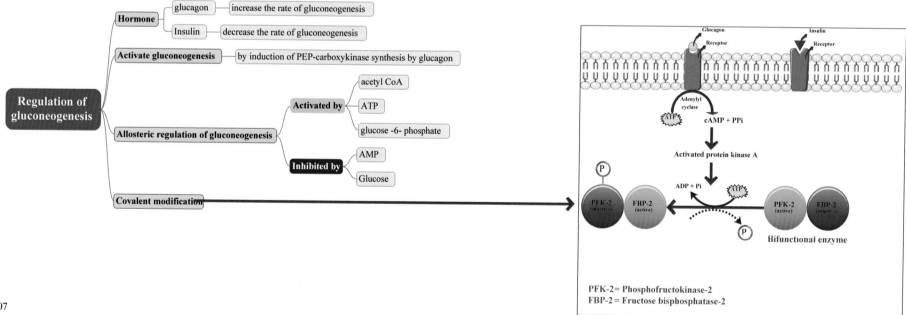

Gluconeogenesis : Exercises

Q 1: Circle the best correct answer:

1.The false statement about matrix of mitochondrial is:

a. Contains electron transport chain

b. Contains circle double stranded DNA

c. Include the enzymes responsible for the oxidation of pyruvate, amino acids,and TCA cycle

d. Gel-like solution in the interior of mitochondria and consist from 50% protein

2.When..................the reaction goes spontaneously (exergonic) from A →B:

a. ΔG negative

b. ΔGo negative

c. ΔS negative

d. ΔH positive

3.Which of the following statements about inner mitochondrial membrane is incorrect?

a. It is impermeable to most small ions

b. rich in protein such as electron transport chain

c. The convolutions, increase the surface area of the inner membrane.

d. permeable to most ions and small molecules

4.ATP has ....high-energy bonds:

a. One phosphate bond

b. Two phosphate bond

c. Two glycosidic bond

d. Two covalent bond

5.Glucose and mannose are an example of:

a. Isomers

b. Enantiomers

c. Epimers

d. all of these

6.Isomaltase cleaves the............................bond in isomaltose.

a. α(1→6)

b. α(1→4)

c. β(1→6)

d. β(1→4)

7.Sucrose is disaccharide that is consist from:

a. Glucose and fructose

b. Galactose and glucose

c. Only glucose

d. Only fructose

8.Glucose enters into the cells by............

a. Sodium-independent facilitated diffusion transport

b. Sodium-dependent glucose cotransporter 1 (SGLT-1)

c. GLUT-5

d. both a and b

9.Glucose and fructose are an example of.........

a. Isomers

b. Enantiomers

c. Epimers

d. all of these

10.Salivary α-amylase is hydrolyzing random:

a. α(1→6) glycosidic bond

b. α(1→4) glycosidic bond

c. β(1→4) glycosidic bond

d. Peptide bond

11.Lactose is disaccharide that is consist from:

a. Glucose and fructose

b. Galactose and glucose

c. Only glucose

d. Only fructose

12.Fructose enters into the cells by......

a. Sodium-independent facilitated diffusion transport

b. sodium-dependent glucose cotransporter 1 (SGLT-1)

c. sodium-independent monosaccharide transporter GLUT-5

d. both a and b

Gluconeogenesis : Exercises

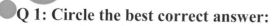

Q 1: Circle the best correct answer:

15. The reaction of substrate level phosphorylation in glycolysis is catalyzed by:
a. PFK-1
b. Phosphoglycerate dehydrogenase
c. pyruvate kinase
d. pyruvate Carboxylase

16. Dehydration of 2-phosphoglycerate to phosphoenolpyruvate (PEP) in glycolysis by:
a. Aldolase
b. Enolase
c. Enolase
d. phosphoglycerate mutase

17. Glycolysis is an example of.......................
a. Catabolism
b. Anabolism
c. Glucose synthesis
d. Glycogen synthesis

18. In anaerobic glycolysis, one mole of glucose is produced:
a. 2 NADH
b. 2 NADH & 2 ATP
c. 2 ATP
d. 4 ATP

19. The first step of metabolism for monosaccharide such as glucose, fructose, mannose, galactose is:
a. Phosphorylation
b. Carboxylation
c. Dehydration
d. Deamination

20. The bifunctional PFK2 are:
a. It has carboxylase activity and dehydrogenase activity
b. It has carboxylase activity and phosphatase activity
c. It has decarboxylase activity and kinase activity
d. It has kinase activity and phosphatase activity

21. The allosteric activator of (PFK-1) are:
a. ATP
b. Citrate
c. Fructose 2,6 bisphosphate & AMP
d. both a and b

22. Glucose is phosphorylated during fasting by:
a. Aldolase
b. Phosphoglucose isomerase
c. Glucokinase
d. Hexokinase

23. Which of the following enzyme are responsible for interconverts
dihydroxyacetone phosphate and glyceraldehyde 3-phosphate.
a. Aldolase
b. Triose phosphate isomerase
c. Phosphoglycerate kinase
d. Pyruvate kinase

24. Which one of the following about anaerobic glycolysis is true?
a. produced lactate and 2ATP
b. produced lactate and 2NADH
c. Produce 4 ATP
d. All of these

25. Pyruvate kinase is regulated by:
a. Allosteric effect by fructose 1,6-bisphosphate
b. Phosphorylation
c. Activated by acetyl CoA
d. Both a& b

26. The glycolysis and gluconeogenesis occurs mainly in......of the cells:
a. Cytosol
b. Golgi body
c. Nucleus
d. Mitochondria

Gluconeogenesis : Exercises

Q 1: Circle the best correct answer:

27.Glycolysis is increased by:
a. Glucagon
b. Epinephrine
c. Glucocorticoids
d. Insulin

28.The breakdown of glucose to pyruvate is termed:
a. Glycolysis
b. Oxidative decarboxylation
c. Specific dynamic action
d. Gluconeogenesis

29.Which of the following is an enzyme required for glycolysis?
a. Pyruvate kinase
b. Pyruvate carboxylase
c. Glucose-6-phosphatase
d. PEP carboxykinase

30.During glycolysis, Fructose 1, 6 Bisphosphate is decomposed to trioses sugar by the enzyme called:
a. Enolase
b. Fructokinase
c. Aldolase
d. Diphosphofructophosphatose

31.The glycolysis is regulated by:
a. Hexokinase
b. Phosphofructokinase-1 (PFK1)
c. Pyruvate kinase
d. All of these

32.Phosphofructokinase1 (PFK1) is allosterically inhibited by......
a. AMP, Fructose 2,6 bisphosphate
b. Citrate, ATP
c. Pyruvate, PEP
d. G6-P, F6-P

33. In diabetes patient, the glucose converted to......which is caused several disease.
a. Acetyl CoA
b. Sorbitol
c. Ethanol
d. Glyceraldehyde

34.Regulation of glycolysis involves:
a. Allosteric activation by ADP
b. Allosteric inhibition by ATP
c. Hormonal activation by insulin
d. All of these

35.The sites for gluconeogenesis are:
a. Liver and kidney
b. Skin and pancreas
c. Lung and brain
d. Intestine and lens of eye

36.Which one of the following statements about galactose are incorrect?
a. The source of galactose is lactose
b. Entry of galactose into cells is not insulin dependent
c. galactose phosphorylated by galactokinase to galactose 6-phosphate
d. galactose metabolism is important for lactose synthesis

37.Which one of the following statements about fructose areincorrect?
a. Fructose metabolism is lower than glucose metabolism
b. Entry of fructose into cells is not insulin dependent
c. deficiency of fructokinase and aldolase B lead to heredity fructose intolerance
d. Fructose phosphorylated to fructose 1-phosphate

38. The cori cycle is:
a. Involved glycogen synthesis and breakdown
b. Does not involved the reaction of lactate to pyruvate
c. Involves glycolysis and gluconeogenesis
d. Take place exclusive in the liver

Gluconeogenesis : Exercises

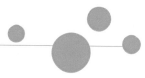

Q 1: Circle the best correct answer:

39.The coenzyme for Pyruvate carboxylase is:
a. Thiamine
b. Lipoic acid
c. FMN
d. Biotin

40.In gluconeogenesis, Conversion of oxaloacetate into phosphoenolpyruvate (PEP) are catalyzed by:
a. Required GTP
b. Required PEP carboxykinase
c. It involves decarboxylation and phosphorylation
d. All of these

41.The bifunctional PEP carboxykinase are:
a. It has carboxylase activity and dehydrogenase activity
b. It has carboxylase activity and phosphatase activity
c. It has decarboxylase activity and phosphorylation activity
d. It has kinase activity and phosphatase activity

42.Types of gluconeogenesis Regulation are:
a. Glucagon increase cAMP that activated fructose 1, 6 bisphosphatase so increase gluconeogenesis.
b. gluconeogenesis activated by ATP and NADH
c. Allosteric activation by acetyl CoA
d. All of these

43.The false statements about glucose 6-phosphatase is:
a. Glucose 6-phosphatase removes the phosphate and producing free glucose
b. Present in Liver and kidney
c. present in mitochondria
d. present in endoplasmic reticulum

44.Produce 1 mole of glucose from 2 mole of pyruvate are need:
a. 4 ATP
b. 2 GTP
c. 2 NADH
d. All of these

45.Which one of the following enzymes are NOT regulatory enzyme of gluconeogenesis?
a. Glucose 6-phosphatase
b. Glucokinase
c. Fructose 1,6 bisphosphatase
d. Pyruvate carboxylase and PEP carboxykinase

46.Pyruvate dehydrogenase complex require the following for their oxidative decarboxylation:
a. CoA and Lipoic acid
b. NAD^+ and FAD
c. CoA and TPP
d. CoA, TPP, NAD^+, FAD, Lipoic acid

47.Pyruvate dehydrogenase a multienzyme complex is required for the production of:
a. Acetyl-CoA
b. Lactate
c. Phosphoenolpyruvate
d. PEP

48.Pyruvate dehydrogenase activity is activated by:
a. Mercury
b. Zinc
c. Calcium
d. Sodium

49.Biotin is a coenzyme for:
a. Pyruvate dehydrogenase
b. Pyruvate carboxylase
c. PEP carboxykinase
d. Glutamate pyruvate transaminase

50. Conversion of pyruvate into acetyl CoA is catalysed by:
a. Pyruvate dehydrogenase
b. Didrolipoyl acetyl transferase
c. Dihydrolipoyl dehydrogenase
d. All of these

Gluconeogenesis : Exercises

Q 1: Circle the best correct answer:

51. Which of the following about pyruvate carboxylase is false?
a. Need ATP and biotin as coenzyme
b. Added carboxyl group
c. Activated by Acetyl CoA
d. Activated by pyruvate

52. Which of the following enzymes remove the phosphate group in gluconeogenesis?
a. Hexokinase, phosphofructokinase
b. Phosphenol pyruvate carboxy kinase, aldolase A
c. Fructose1,6 phosphatase, glucose 6 phosphatase
d. PEP carboxykinase and hexokinase

53. Which of the following enzymes is important in reciprocal regulation of glycolysis and gluconeogenesis?
a. PEP Carboxykinas
b. PFK2-FBP2
c. Aldolase
d. Hexokinase

54. Which of the following statements about Regulation of gluconeogenesis is true?
a. Gluconeogenesis increased by Glucagon .
b. Gluconeogenesis activated by ATP and NADH
c. Allosteric activation by acetyl CoA
d. All of these

55. Gluconeogenesis is decreased by:
a. Glucagon
b. Epinephrine
c. Glucocorticoids
d. Insulin

56. Pyruvate transfer from mitochondrial to cytosol in gluconeogenesis as:
a. Oxaloacetate
b. Phosphoenol pyruvate
c. Malate
d. Lactate

57. Which of the following compounds are not substrate for glucose synthesis?
a. Pyruvate & Lactate
b. Glycerol
c. α-ketoglutarate
d. Oxaloacetate

58. Glucose 6-phosphatase present in.........................
a. Endoplasmic reticulum
b. Cytosol
c. Mitochondria
d. Nucleus

59. The positive allosteric regulator of pyruvate carboxylase is:
a. ATP
b. Acetyl Co-A
c. Oxaloacetate
d. fructose 1-phosphate

60. Deficiency of biotin will affect the activity of:
a. Phosphoenol pyruvate carboxy kinase
b. Pyruvate kinase
c. Fructose 1,6 bisphosphatase
d. pyruvate carboxylase

61. Which one of the following are not regulatory enzymes in glycolysis?
a. PFK-1
b. Pyruvate kinase
c. Glucokinase or hexokinase
d. Phosphoglycerate kinase

62. Which one of the following enzymes are not involve in the regulation of gluconeogenesis?
a. glucose 6-phosphatase
b. Glucokinase
c. Fructose 1,6 bisphosphatase
d. Pyruvate carboxylase
e. PEP carboxykinase

63. PFK2/FBP2 enzymes are important in reciprocal regulation of:
a. glycolysis/gluconeogenesis
b. TCA/gluconeogenesis
c. Cori cycle/glycolysis
d. Lactate/pyruvate cycle
e. Oxidative phosphorylation/ electron transport cycle

Gluconeogenesis : Exercises

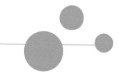

Q 2: Write short notes on:

Explain:

1. The first step of glycolysis is phosphorylation.
2. The fates of pyruvate.
3. The function of enolase.
4. The importance of glycolysis.
5. The importance of gluconeogenesis.
6. The difference between hexokinase and glucokinase?
7. The regulatory enzymes for glycolysis.
8. The effects of insulin on glycolysis.
9. Explain:
In the first step of gluconeogenesis, pyruvate converted to malate. (write the reaction)

10. Describe:
the regulation of pyruvate kinase.

11. Describe :
glycolysis and its regulation.

Explain:
the energetics of aerobic and anaerobic glycolysis.

12. Describe:
gluconeogenesis,.

13. Describe:
the reciprocal regulation of glycolysis and gluconeogenesis.

14. Cori cycle

15. Describe: the regulation of pyruvate dehydrogenase complex.

16. precursors of gluconeogenesis.

17. Explain:
In mitochondria, pyruvate is converted to malate in gluconeogenes

18. Explain:
glycolysis and gluconeogenesis do not occur at the same time, they are reciprocally regulated.

OVERVIEW

Every cell of the human body requires energy to perform the metabolic functions that sustain life. Glucose is a small, simple sugar that serves as a primary fuel for energy production, especially for the brain, mature erythrocyte (no mitochondria) muscles where it is the substrate for anaerobic glycolysis and several other body organs and tissues. Blood glucose can be obtained from three primary sources: the diet, degradation of glycogen, and gluconeogenesis. Dietary intake of glucose and polysaccharide, such as starch, is sporadic and, depending on the diet, is not always a reliable source of blood glucose. In contrast, gluconeogenesis can provide sustained synthesis of glucose, but it is somewhat slow in responding to a falling blood glucose level. Therefore, the body has developed mechanisms for storing a supply of glucose in a rapidly mobilizable form, namely, glycogen. In the absence of a dietary source of glucose, Glycogen in liver and kidney role in maintaining blood-glucose levels is especially important because glucose is virtually the only fuel used by the brain, except during prolonged starvation. Moreover, the glucose from glycogen is readily mobilized and is therefore a good source of energy for sudden, strenuous activity, muscle glycogen is degraded in muscle for ATP synthesis.

Chapter 11 : Glycogen Metabolism

11.1. Glycogen

In humans, glycogen is made and stored primarily in the cells of the liver and skeletal muscle. Glycogen is composed of units of glucose linked alpha (1-4) with branches occurring alpha (1-6) approximately every 8-12 residues. In the liver, glycogen can make up from 10% of weight of liver can store roughly 100 grams of glycogen. In skeletal muscle, glycogen is found in a low concentration (1–2% of the muscle mass) and the skeletal muscle stores roughly 400 grams of glycogen, therefore the total amount of glycogen in adult human body roughly 500 grams. The glycogen store in liver, kidney, and skeletal muscle. liver glycogen is the primary source of blood glucose used by the rest of the body for fuel so it can maintain the glucose level in blood but glycogen in liver used to synthesis of ATP. As muscle cells lack glucose-6-phosphatase, which is required to pass glucose into the blood.

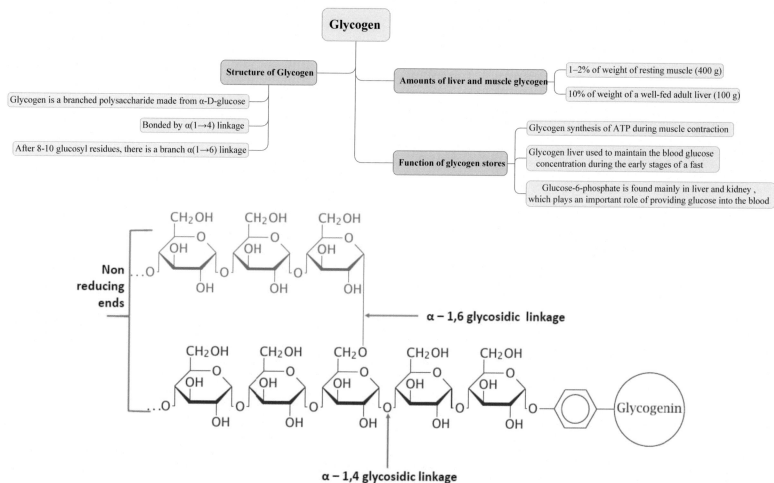

Chapter 11 : Glycogen Metabolism

11.2.Glycogen synthesis (Glycogenesis) : Glycogen synthesis is glycogen synthesis from glucose. The energy for glycogen synthesis comes from uridine triphosphate (UTP), which reacts with glucose-1-phosphate, forming UDP-glucose by UDP-glucose pyrophosphorylase. Glycogen is synthesized from UDP-glucose initially by the protein glycogenin, which has two tyrosine to accept of glucose residues from UDP-glucose. The elongation of a glycogen by transfer of glucose from UDP-glucose to the non-reducing end of the growing chain by glycogen synthase that is making the α(1→4) linkages. The glycogen branching enzyme transfer of a terminal fragment of six or eight glucose residues from a non-reducing end to the C-6 hydroxyl group of a glucose residue deeper into the interior of the glycogen molecule

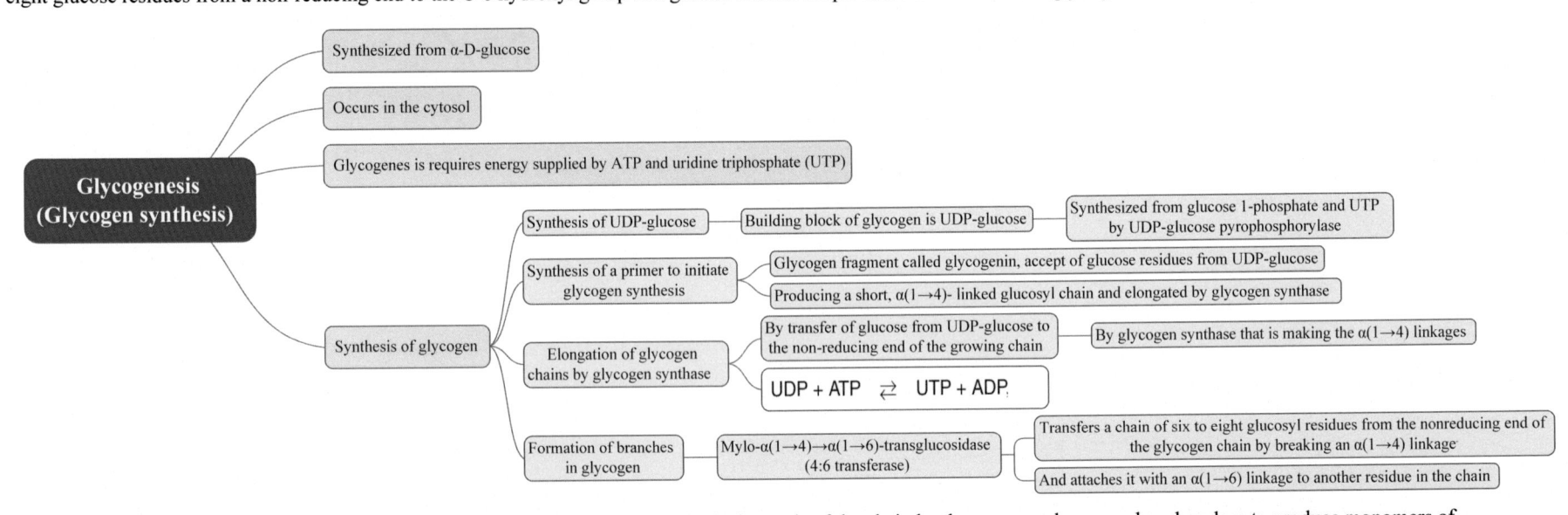

11.3.Glycogenlysis (glycogen degradation) :Glycogen is cleaved from the non-reducing ends of the chain by the enzyme glycogen phosphorylase to produce monomers of glucose-1-phosphate. Glucose-1-phosphate is then converted to glucose 6-phosphate (G6P) by phosphoglucomutase. A special debranching enzyme has two activity, the first activity (4:4 transferase activity; break α (1→4) and make α (1→4) remove the three of four glycosyl residue attached to the branch then transfers them to the non-reducing end. The second activity is 1:6 glucosidase activity; break α (1→6) removed glucose residue attached in an α(1→6) linkage, and also 1-3% of glycogen degraded by lysosomal enzyme (α(1→4)-glucosidase (acid maltase).

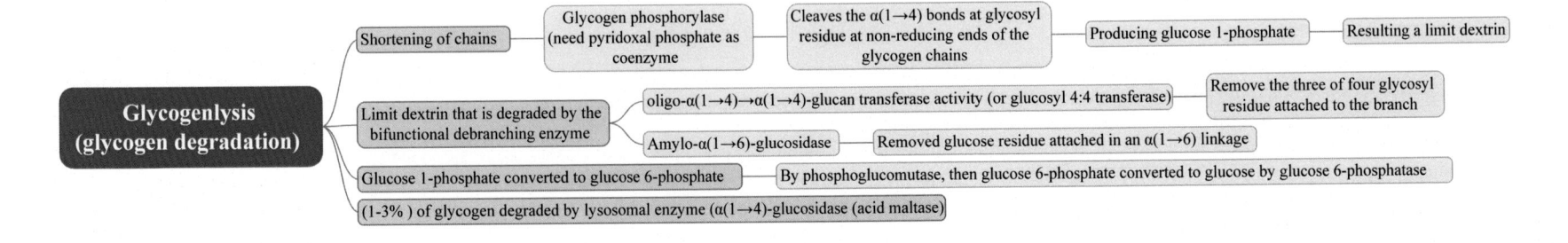

Chapter 11 : Glycogen Metabolism

11.4.Regulation of glycogenesis (glycogen synthesis)

The reaction is highly regulated by allosteric effectors such as glucose-6-phosphate (activator) and by covalent modification, glucagon enhance phosphorylation of glycogen synthase results deactivating of glycogenesis. On other hand, insulin enhance dephosphorylation of glycogen synthase results activating of glycogenesis.

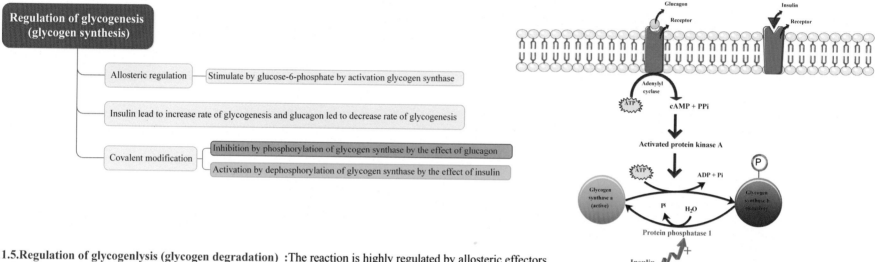

Regulation of glycogenesis (glycogen synthesis)
- Allosteric regulation — Stimulate by glucose-6-phosphate by activation glycogen synthase
- Insulin lead to increase rate of glycogenesis and glucagon led to decrease rate of glycogenesis
- Covalent modification
  - Inhibition by phosphorylation of glycogen synthase by the effect of glucagon
  - Activation by dephosphorylation of glycogen synthase by the effect of insulin

11.5.Regulation of glycogenlysis (glycogen degradation)

The reaction is highly regulated by allosteric effectors such as glucose-6-phosphate (activator) and by covalent modification, glucagon enhance phosphorylation of glycogen synthase results deactivating of glycogenesis. On other hand, insulin enhance dephosphorylating of glycogen synthase results activating of glycogenesis.

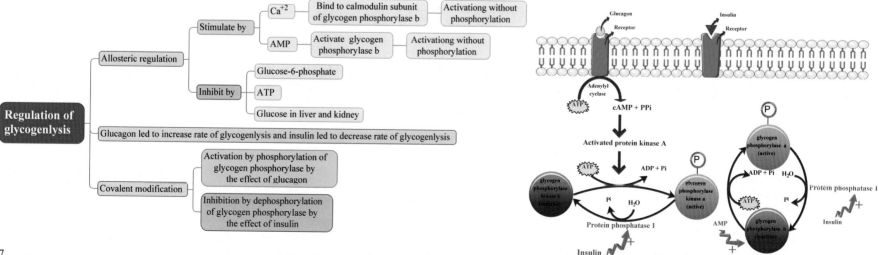

Regulation of glycogenlysis
- Allosteric regulation
  - Stimulate by
    - Ca^{+2} — Bind to calmodulin subunit of glycogen phosphorylase b — Activationg without phosphorylation
    - AMP — Activate glycogen phosphorylase b — Activationg without phosphorylation
  - Inhibit by
    - Glucose-6-phosphate
    - ATP
    - Glucose in liver and kidney
- Glucagon led to increase rate of glycogenlysis and insulin led to decrease rate of glycogenlysis
- Covalent modification
  - Activation by phosphorylation of glycogen phosphorylase by the effect of glucagon
  - Inhibition by dephosphorylation of glycogen phosphorylase by the effect of insulin

11.6.Pathways involved in the regulation of glycogen phosphorylase by epinephrine activation of α-adrenergic receptors
PLC-β is phospholipase C-β. The substrate for PLC-β is phosphatidylinositol-4,5-bisphosphate (PIP2) and the products are IP3 (inositol-1,4,5-trisphosphate) and DAG (diacylglycerol). GS-GP kinase is glycogen synthase-glycogen phosphorylase kinase, often just referred to as phosphorylase kinase, PHK. +ve refers to positive effect

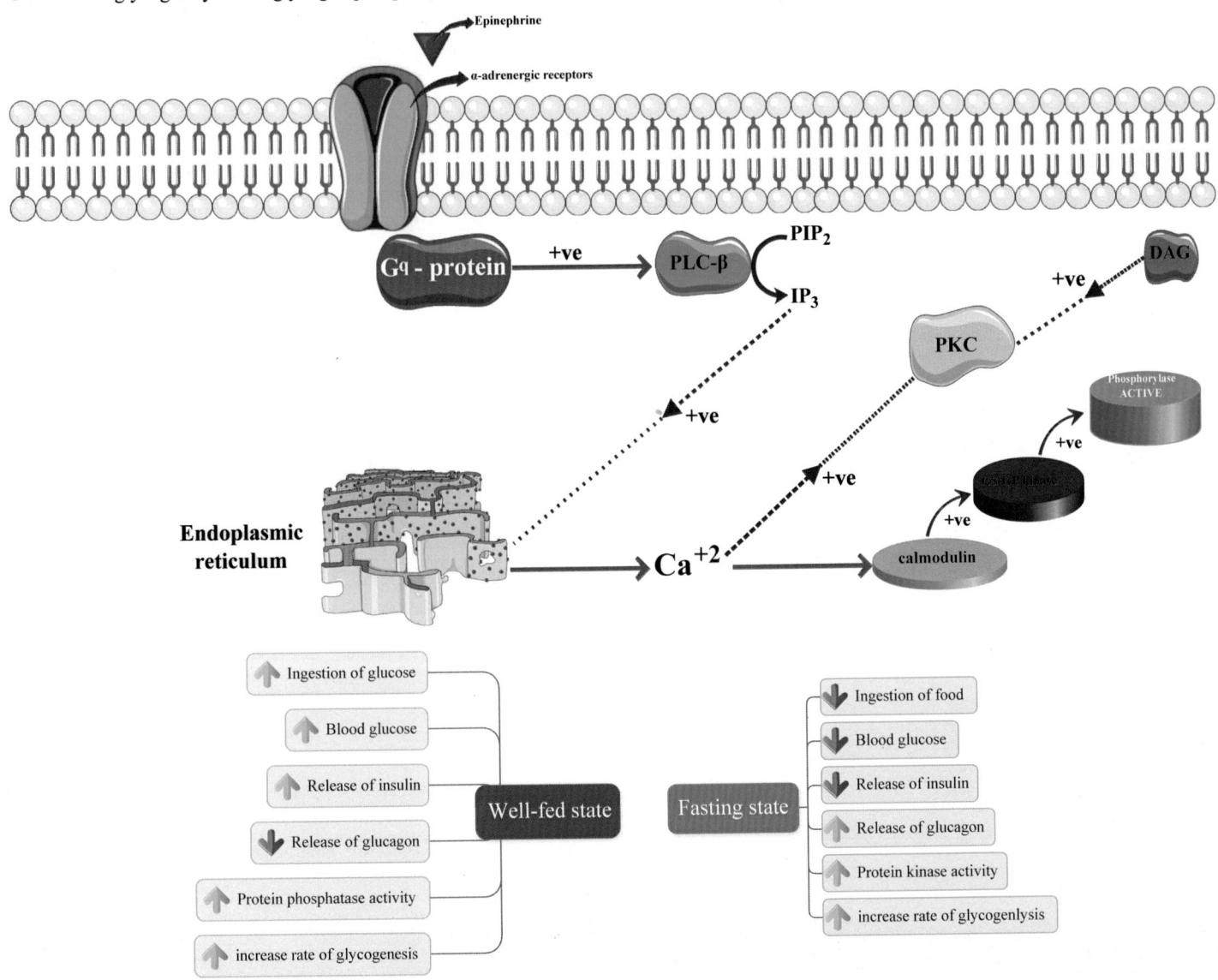

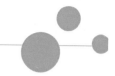

Glycogen Metabolism : Exercises

Q 1: Circle the best correct answer:

1.Insulin increases :
a. Glycogenesis (glycogen synthesis)
b. Glycogenlysis (glycogen degradation)
c. glycogen phosphorylase activity
d. debranching enzyme activity

2.Which of the following statements about branching enzyme is false?
a. Make α-1-4 glyosidic bond
b. Break α-1-4 glyosidic bond, and Make α-1-6
c. Make α-1-4 glyosidic bond break α-1-6
d. Make α-1-6 glyosidic bond

3.The regulatory enzyme in glycogenesis (glycogen synthesis) is:
a. UDP-glucose phosphorylase
b. Glycogen synthase
c. Glycogen phosphorylase
d. Debranching enzyme

4.All the following compounds are activated glycogen degradation except:
a. Glucagon and adrenalin
b. Ca^{2+}
c. AMP
d. ATP

5.Glycogenesis requires:
a. GTP
b. CTP
c. UTP
d. ATP

6.Glycogen stores in:
a. Muscle only
b. Liver only
c. liver and muscle
d. Brain and Kidney

7.Glycogen phosphorylase generates the following from glycogen:
a. Glucose
b. Glucose-6-phosphate
c. Glucose-1-phosphate
d. Maltose

8.Glycogenin is :
a. Uncouplers of oxidative phosphorylation
b. Polymer of glycogen molecules
c. Protein primer provided hydroxyl group for glycogen synthesis
d. Intermediate in glycogen breakdown

9.Debranching enzyme is absent in:
a. Cori's disease
b. Andersen's disease
c. Von Gierke's disease
d. Her's disease

10.Glucose 6-phosphatase deficiency cause glycogen storage disease:
a. Type III (Pomp disease)
b. Type I (Von Gierke disease)
c. Type V (Mcardle syndrome)
d. None of the above

11.In presence of glucagon:
a. Glycogen phosphorylase inactive and glycogen synthase active
b. Glycogen phosphorylase active and glycogen synthase inactive
c. Glycogen phosphorylase and glycogen synthase are inactive
d. Glycogen phosphorylase and glycogen synthase are active

12. Active G-protein →active adenylyl cyclase →C-AMP activate Protein kinase A →.......
a. Phosphorylate glycogen phosphorylase kinase→inhibit glycogen degradation
b. Activate protein phosphatase → inhibit glycogen degradation
c. Phosphorylate glycogen synthase kinase → inhibit glycogen synthesis
d. Phosphorylate glycogen synthase → activate glycogen synthesis

Glycogen Metabolism : Exercises

Q 1: Circle the best correct answer:

13.Glycogen synthase add the glucose to:
a. Glycogen fragment
b. Glycogenin primer
c. Any glucose unit
d. both a and b

14. Liver glycogen function is
a. Maintenance of blood glucose
b. ATP synthesis
c. Both A and B
d. Precursor for triacylglycerol

15.Which enzyme is the direct activator of glycogen phosphorylase?
a. Protein kinase A
b. Glycogen phosphorylase kinase a
c. Protein kinase C
d. Protein kinase B

16.The inactive form of glycogen ……… is phosphorylated and the active form of glycogen …… is dephosphorylated.
a. Hydrolase; dehydrogenase
b. Dehydrogenase; hydrolase
c. Phosphorylase; synthase
d. Synthase; phosphorylase

17.Protein phosphatase 1 in muscles:
a. Converts glycogen phosphorylase a to b
b. Converts glycogen phosphorylase kinase a to b
c. Converts glycogen synthase a to b
b. A and C

21.Glucose is an allosteric inhibitor in liver to:
a. Glycogen synthase b
b. Glycogen synthase a
c. Glycogen phosphorylase a
d. Glycogen phosphorylase b

18.Glycogen is converted to glucose-1- phosphate by:
a. UDP-glucose transferase
b. Branching enzyme
c. Glycogen Phosphorylase
d. Glucose Phosphatase

19.For glycogenesis, Glucose should be converted to:
a. Glucuronic acid
b. Pyruvic acid
c. UDP glucose
d. Sorbitol

20.The total glycogen content of the body is about _____ grams.
a. 100
b. 300
c. 400
d. 500

Q 2: Write short notes on:

1.The importance of glycogen in liver and in muscle.
2.The activity of debranching enzyme.
3.The activity of branching enzyme.
4.Describe glycogen degradation and its regulation.
5.Describe glycogenesis and its regulation.
6.Describe the regulation of blood glucose concentration.
7.Explain the reciprocal regulation of gluconeogenesis and glycolysis.
8.Glycogen storage diseases.
9.Explain:
The function of glycogen in muscle is only produce energy.

OVERVIEW

Fuel for Metabolism. One major function of a monosaccharide is its use for energy within a living organism. Glucose is a commonly known carbohydrate that is metabolized within cells to create fuel. In the presence of oxygen, glucose breaks down into carbon dioxide and water, and energy is released as a byproduct. However, two other monosaccharides such as fructose and galactose occur in significant amounts in the diet (primarily in disaccharides), and make important contributions to energy metabolism. In addition, galactose is an important component of cell structural carbohydrates.

Chapter 12 : Metabolism of Monosaccharides and Disaccharides

12.1.Lactose synthesis : Lactose is a type of sugar found naturally in the milk of most mammals. Lactose intolerance is a condition characterized by symptoms such as stomach pain, bloating, gas and diarrhea, which are caused by lactose malabsorption. In humans, an enzyme known as lactase is responsible for breaking down lactose for digestion. Lactose is synthesized by lactose synthase (UDP- galactose:glucose galactosyltransferase), from UDP-galactose and glucose in the lactating mammary gland.

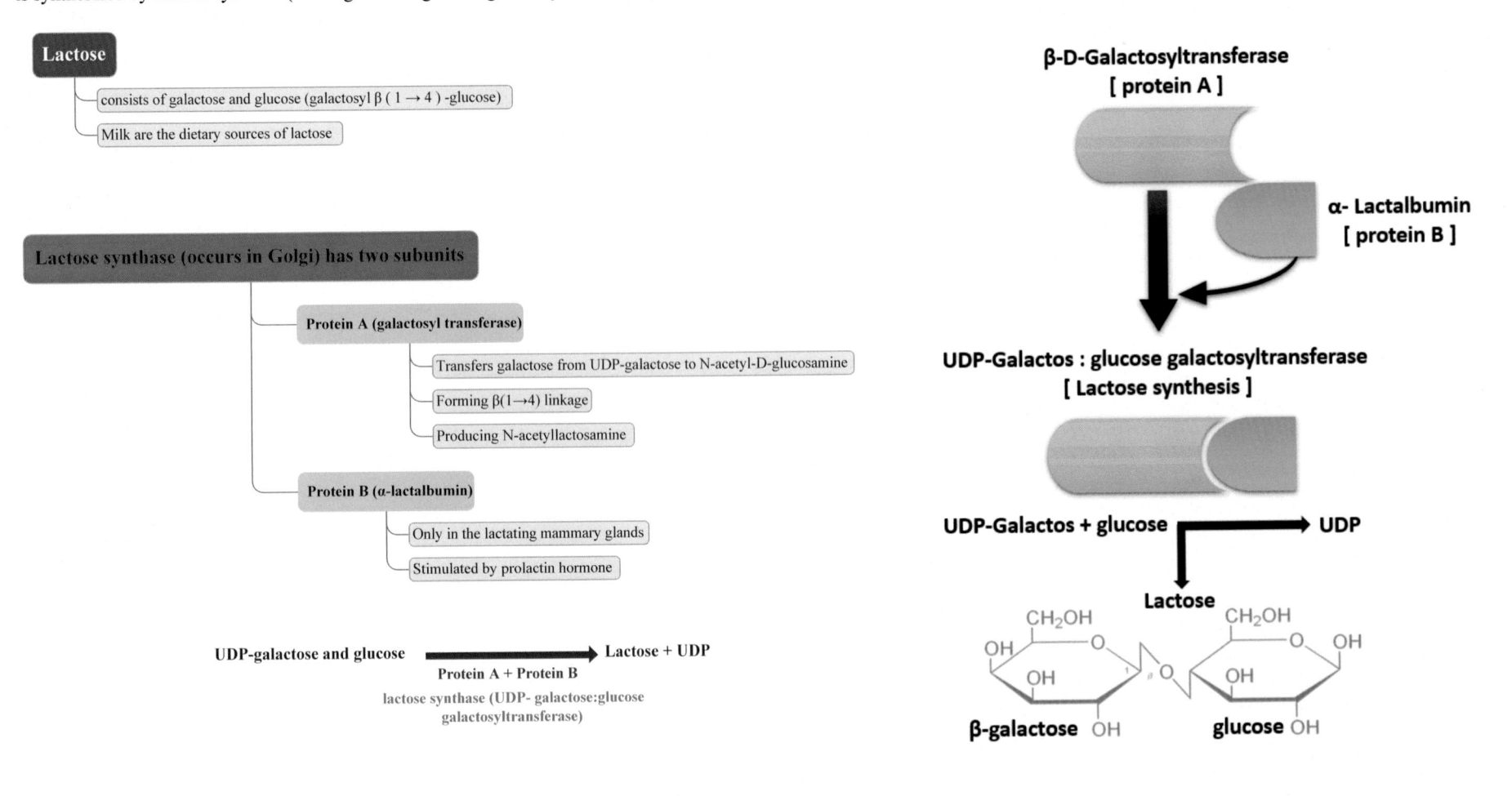

12.2.Mannose metabolism : Mannose, packaged as the nutritional supplement "d-mannose", is a sugar monomer of the aldohexose series of carbohydrates. Mannose is a C-2 epimer of glucose. Mannose is important in human metabolism, especially in the glycosylation of certain proteins.

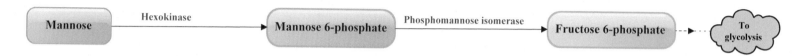

12.3.Fructose: Fructose: is a simple ketone monosaccharide found in many plants, where it is often bonded to glucose to form the disaccharide sucrose. It is one of the three dietary monosaccharides, along with glucose and galactose, that are absorbed directly into blood during digestion.

12.4.Sorbitol synthesis: Sorbitol may be synthesised via a glucose reduction by the aldehyde group is converted into a hydroxyl group. The reaction requires NADPH and is catalyzed by aldose reductase.

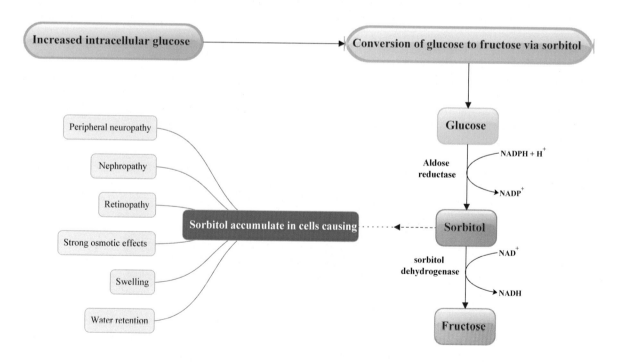

12.5. Important dietary monosaccharides

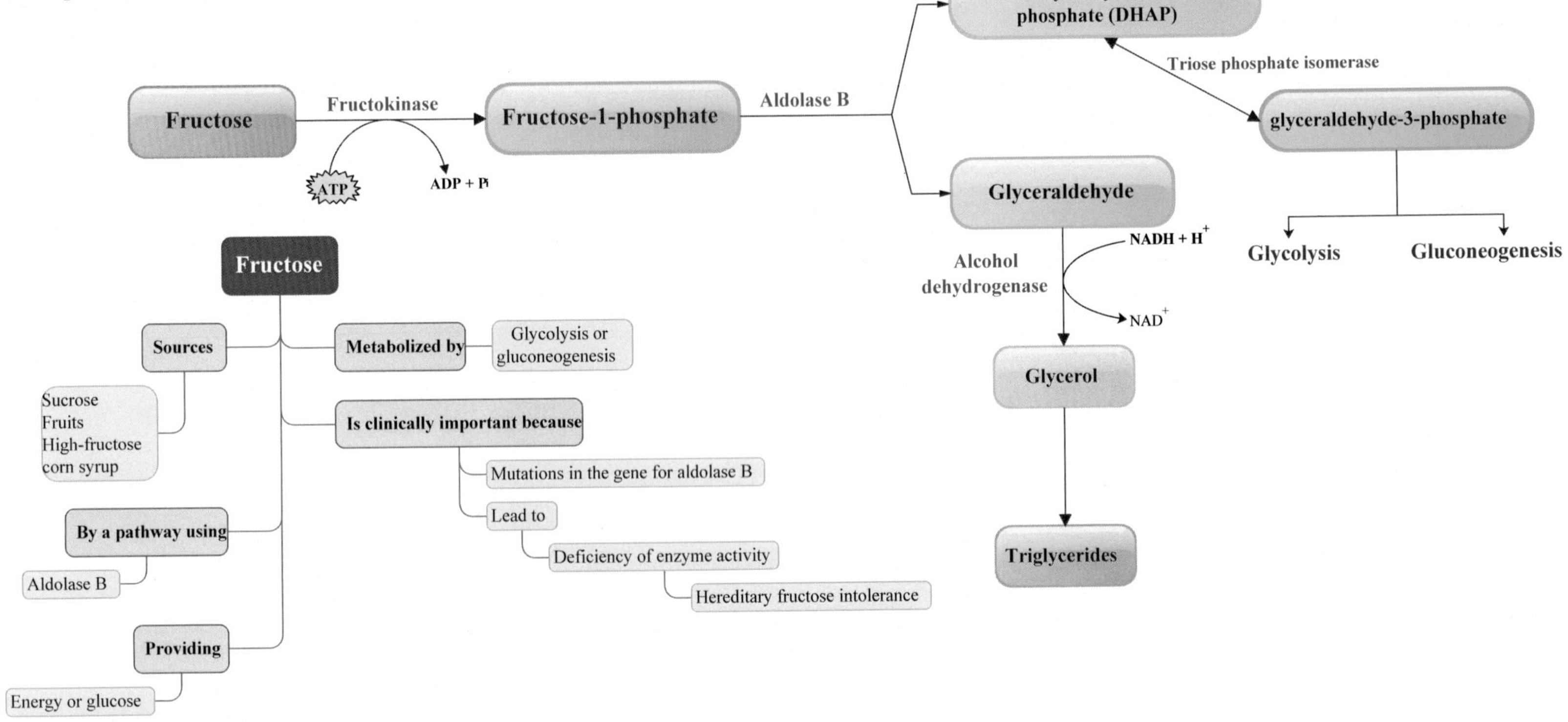

Fructose →(Fructokinase)→ Fructose-1-phosphate →(Aldolase B)→ Dihydroxyacetone phosphate (DHAP), Glyceraldehyde

ATP → ADP + Pi

Dihydroxyacetone phosphate (DHAP) ↔(Triose phosphate isomerase)↔ glyceraldehyde-3-phosphate

glyceraldehyde-3-phosphate → Glycolysis, Gluconeogenesis

Glyceraldehyde →(Alcohol dehydrogenase; NADH + H$^+$ → NAD$^+$)→ Glycerol → Triglycerides

Fructose
- Sources
  - Sucrose
  - Fruits
  - High-fructose corn syrup
- Metabolized by — Glycolysis or gluconeogenesis
- Is clinically important because
  - Mutations in the gene for aldolase B
  - Lead to
    - Deficiency of enzyme activity
      - Hereditary fructose intolerance
- By a pathway using
  - Aldolase B
- Providing
  - Energy or glucose

12.6. Galactose: is a monosaccharide and also the source of galactose is lactose obtained from milk. The entry of galactose into cells is not insulin dependent.

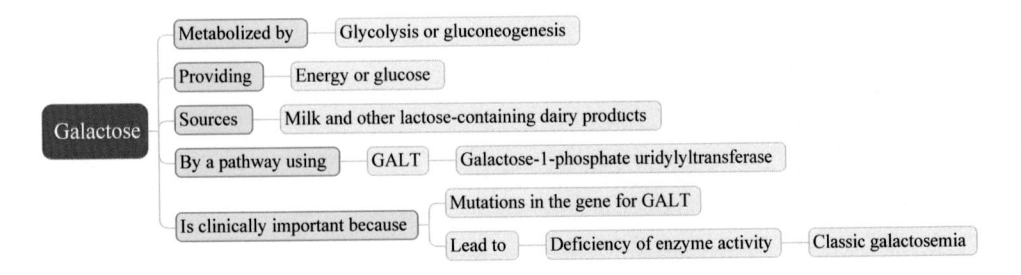

Galactose
- Metabolized by — Glycolysis or gluconeogenesis
- Providing — Energy or glucose
- Sources — Milk and other lactose-containing dairy products
- By a pathway using — GALT — Galactose-1-phosphate uridylyltransferase
- Is clinically important because
  - Mutations in the gene for GALT
  - Lead to — Deficiency of enzyme activity — Classic galactosemia

OVERVIEW

The pentose phosphate pathway (also called the hexose monophosphate pathway, or 6 phosphogluconate pathway) occurs in the cytosol of the cell. It includes two, irreversible oxidative reactions, followed by a series of reversible sugar–phosphate interconversions . No ATP is directly consumed or produced in the cycle. Carbon 1 of glucose 6-phosphate is released as CO_2, and two NADPH are produced for each glucose 6-phosphate molecule entering the oxidative part of the pathway. The rate and direction of the reversible reactions of the pentose phosphate pathway are determined by the supply of and demand for intermediates of the cycle. The pathway provides a major portion of the body's NADPH, which functions as a biochemical reductant. It also produces ribose 5-phosphate, required for the biosynthesis of nucleotides, and provides a mechanism for the metabolic use of five-carbon sugars obtained from the diet or the degradation of structural carbohydrates in the body.

Chapter 13 : Pentose Phosphate Pathway and NADPH

13.1.pentose phosphate pathway consists of two phases:

A. Irreversible oxidative reaction

Glucose 6-P +2NADP+ +H $_2$O →Ribulose-5-phosphate + 2NADPH + CO $_2$+ 2H$^+$

B. Reversible nonoxidative reactions

Ribose5-phosphate → Synthesis of Ribose-5-phosphate to synthesis (DNA, RNA, ATP, NADH, FAD, and CoA) OR synthesis intermediates for glycolysis

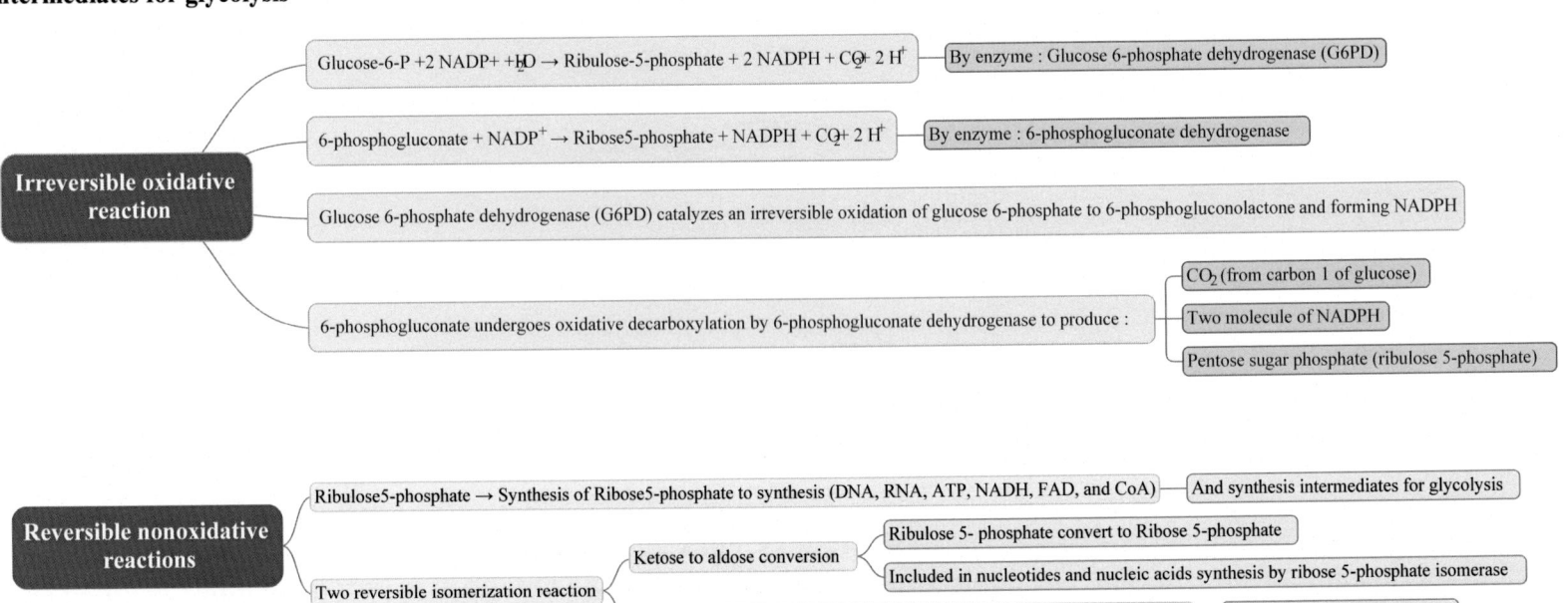

Irreversible oxidative reaction

- Glucose-6-P +2 NADP+ +H$_2$D → Ribulose-5-phosphate + 2 NADPH + CO$_2$+ 2 H$^+$ — By enzyme : Glucose 6-phosphate dehydrogenase (G6PD)
- 6-phosphogluconate + NADP$^+$ → Ribose5-phosphate + NADPH + CO$_2$+ 2 H$^+$ — By enzyme : 6-phosphogluconate dehydrogenase
- Glucose 6-phosphate dehydrogenase (G6PD) catalyzes an irreversible oxidation of glucose 6-phosphate to 6-phosphogluconolactone and forming NADPH
- 6-phosphogluconate undergoes oxidative decarboxylation by 6-phosphogluconate dehydrogenase to produce :
  - CO$_2$ (from carbon 1 of glucose)
  - Two molecule of NADPH
  - Pentose sugar phosphate (ribulose 5-phosphate)

Reversible nonoxidative reactions

- Ribulose5-phosphate → Synthesis of Ribose5-phosphate to synthesis (DNA, RNA, ATP, NADH, FAD, and CoA) — And synthesis intermediates for glycolysis
- Two reversible isomerization reaction
  - Ketose to aldose conversion
    - Ribulose 5- phosphate convert to Ribose 5-phosphate
    - Included in nucleotides and nucleic acids synthesis by ribose 5-phosphate isomerase
  - Inversion configuration of Ribulose 5- phosphate to xylulose 5- phosphate — By phosphopentose epimeras

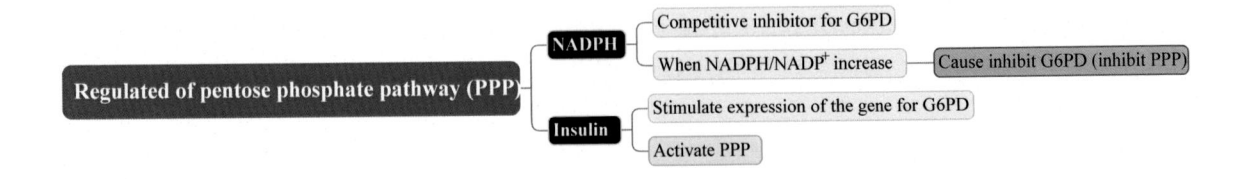

Regulated of pentose phosphate pathway (PPP)

- **NADPH**
  - Competitive inhibitor for G6PD
  - When NADPH/NADP$^+$ increase — Cause inhibit G6PD (inhibit PPP)
- **Insulin**
  - Stimulate expression of the gene for G6PD
  - Activate PPP

Chapter 13 : Pentose Phosphate Pathway and NADPH

Transketolase reaction I — Transketolase catalyse by coenzyme thiamine pyrophosphate (TPP)
- To transfer 2 carbon from xylulose 5-phosphate to Ribose5-phosphate
- Produce glyceraldehyde 3-phosphate and seven carbons sugar

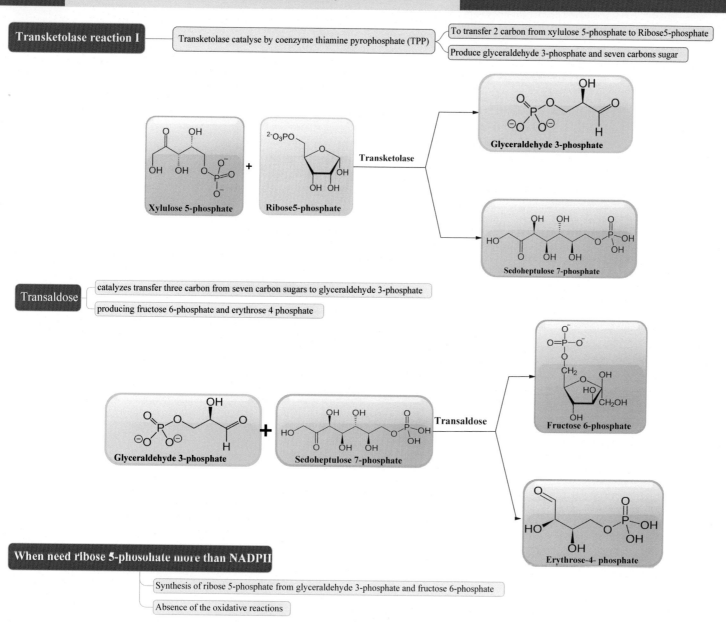

Transaldose
- catalyzes transfer three carbon from seven carbon sugars to glyceraldehyde 3-phosphate
- producing fructose 6-phosphate and erythrose 4 phosphate

When need ribose 5-phosphate more than NADPH
- Synthesis of ribose 5-phosphate from glyceraldehyde 3-phosphate and fructose 6-phosphate
- Absence of the oxidative reactions

The sequence of reactions are divided into two types

oxidative reaction phase

1st reaction:
Conversion of glucose to glucose-6 phosphate

Ccatalyzed by the enzyme hexokinase and a molecule of ATP is utilized

This reaction is actually a primary step of glycolysis

2nd reaction:
Conversion of glucose-6 phosphate to 6-phosphogluconolactone

Catalyzed by an enzyme glucose-6 phosphate dehydrogenase (G6PD) in the presence of Mg^{++} ion

In this reaction a molecule of NADPH is produced

3rd reaction:
Conversion of 6-phosphogluconolactone to 6-phosphogluconate

This reaction is a hydrolysis reaction catalyzed by hydrolase enzyme

4th reaction:
Conversion of 6-phosphogluconate to ribulose-5 phosphate

Catalyzed by the enzyme 6-phosphogluconate dehydrogenase to produce 3-keto-6-phosphogluconate which undergoes decarboxylation to produce ribulose-5 phosphate

In this reaction a molecule of NADPH is generated

Non-oxidative reaction phase

Oxidative reactions is followed by a series reversible sugar phosphate inter-conversion reaction

Ribulose-5-phosphate is epimerized to produce xylulose 5-phosphate in the presence of enzyme phosphor pentose epimerase

Similarly ribulose-5-phosphate is also keto-isomerized into ribose 5-phosphate

Xylulose-5-phsphate transfer two carbon moiety to ribose 5-phospahate in the presence of enzyme transketolase to form sedoheptulose-7-phosphate and glyceraldehyde 3-phosphate

Sedoheptulose -7-phosphate transfer three carbon moiety to glyceraldehyde -3-phosphate to form fructose 6-phopsphate and erythrose 4-phosphate in the presence of enzyme transaldolase

Transketolase enzyme catalyse the transfer of two carbon moiety from Xylulose-5-phsphate to erythrose-4- phosphate to form fructose-6-phosphate and glyceraldehyde-3-phosphate

Fructose-6-phosphate and glyceraldehyde-3-phosphate is later enter into glycolysis and kreb's cycle

The rate and direction of reversible reaction depends upon the needs of cell

If cell needs only NADPH then fructose-phosphate and glyceraldehyde-3-phosphate are converted back to glucose by reverse glycolysis

Otherwise converted to pyruvate and enter TCA cycle generating ATPs

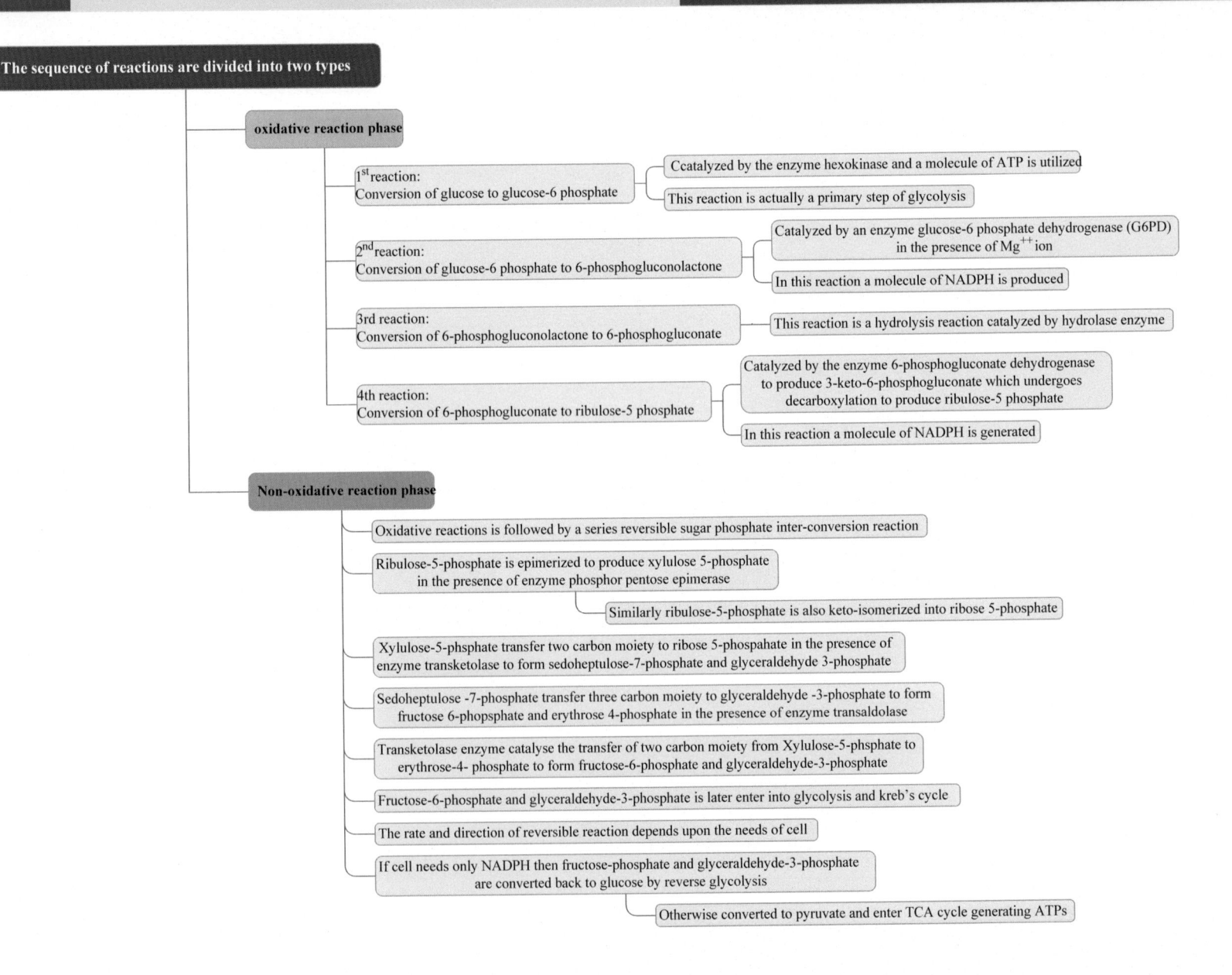

Oxidative reaction phase

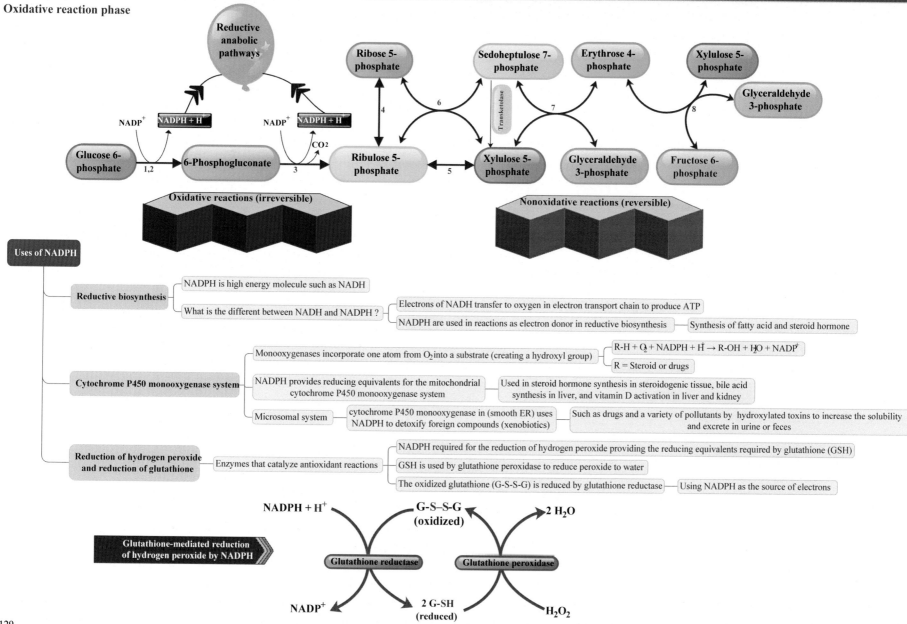

Uses of NADPH

Reductive biosynthesis
- NADPH is high energy molecule such as NADH
- What is the different between NADH and NADPH ?
  - Electrons of NADH transfer to oxygen in electron transport chain to produce ATP
  - NADPH are used in reactions as electron donor in reductive biosynthesis — Synthesis of fatty acid and steroid hormone

Cytochrome P450 monooxygenase system
- Monooxygenases incorporate one atom from O_2 into a substrate (creating a hydroxyl group)
  - $R-H + O_2 + NADPH + H^+ \rightarrow R-OH + H_2O + NADP^+$
  - R = Steroid or drugs
- NADPH provides reducing equivalents for the mitochondrial cytochrome P450 monooxygenase system — Used in steroid hormone synthesis in steroidogenic tissue, bile acid synthesis in liver, and vitamin D activation in liver and kidney
- Microsomal system — cytochrome P450 monooxygenase in (smooth ER) uses NADPH to detoxify foreign compounds (xenobiotics) — Such as drugs and a variety of pollutants by hydroxylated toxins to increase the solubility and excrete in urine or feces

Reduction of hydrogen peroxide and reduction of glutathione
- Enzymes that catalyze antioxidant reactions
  - NADPH required for the reduction of hydrogen peroxide providing the reducing equivalents required by glutathione (GSH)
  - GSH is used by glutathione peroxidase to reduce peroxide to water
  - The oxidized glutathione (G-S-S-G) is reduced by glutathione reductase — Using NADPH as the source of electrons

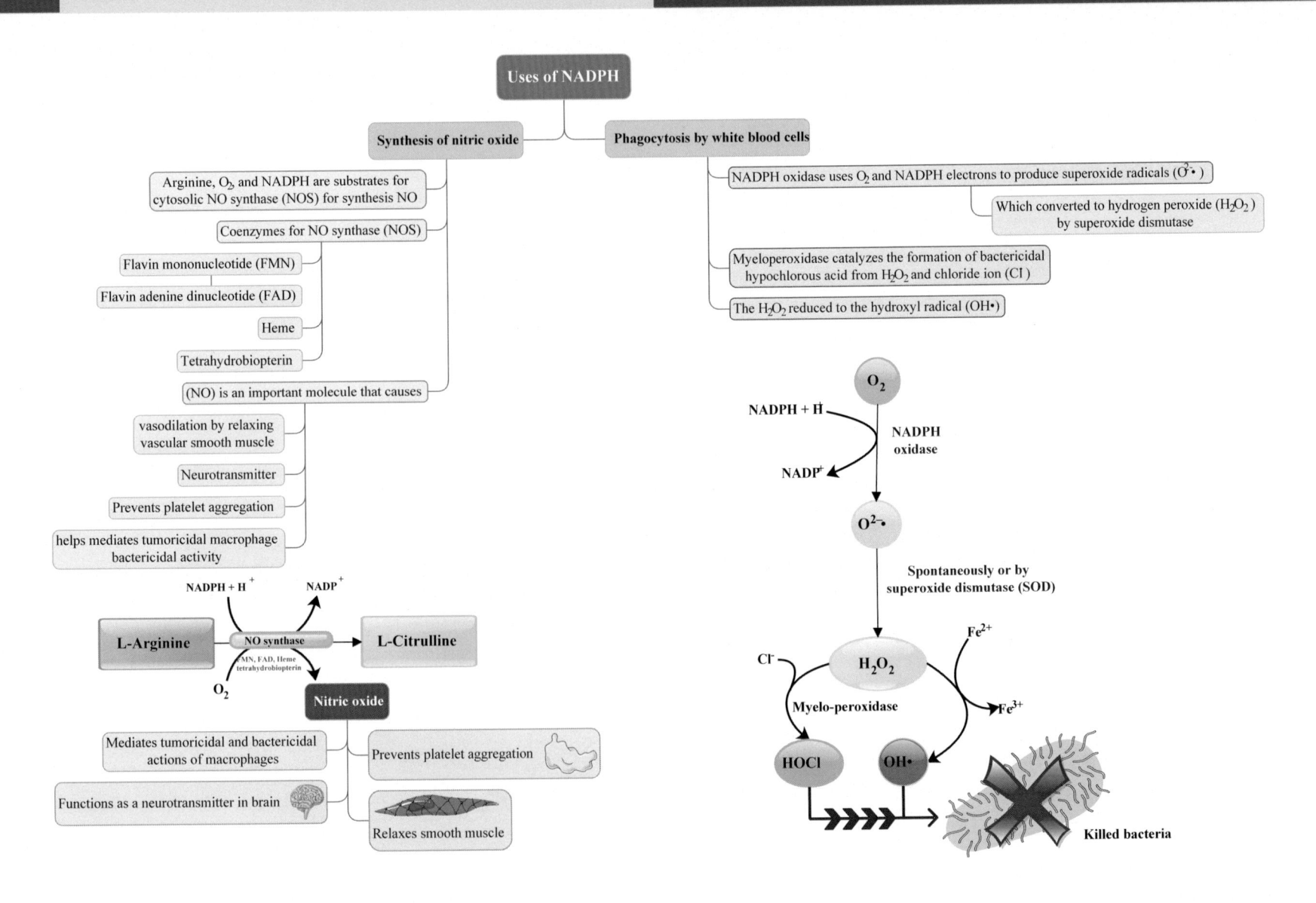

13.2.Glucose 6-phosphate dehydrogenase deficiency

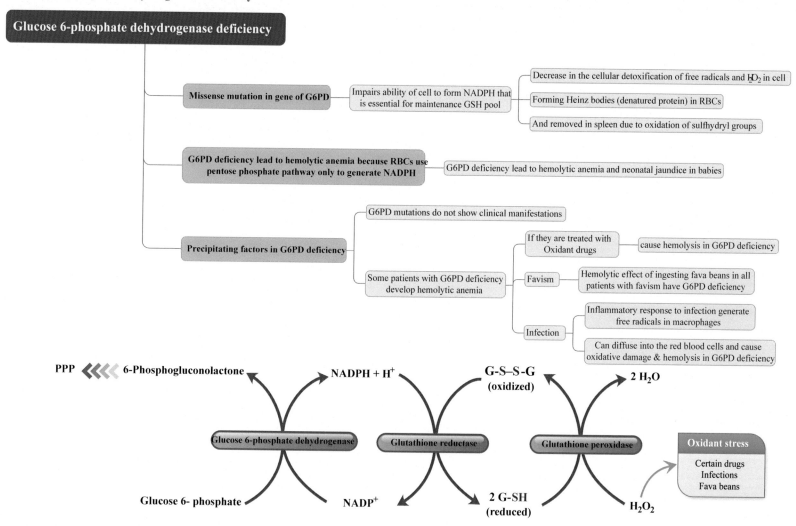

Glucose 6-phosphate dehydrogenase deficiency

- **Missense mutation in gene of G6PD** → Impairs ability of cell to form NADPH that is essential for maintenance GSH pool →
  - Decrease in the cellular detoxification of free radicals and H_2O_2 in cell
  - Forming Heinz bodies (denatured protein) in RBCs
  - And removed in spleen due to oxidation of sulfhydryl groups

- **G6PD deficiency lead to hemolytic anemia because RBCs use pentose phosphate pathway only to generate NADPH** → G6PD deficiency lead to hemolytic anemia and neonatal jaundice in babies

- **Precipitating factors in G6PD deficiency**
  - G6PD mutations do not show clinical manifestations
  - Some patients with G6PD deficiency develop hemolytic anemia
    - If they are treated with Oxidant drugs → cause hemolysis in G6PD deficiency
    - Favism → Hemolytic effect of ingesting fava beans in all patients with favism have G6PD deficiency
    - Infection
      - Inflammatory response to infection generate free radicals in macrophages
      - Can diffuse into the red blood cells and cause oxidative damage & hemolysis in G6PD deficiency

PPP ⋘ 6-Phosphogluconolactone   NADPH + H⁺   G-S–S-G (oxidized)   2 H₂O

Glucose 6-phosphate dehydrogenase   Glutathione reductase   Glutathione peroxidase   **Oxidant stress**
Certain drugs
Infections
Fava beans

Glucose 6- phosphate   NADP⁺   2 G-SH (reduced)   H₂O₂

Glucose 6-phosphate dehydrogenase deficiency pathophysiology

G6PD converts glucose-6-phosphate into 6-phosphoglucono-δ-lactone and is the rate-limiting enzyme of this metabolic pathway that supplies reducing energy to cells

By maintaining the level of the reduced form of the co-enzyme nicotinamide adenine dinucleotide phosphate (NADPH)

The NADPH in turn maintains the supply of reduced glutathione in the cells that is used to mop up free radicals that cause oxidative damage

The G6PD / NADPH pathway is the only source of reduced glutathione in red blood cells (erythrocytes)

People with G6PD deficiency are therefore at risk of hemolytic anemia in states of oxidative stress

Oxidative stress can result from infection and from chemical exposure to medication and certain foods

Fava beans

Contain high levels of vicine, divicine, convicine and isouramil, all of which create oxidants

When all remaining reduced glutathione is consumed, enzymes and other proteins (including hemoglobin)

Are subsequently damaged by the oxidants, leading to cross-bonding and protein deposition in the red cell membranes

Damaged red cells are phagocytosed and sequestered (taken out of circulation) in the spleen

The hemoglobin is metabolized to bilirubin (causing jaundice at high concentrations)

The red cells rarely disintegrate in the circulation, so hemoglobin is rarely excreted directly by the kidney, but this can occur in severe cases, causing acute renal failure

Deficiency of G6PD in the alternative pathway causes the buildup of glucose and thus there is an increase of advanced glycation endproducts (AGE)

The deficiency also reduces the amount of NADPH, which is required for the formation of nitric oxide (NO)

The high prevalence of diabetes mellitus type 2 and hypertension in Afro-Caribbeans in the West could be directly related to the incidence of G6PD deficiency in those populations

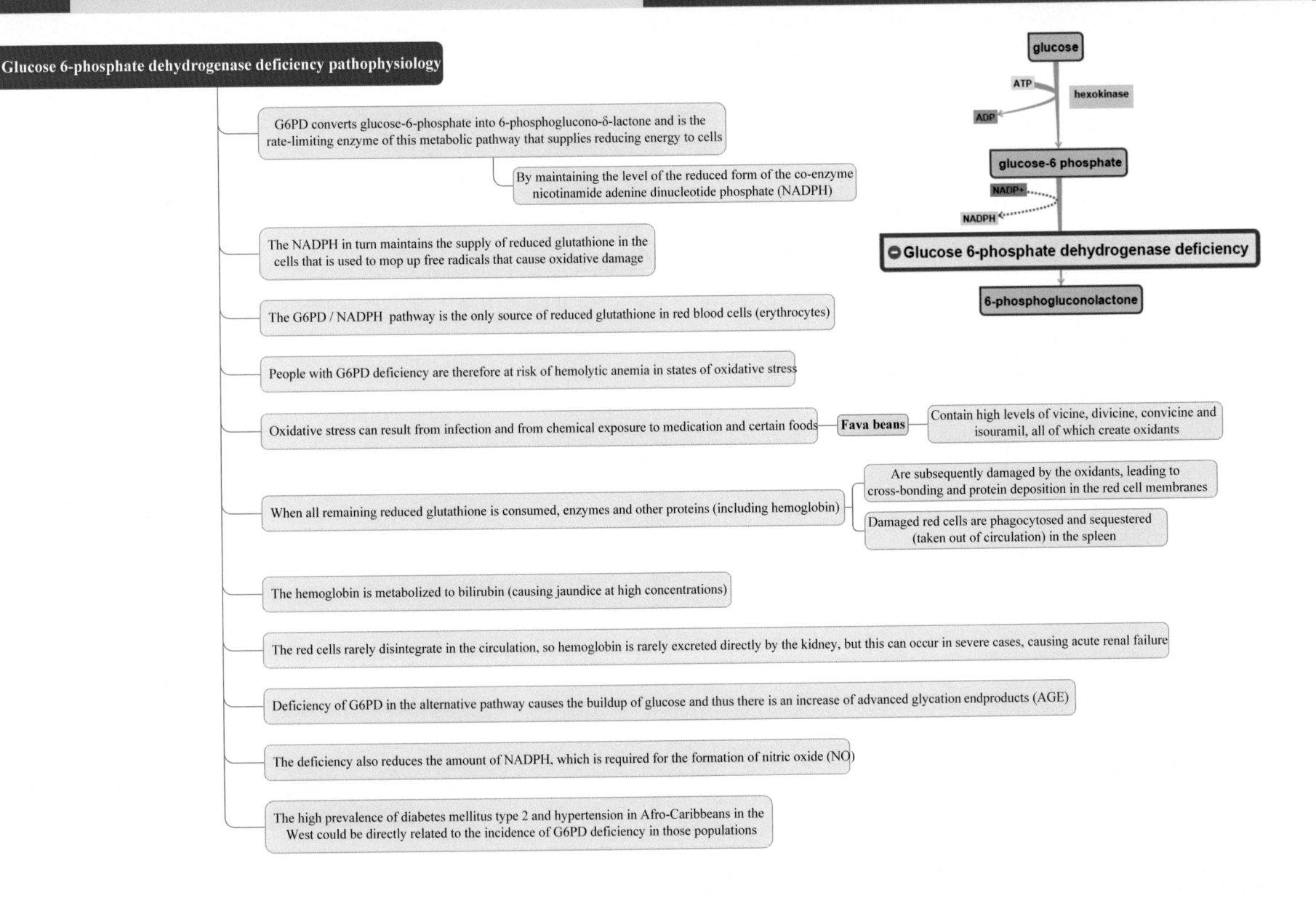

13.2.Glucose 6-phosphate dehydrogenase deficiency

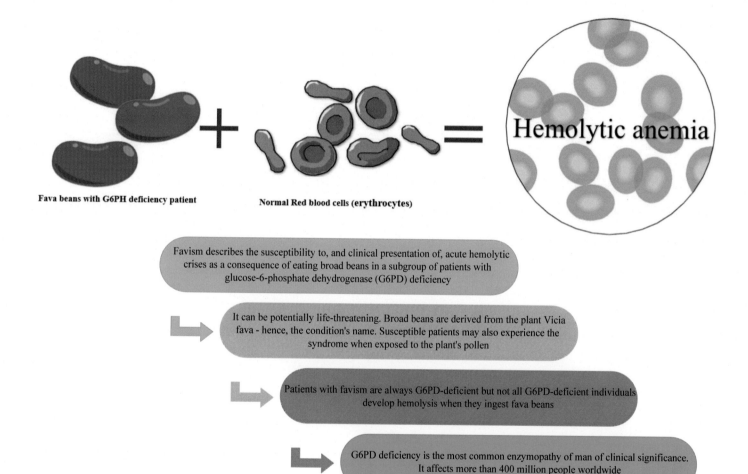

Fava beans with G6PH deficiency patient   Normal Red blood cells (erythrocytes)   Hemolytic anemia

Favism describes the susceptibility to, and clinical presentation of, acute hemolytic crises as a consequence of eating broad beans in a subgroup of patients with glucose-6-phosphate dehydrogenase (G6PD) deficiency

It can be potentially life-threatening. Broad beans are derived from the plant Vicia fava - hence, the condition's name. Susceptible patients may also experience the syndrome when exposed to the plant's pollen

Patients with favism are always G6PD-deficient but not all G6PD-deficient individuals develop hemolysis when they ingest fava beans

G6PD deficiency is the most common enzymopathy of man of clinical significance. It affects more than 400 million people worldwide

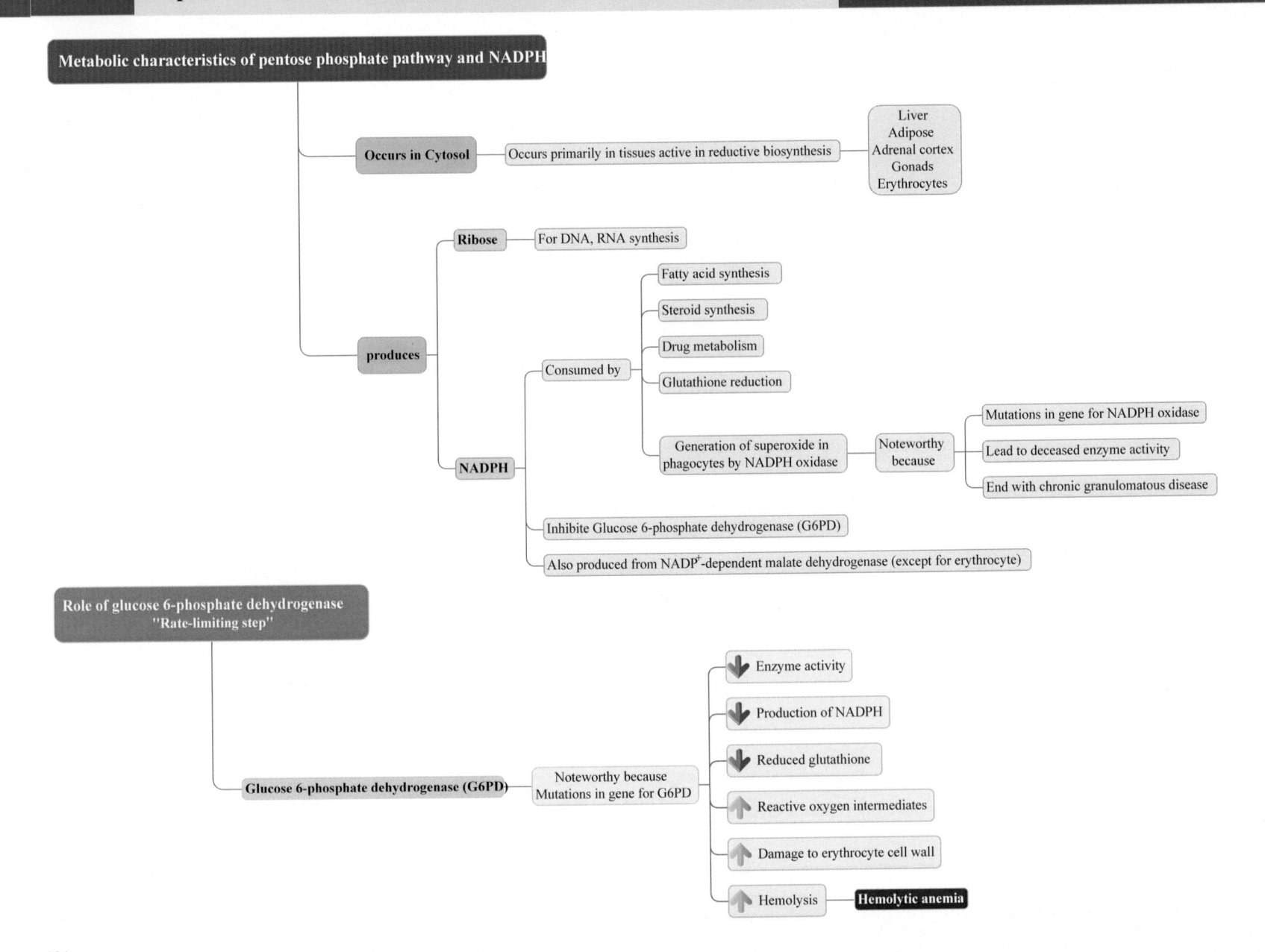

Metabolic characteristics of pentose phosphate pathway and NADPH

Occurs in Cytosol — Occurs primarily in tissues active in reductive biosynthesis — Liver / Adipose / Adrenal cortex / Gonads / Erythrocytes

produces

Ribose — For DNA, RNA synthesis

NADPH — Consumed by:
- Fatty acid synthesis
- Steroid synthesis
- Drug metabolism
- Glutathione reduction
- Generation of superoxide in phagocytes by NADPH oxidase — Noteworthy because:
  - Mutations in gene for NADPH oxidase
  - Lead to deceased enzyme activity
  - End with chronic granulomatous disease

Inhibite Glucose 6-phosphate dehydrogenase (G6PD)

Also produced from $NADP^+$-dependent malate dehydrogenase (except for erythrocyte)

Role of glucose 6-phosphate dehydrogenase "Rate-limiting step"

Glucose 6-phosphate dehydrogenase (G6PD) — Noteworthy because Mutations in gene for G6PD:
- ↓ Enzyme activity
- ↓ Production of NADPH
- ↓ Reduced glutathione
- ↑ Reactive oxygen intermediates
- ↑ Damage to erythrocyte cell wall
- ↑ Hemolysis — **Hemolytic anemia**

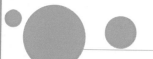

Pentose Phosphate Pathway : Exercises

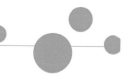

Q 1: Circle the best correct answer:

1.Which of the following is required as a reductant in fatty acid synthesis?
a. NADH
b. NADPH
c. $FADH_2$
d. $FMNH_2$

2.$NADP^+$ is required as a coenzyme in:
a. Glycolysis
b. Citric acid cycle
c. PPP
d. Gluconeogenesis

3.The decarboxylation reaction in PPP is catalyzed by:
a. Gluconolactone hydrolase
b. 6-Phosphogluconate dehydrogenase
c. Glucose 6-phosphate dehydrogenase
d. Transaldolase

4.The first pentose formed in Irreversible oxidative reaction of PPP is:
a. Ribose-5-phosphate
b. Ribulose-5-phosphate
c. Xylose-5-phosphate
d. Xylulose-5-phosphate

5.The regulatory enzyme in PPP is:
a. Glucose-6-phosphate dehydrogenase
b. 6-Phosphogluconate dehydrogenase
c. Transketolase
d. Transaldose

6.The rate of PPP reactions is
a. Increased by Insulin
b. Increased in growth hormone
c. Increased by glucagon
d. Increased in starvation

7.Two important by products of PPP are:
a. NADH and pentose sugars
b. NADPH and pentose sugars
c. Pentose sugars and $FADH_2$
d. Pentose sugars and sedoheptulose

8.One molecule of glucose gives………molecules of CO_2 in one round of PPP.
a. 6
b. 1
c. 2
d. 3

9.Which of the following enzymes is not involved in PPP?
a. Glyceraldehyde-3-p dehydrogenase
b. Glucose-6-p-dehydrogenase
c. Transketolase
d. Phosphogluconate dehydrogenase

10.Reduced glutathione functions in R.B.Cs to:
a. Produce NADPH
b. Reduce methemoglobin to hemoglobin
c. Produce NADH
d. Reduce oxidizing agents such as H_2O_2

11.The main source of reducing equivalents (NADPH) for lipogenesis is:
a. Pentose phosphate pathway
b. Citric acid cycle
c. Glycolysis
d. Glycogenolysis

12.The PPP includes the enzyme:
a. Maltase dehydrogenase
b. Hexokinase
c. α-Ketoglutarate dehydrogenase
d. Glucose-6-phosphate dehydrogenase

Q 1: Circle the best correct answer:

13.Hemolytic anemia is caused by the deficiency of certain enzymes of the pentose phosphate pathway, the principal enzyme involved is:
a. Glucose-6-phosphate dehydrogenase
b. Aldolase
c. Fructose 1, 6-bisphosphatase
d. Phosphohexose isomerase

14.In microsomal system: cytochrome P450 monooxygenase in (smooth ER) uses NADPH to:
a. Synthesis of steroid hormone, fatty acids and nitric oxide
b. Regeneration of reduced glutathione.
c. Drugs detoxification
d. Produce 3 ATP.

15.Mitochondrial cytochrome P450 monooxygenase system uses NADPH to:
a. Synthesis of steroid hormone, fatty acids and nitric oxide
b. regeneration of reduced glutathione.
c. Drugs detoxification
d. Produce 3 ATP

16.(NADPH and NADP $^+$) is maintained at a high level in cells primarily by:
a. Combined actions of glucose-6-phosphate dehydrogenase and 6-phosphogluconate dehydrogenase
b. Combined actions of transketolase and transaldolase
c. The action of electron transport chain
d. Myeloperoxidase

17.Regulated of pentose phosphate pathway (PPP):
a. NADH is inhibitor for G6PD and glucagon stimulate synthesis of G6PD
b. NADPH is a competitive inhibitor for G6PD and Insulin stimulate synthesis of G6PD
c. NADPH is inhibitor for transketolase
d. NADH is inhibitor for transaldolase

18.Which of the following statements about the use of the NADPH generated from the pentose phosphate pathway is false?
a. NADPH is used for synthesis of steroid hormone, fatty acids and nitric oxide
b. NADPH is used for the regeneration of reduced glutathione.
c. NADPH and cytochrome P450 monooxygenase system used for drugs detoxification
d. NADPH and NADH is metabolically interchangeable and produce 3 ATP.

19.The important of irreversible oxidative section of the pentose phosphate pathway is:
a. Synthesis of ribose-5-phosphate
b. synthesis intermediates for glycolysis
c. Generate NADPH and supplies ribulose-5-phosphate.
d. Generate 3ATP, 2NADH and FADH$_2$

20.Which of the following statements about pentose phosphate pathway is false?
a. Synthesis of ribose-5-phosphate and generate NADPH
b. Isomerization of ribose-5-phosphate to C4 and C7 sugars
c. Synthesis intermediates for glycolysis
d. The rate-limiting reaction is catalyzed by glucose-6-phosphatase

21.Which of the following statements about the Glucose 6-phosphate dehydrogenase (G6PD) is false?
a. G6PD deficiency lead to hemolytic anemia
b. Forming Heinz bodies in RBCs
c. G6PD generate NADH
d. G6PD deficiency impairs ability of cell to form NADPH

22.The false statement about microsomal system of cytochrome P450 is :
a. Found in smooth endoplasmic reticulum
b. Used NADPH to steroid hormone synthesis and vitamin D synthesis
c. Uses NADPH to detoxify drugs and toxin
d. Hydroxylated toxins to increase the solubility and excrete in urine

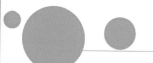

Pentose Phosphate Pathway : Exercises

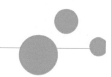

Q 1: Circle the best correct answer:

23.The true statement about the reaction catalyzed by transketolase is:

a. Require thiamine pyrophosphate (TPP)

b. Transfer a 3Cgroup

c. Produce a six-carbon and 4-carbon sugar phosphate

d. Act only on5-C sugar phosphate

24.The generation of reduced glutathione (G-SH) is needed to:

a. Catalase and superoxide dismutase

b. $NADP^+$ and glutathione peroxidase

c. NADPH and glutathione reductase

d. NADH

25.Transketolase has the coenzyme:

a. NAD^+

b. Riboflavin

c. Thiamin pyrophosphate (TPP)

d. Pyridoxol phosphate

Q 2 : Write short notes on:

1.Describe pentose phosphate pathway and its importance.

2.Describe the regulation of pentose phosphate pathway.

3.The difference between NADPH and NADH

4.The function of mitochondrial cytochrome P450 monooxygenase system.

5.The function of microsomal cytochrome P450 monooxygenase system.

6.The important of glycogenin in synthesis of glycogen.

7.Describe the pathological mechanism (pathomechanism) of favism disease.

8.Uses of NADPH.

OVERVIEW

Glycosaminoglycans are large complexes of negatively charged hetero -polysaccharide chains. They are generally associated with a small amount of protein, forming proteoglycans, which typically consist of over 95% carbohydrate. [Note: This is in comparison to the glyco proteins, which consist primarily of protein with a small amount of carbohydrate] Glycosaminoglycans have the special ability to bind large amounts of water, thereby producing the gel-like matrix that forms the basis of the body's ground substance, which, along with fibrous structural proteins such as collagen and elastin, and adhesive proteins such as fibronectin, make up the extracellular matrix (ECM). The hydrated glycosaminoglycans serve as a flexible support for the ECM, interacting with the structural and adhesive proteins, and as a molecular sieve, influencing movement of materials through the ECM.

Chapter 14 : Glycosaminoglycans, Proteoglycans, and Glycoproteins

14.1.Glycosaminoglycans (GAGs) or mucopolysaccharides

Are long unbranched polysaccharide consisting of a repeating disaccharide unit. The repeating unit (except for keratan) consists of an amino sugar (N-acetylglucosamine or N-acetylgalactosamine) along with a uronic sugar (glucuronic acid or iduronic acid) or galactose. Glycosaminoglycans are highly polar and attract water. They are therefore useful to the body as a lubricant or as a shock absorber.

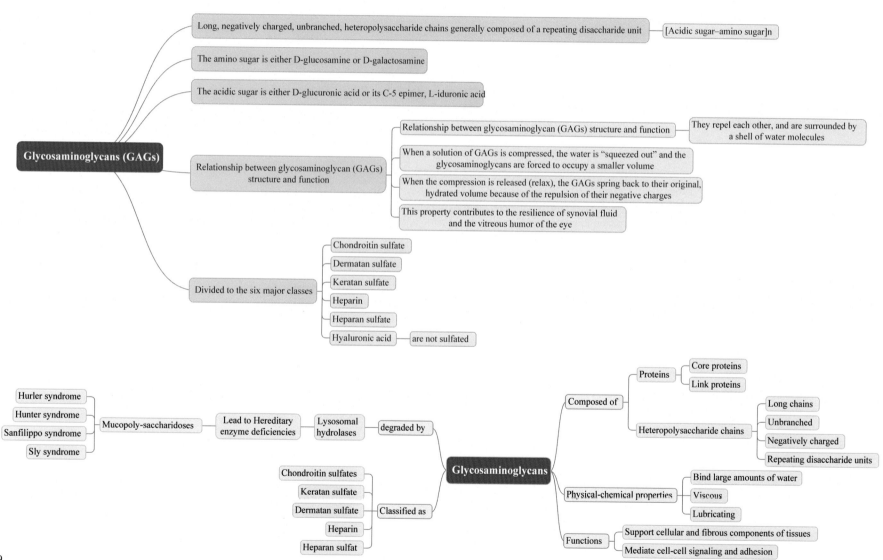

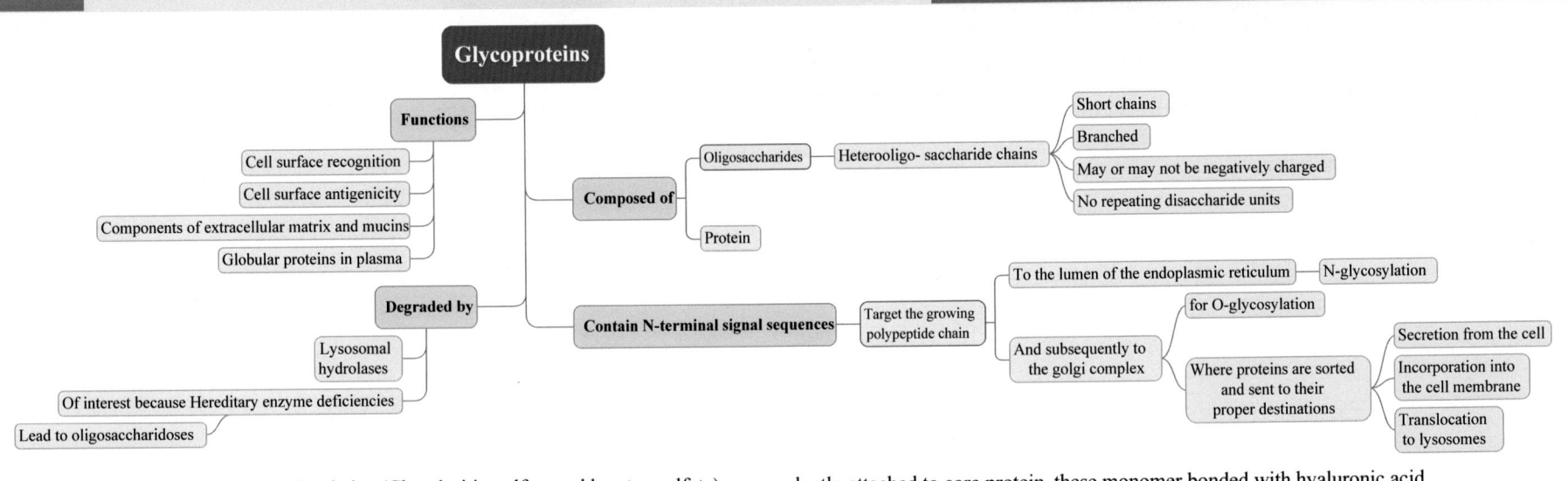

proteoglycan monomer, is linear GAGs chains (Chondroitin sulfate and keratan sulfate) are covalently attached to core protein. these monomer bonded with hyaluronic acid through ionic interaction and stabilize by link proteins. Each chains, composed of more than 100 monosaccharides, extend out from the core protein, and remain separated from each other because of charge repulsion. The resulting structure resembles a "bottle brush". The linkage between the carbohydrate chain and the protein: This linkage through a trihexoside (galactose-galactose- xylose) and a serine residue, respectively. An O-glycosidic bond is formed between the xylose and the hydroxyl group of the serine

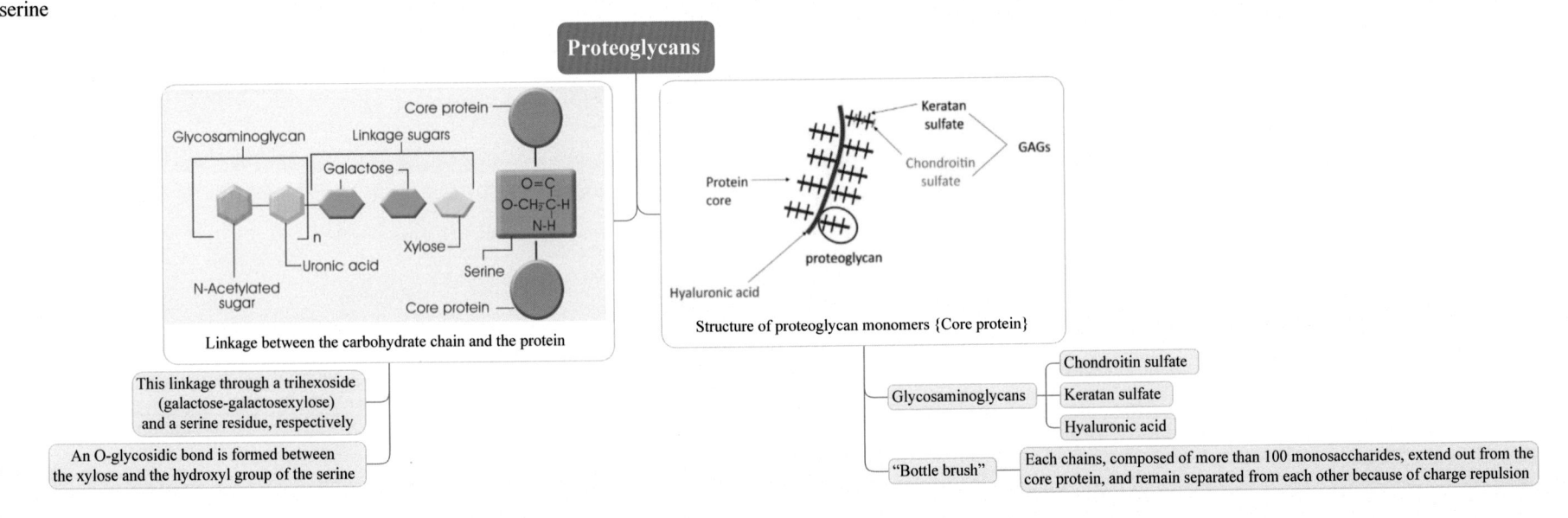

Glycoproteins are proteins to which oligosaccharides are covalently attached. They differ from the proteoglycans in that the length of the glycoprotein's carbohydrate chain is relatively short. Glycoproteins contain highly variable amounts of carbohydrate. For example, immunoglobulin IgG (<4%), human gastric glycoprotein (mucin) >80%. Membrane-bound glycoproteins participate in a broad range of cellular phenomena, including

1.Cell surface recognition (by other cells, hormones, and viruses),

2.Cell surface antigenicity (such as the blood group antigens).

3.Components of the extracellular matrix.

4.Components of the mucins of the gastrointestinal and urogenital tracts, where they act as protective biologic lubricants. almost all of the   globular proteins present in human plasma are glycoproteins

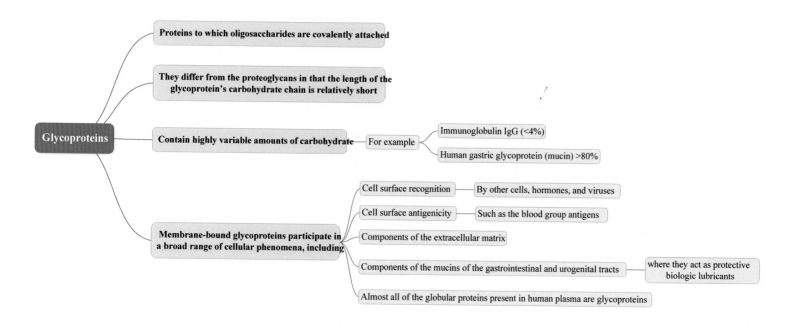

OVERVIEW

Lipid: Another word for "fat". A lipid is chemically defined as a substance that is insoluble in water and soluble in alcohol, ether, and chloroform. Because of their insolubility in aqueous solutions, body lipids are generally found compartmentalized, as in the case of membrane-associated lipids or droplets of triacylglycerol in white adipocytes, or transported in plasma in association with protein, as in lipoprotein particles, or on albumin. Lipids are an important component of living cells. Together with carbohydrates and proteins, lipids are the main constituents of plant and animal cells. Cholesterol and triglycerides are lipids. Lipids are easily stored in the body. They serve as a source of fuel and are an important constituent of the structure of cells, and they also provide the hydrophobic barrier that permits partitioning of the aqueous contents of cells and subcellular structures. Lipids serve additional functions in the body, for example,Fat-soluble vitamins - A, D, E, and K - dissolve in fat and can be stored in your liver and fat tissue until needed. Fat-soluble vitamins have a multitude of functions from keeping your bones strong to helping your muscles move and alsovitamins have regulatory or coenzyme functions, and the prostaglandins and steroid hormones play major roles in the control of the body's homeostasis. Not surprisingly, deficiencies or imbalances of lipid metabolism can lead to some of the major clinical problems encountered by physicians, such as atherosclerosis and obesity.

Introduction: Simplest lipids, fatty acids (esters of fatty acids with alcohol), have general formula R-COOH (R represent hydrocarbon chain) therefore They are either hydrophobic (nonpolar) or amphipathic (containing both nonpolar and polar). these can be divided into two groups, Fats (saturated or unsaturated), are the ester of fatty acids with glycerol (oil), triacylglycerols, glycerophospholipids, and sphingolipids and waxes, hormones, and steroids. This feature of lipids allows our bodies to use them as waterproof barriers and as biological membranes. The glycerol backbone and fatty acid tail of a phospholipid.

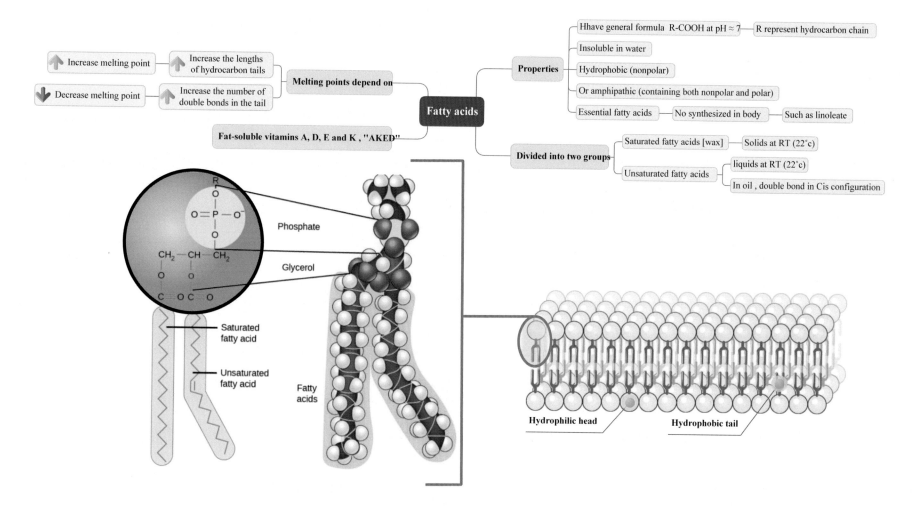

- Increase melting point
- Decrease melting point
- Increase the lengths of hydrocarbon tails
- Increase the number of double bonds in the tail
- Melting points depend on
- Fat-soluble vitamins A, D, E and K , "AKED"

Fatty acids

- **Properties**
  - Hhave general formula R-COOH at pH ≈ 7 — R represent hydrocarbon chain
  - Insoluble in water
  - Hydrophobic (nonpolar)
  - Or amphipathic (containing both nonpolar and polar)
  - Essential fatty acids — No synthesized in body — Such as linoleate
- **Divided into two groups**
  - Saturated fatty acids [wax] — Solids at RT (22°c)
  - Unsaturated fatty acids — liquids at RT (22°c) — In oil , double bond in Cis configuration

Phosphate

Glycerol

Saturated fatty acid

Unsaturated fatty acid

Fatty acids

Hydrophilic head   Hydrophobic tail

Fatty acids are generally stored as neutral lipids called triacylglycerolsTriacylglycerols, also known as triglycerides, are the simplest lipids formed by fatty acids. It is made up of three fatty acids ester linked to a single glycerol. Most triacylglycerols contain two or three different fatty acids. Triacylglycerols are nonpolar, hydrophobic, and insoluble in water

Triacylglycerols
- Storage form of fatty acids
- Very hydrophobic [non polar] — Because of this , it doesn't exist in cell membrane

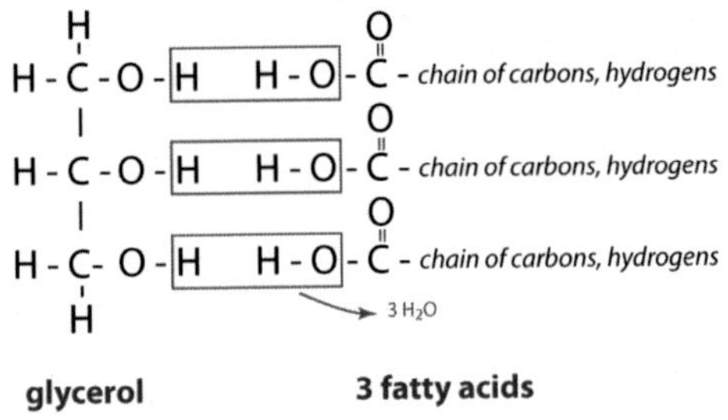

glycerol   3 fatty acids

15.1.Glycerophospholipid
- Amphipathic molecules, with a polar head and long nonpolar tails
- Abundant in the cell membrane
- The simplest Glycerophospholipids (phosphatidates) — Consist of two fatty acyl groups esterified to C-1 and C-2 of glycerol 3-phosphate

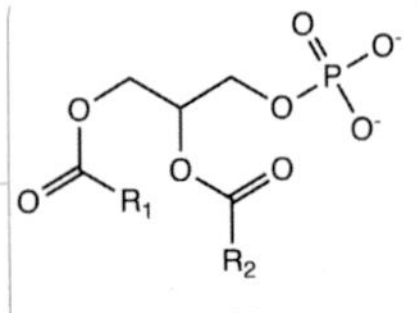

Phosphatidates

- Plasmalogens
  - Is one of the major type of glycerophospholipids
  - Differ from phophatidates in having the hydrocarbon substituent on the C-1 hydroxyl group of glycerol attached by a vinyl ether linkage rather than ester linkage
  - Abundant in the human central nervous system

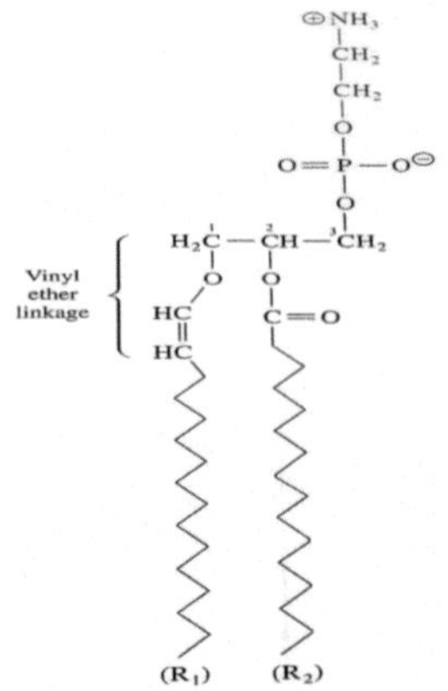

Structure of an enthanolamine plasmolagen

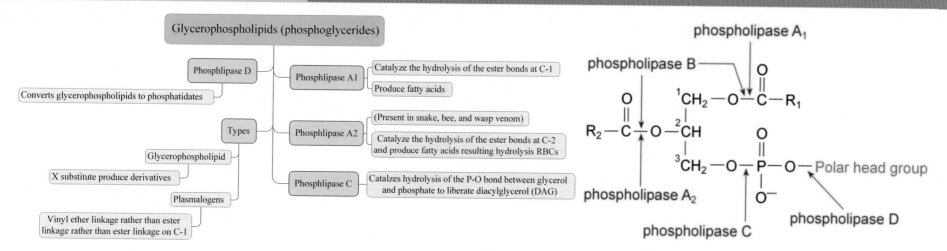

Glycerophospholipids (phosphoglycerides)

Phosphlipase D

Converts glycerophospholipids to phosphatidates

Types

Glycerophospholipid

X substitute produce derivatives

Plasmalogens

Vinyl ether linkage rather than ester linkage rather than ester linkage on C-1

Phosphlipase A1 — Catalyze the hydrolysis of the ester bonds at C-1 / Produce fatty acids

Phosphlipase A2 — (Present in snake, bee, and wasp venom) / Catalyze the hydrolysis of the ester bonds at C-2 and produce fatty acids resulting hydrolysis RBCs

Phosphlipase C — Catalzes hydrolysis of the P-O bond between glycerol and phosphate to liberate diacylglycerol (DAG)

15.2.Sphingolipid , any member of a class of lipids (fat-soluble constituents of living cells) containing the organic aliphatic amino alcohol sphingosine or a substance structurally similar to it. Among the most simple sphingolipids are the ceramides (sphingosine plus a fatty acid), widely distributed in small amounts in plant and animal tissues. The other sphingolipids are derivatives of ceramides.

Sphingolipids — Abundant in the central nervous system, Found in cell membrane, [its amphipathic]

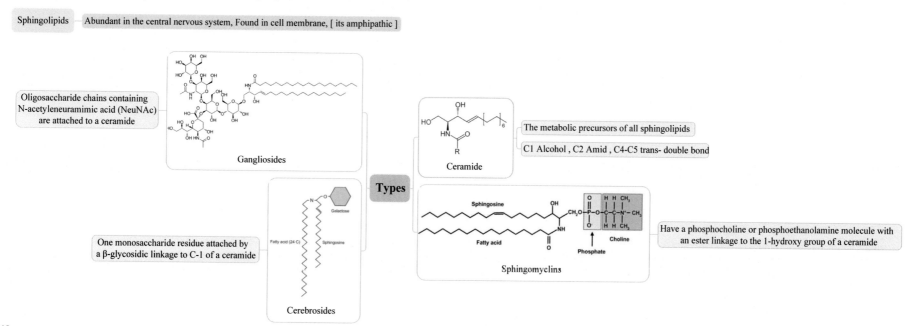

Oligosaccharide chains containing N-acetyleneuramimic acid (NeuNAc) are attached to a ceramide

Gangliosides

One monosaccharide residue attached by a β-glycosidic linkage to C-1 of a ceramide

Cerebrosides

Types

Ceramide — The metabolic precursors of all sphingolipids / C1 Alcohol , C2 Amid , C4-C5 trans- double bond

Sphingomyclins — Have a phosphocholine or phosphoethanolamine molecule with an ester linkage to the 1-hydroxy group of a ceramide

15.3.Steroids: Cholesterol is also a key regulator of membrane fluidity in animals. It is able to insert itself into bilayers perpendicular to the membrane plane. The hydroxyl group forms hydrogen bonds with the carbonyl oxygen of a phospholipid head group while the hydrocarbon tail positions itself in the non-polar core of the bilayer. Since the structure of cholesterol differs from phospholipids, it disrupts the normal reactions between fatty acid chains. Cholesterol is also able to form lipid rafts when it forms specific complexes with certain phospholipids, which results in membranes that are less fluid and less subject to phase transitions. This also increase the permeability of the cell membrane to hydrogen and sodium ions.

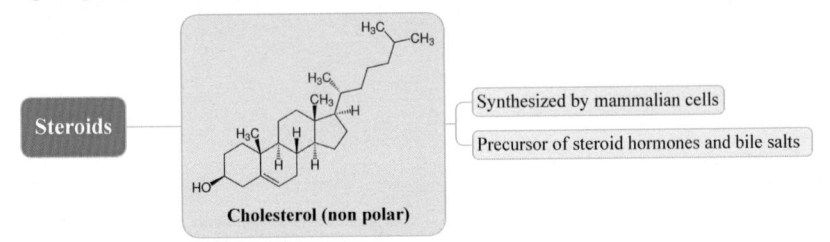

Steroids
- Synthesized by mammalian cells
- Precursor of steroid hormones and bile salts

Cholesterol (non polar)

15.4.A wax is a simple lipid that is an ester of a long-chain alcohol and a fatty acid. The alcohol may be made up of 12-32 carbon atoms.These waxes can be found in nature as coatings on leaves and stems of plants, and prevents the plant from losing excessive amounts of water. Carnuba wax is found on the leaves of Brazilian palm trees and is used in floor and automobile waxes. Lanolin coats lamb's wool. Beeswax is secreted by bees to make cells for honey.

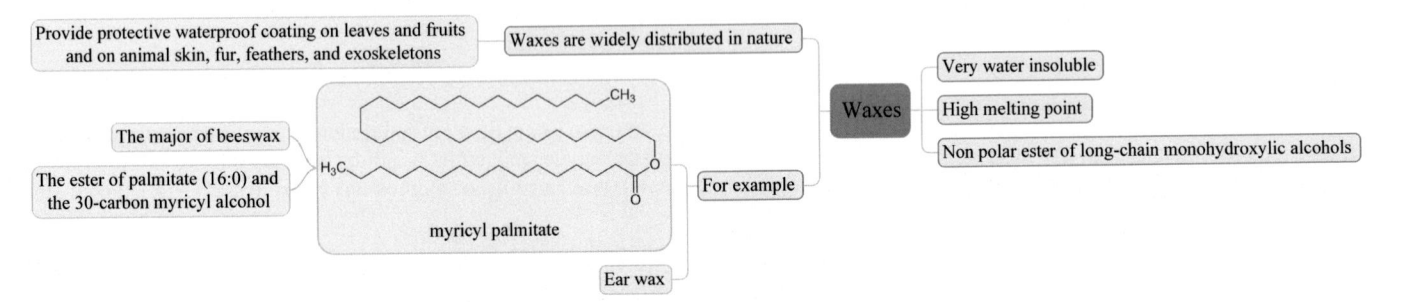

- Provide protective waterproof coating on leaves and fruits and on animal skin, fur, feathers, and exoskeletons
- Waxes are widely distributed in nature
- The major of beeswax
- The ester of palmitate (16:0) and the 30-carbon myricyl alcohol
- For example

myricyl palmitate

- Ear wax

Waxes
- Very water insoluble
- High melting point
- Non polar ester of long-chain monohydroxylic alcohols

15.6.Eicosanoid : any of a class of compounds (such as the prostaglandins) derived from polyunsaturated fatty acids (such as arachidonic acid) and involved in cellular activity , eicosanoids are oxygenated derivatives of C20 polyusaturated fatty acids such asarachidionic acid.

15.7.The prostaglandins (PG) are a group of physiologically active lipid compounds called eicosanoids having diverse hormone-like effects in animals. Prostaglandins have been found in almost every tissue in humans and other animals. They are derived enzymatically from the fatty acid arachidonic acid. Every prostaglandin contains 20 carbon atoms, including a 5-carbon ring. They are a subclass of eicosanoids and of the prostanoid class of fatty acid derivatives.

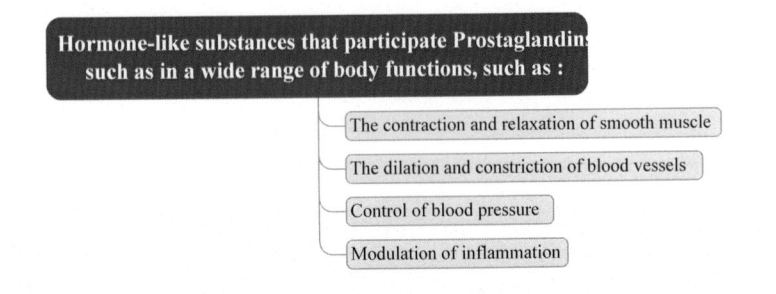

Hormone-like substances that participate Prostaglandins such as in a wide range of body functions, such as :
- The contraction and relaxation of smooth muscle
- The dilation and constriction of blood vessels
- Control of blood pressure
- Modulation of inflammation

15.8.**Biological membranes** are composed of lipid bilayers and proteins Biological membrane define the external boundaries of cells and separate compartments within cells.

Biological membranes function:

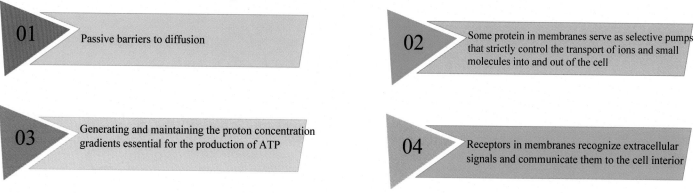

01 Passive barriers to diffusion

02 Some protein in membranes serve as selective pumps that strictly control the transport of ions and small molecules into and out of the cell

03 Generating and maintaining the proton concentration gradients essential for the production of ATP

04 Receptors in membranes recognize extracellular signals and communicate them to the cell interior

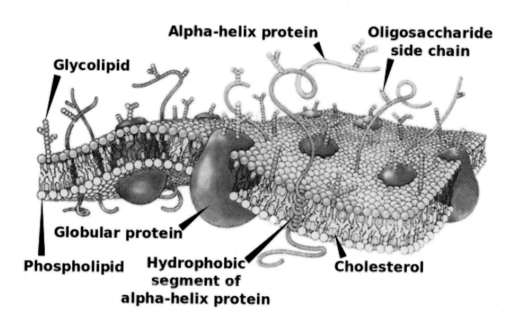

Alpha-helix protein   Oligosaccharide side chain

Glycolipid

Globular protein

Phospholipid   Hydrophobic segment of alpha-helix protein   Cholesterol

Cell-surface (extracellular) receptors:
Tyrosine kinase receptor:
Insulin tyrosine kinase receptor

1. Insulin binds

2. Tyrosine Kinase activation

6. Protein Synthesis
7. Cell Survival
8. Proliferation

4. Translocate GLUT4 transporters

5. Glucose uptake

3. Signaling molecules: IRS, PI3K, PDK1, AKT, AS160 etc.

Metabolism   Storage
Glycolysis   *Glycogenesis*

ATP + Pyruvate   Glycogen

Lipogenesis

Lipids

Insulin tyrosine kinase receptor

The L1, CR, L2, FN III-1 and α-CT are color coded to display their locations in this complex .The insulin molecule is colored in blue and green and its surface is drawn for easy identification. A second chain of the truncated IR protein is shown in ribbon representation and colored grey (except for the α-CT' helix)

FnIII-1   L2   Insulin

αCT   αCT'

L1

CR

Complex of insulin and a truncated version of the insulin receptor shown in ribbon representation
(PDB ID 5kqv , Menting et al., 2013) .

Activation of insulin tyrosine kinase receptor

Insulin bind to receptor tyrosine kinase to activated

Leading to autophosphorylation of insulin-receptor substrates (IRSs) interact with phosphatidylinositide 3-kinase (PI kinase) at the plasma membrane

PI kinase act as effector enzyme, catalyzes phosphorylated PIP_2 to PIP_3

PIP_3 act as a second messenger and activate the protein kinases to phosphorylate the cellular proteins (cellular response)

Biological membranes

Fluid mosaic

Lipid bilayers

Contains about

25%-50% lipid

50%-75% protein by mass

Less than 10% carbohydrate

As a component of glycolipid and glycoproteins

The structure for all biological membranes is the lipid bilayer

Includes amphipathic lipids

Glycerophospholipids

Sphingolipids

Cholesterol

Lipids can diffuse rapidly within a leaflet of the bilayer

The hydrophobic interaction stabilize the bilayer but allow the structure to be flexible and to be self-seal

A lipid bilayer is typically about 5 to 6 nm thick

Consists of two sheets, or monolayers (called leaflets)

In each sheets

The polar head groups of amphipathic lipids are in contact with the aqueous medium

The non polar hydrocarbon tails point toward the interior of the bilayer

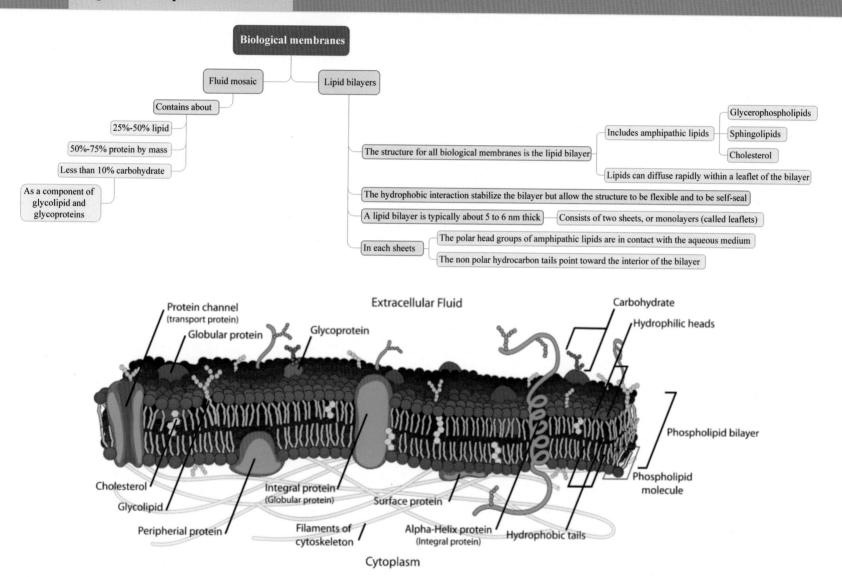

Extracellular Fluid

Protein channel
(transport protein)

Globular protein

Glycoprotein

Carbohydrate

Hydrophilic heads

Phospholipid bilayer

Phospholipid molecule

Cholesterol

Glycolipid

Integral protein
(Globular protein)

Surface protein

Hydrophobic tails

Peripherial protein

Filaments of cytoskeleton

Alpha-Helix protein
(Integral protein)

Cytoplasm

Chapter 15 : Lipid Metabolism

Lipid bilayers and membranes are dynamic structures

Both proteins and lipids are free to move laterally in the plane of the bilayer (lateral diffusion)

but movement of either from one face of the bilayer to the other is restricted (transversed diffusion, or flip-flop)

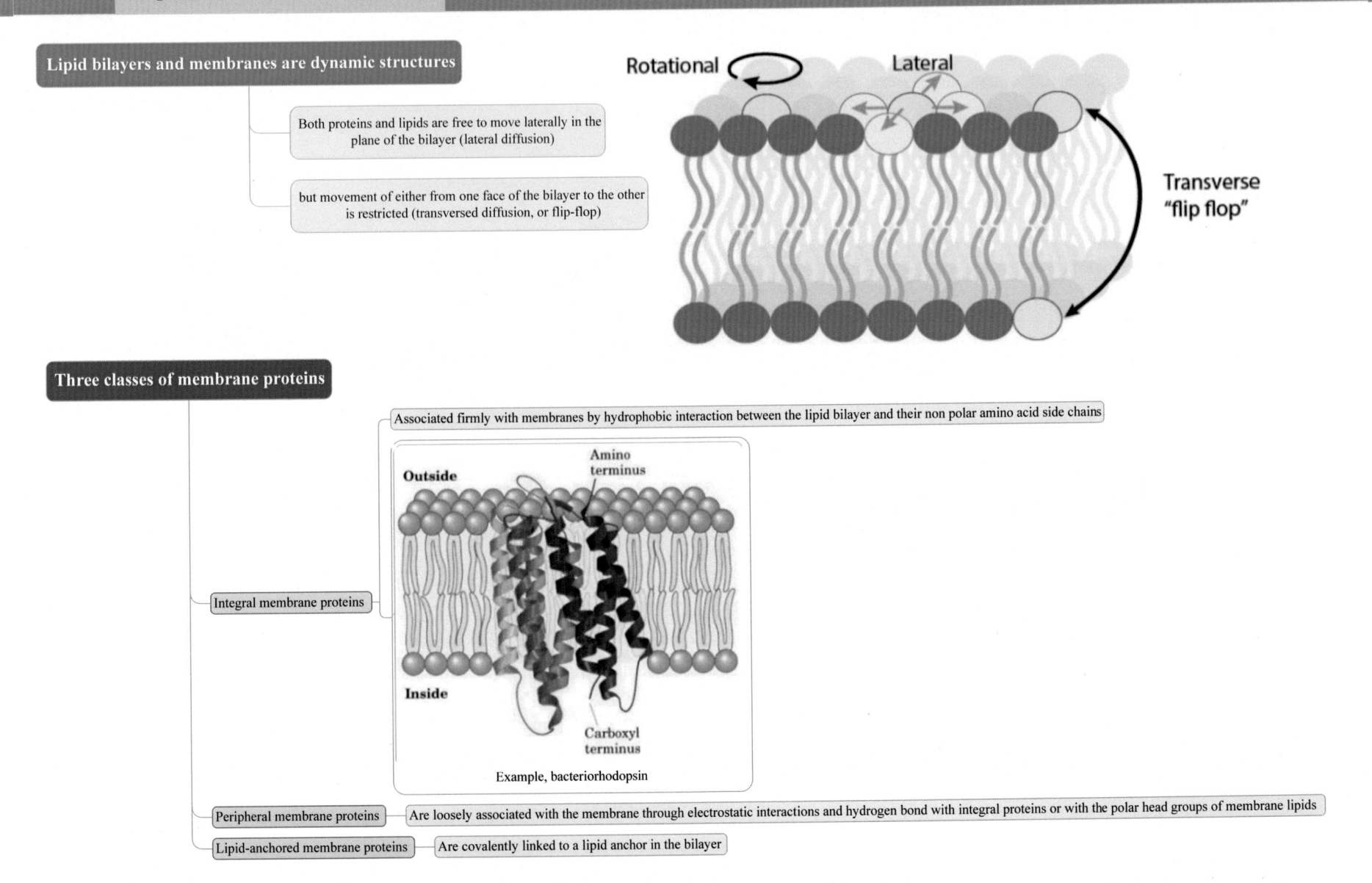

Rotational   Lateral

Transverse "flip flop"

Three classes of membrane proteins

Integral membrane proteins

Associated firmly with membranes by hydrophobic interaction between the lipid bilayer and their non polar amino acid side chains

Outside — Amino terminus

Inside

Carboxyl terminus

Example, bacteriorhodopsin

Peripheral membrane proteins — Are loosely associated with the membrane through electrostatic interactions and hydrogen bond with integral proteins or with the polar head groups of membrane lipids

Lipid-anchored membrane proteins — Are covalently linked to a lipid anchor in the bilayer

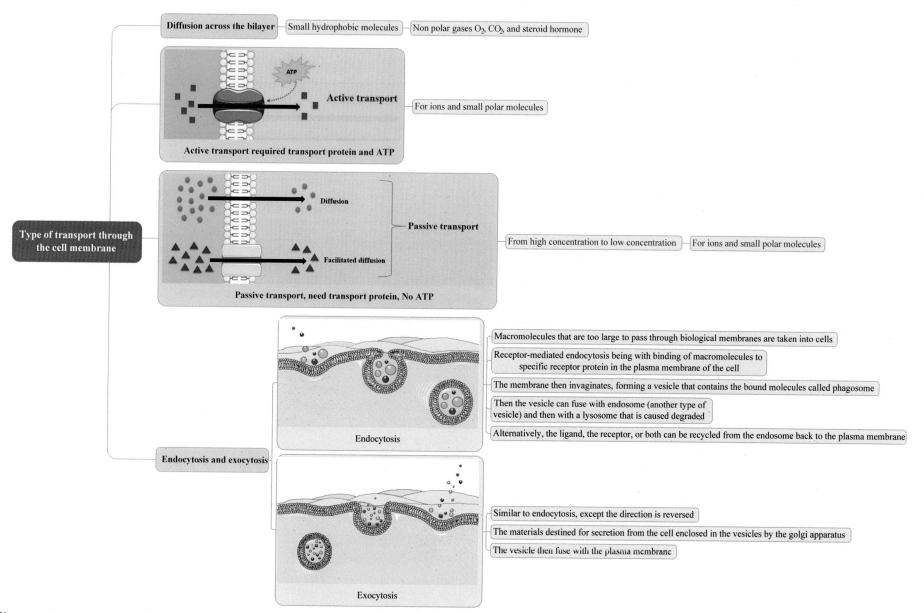

Diffusion across the bilayer — Small hydrophobic molecules — Non polar gases O_2, CO_2, and steroid hormone

Active transport

Active transport required transport protein and ATP

For ions and small polar molecules

Diffusion

Passive transport

Facilitated diffusion

Passive transport, need transport protein, No ATP

From high concentration to low concentration — For ions and small polar molecules

Type of transport through the cell membrane

Endocytosis and exocytosis

Endocytosis

Macromolecules that are too large to pass through biological membranes are taken into cells

Receptor-mediated endocytosis being with binding of macromolecules to specific receptor protein in the plasma membrane of the cell

The membrane then invaginates, forming a vesicle that contains the bound molecules called phagosome

Then the vesicle can fuse with endosome (another type of vesicle) and then with a lysosome that is caused degraded

Alternatively, the ligand, the receptor, or both can be recycled from the endosome back to the plasma membrane

Exocytosis

Similar to endocytosis, except the direction is reversed

The materials destined for secretion from the cell enclosed in the vesicles by the golgi apparatus

The vesicle then fuse with the plasma membrane

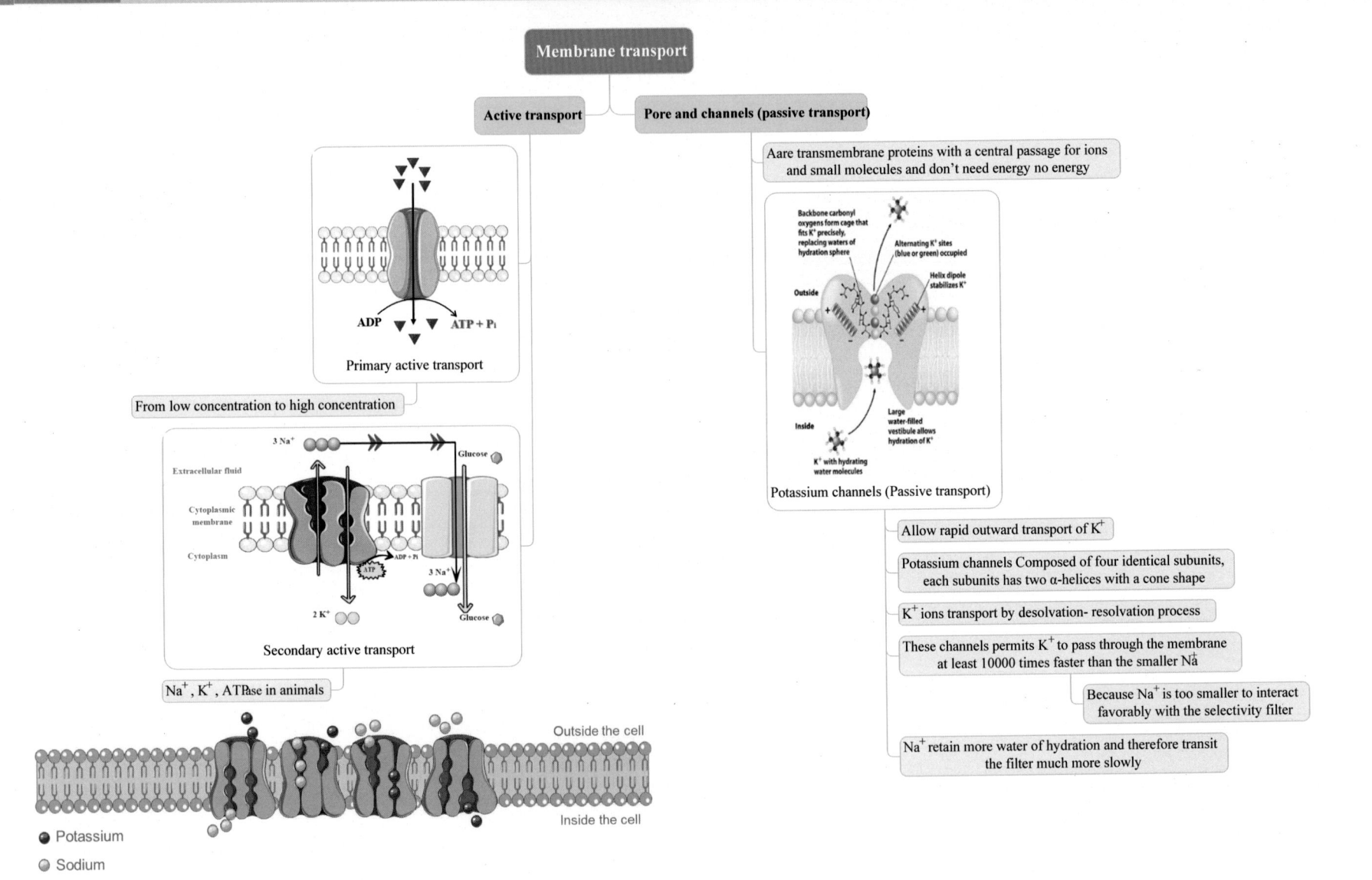

Membrane transport

Active transport

Primary active transport

From low concentration to high concentration

Secondary active transport

Na$^+$, K$^+$, ATPase in animals

- Potassium
- Sodium

Outside the cell

Inside the cell

Pore and channels (passive transport)

Aare transmembrane proteins with a central passage for ions and small molecules and don't need energy no energy

Potassium channels (Passive transport)

Allow rapid outward transport of K$^+$

Potassium channels Composed of four identical subunits, each subunits has two α-helices with a cone shape

K$^+$ ions transport by desolvation- resolvation process

These channels permits K$^+$ to pass through the membrane at least 10000 times faster than the smaller Na$^+$

Because Na$^+$ is too smaller to interact favorably with the selectivity filter

Na$^+$ retain more water of hydration and therefore transit the filter much more slowly

15.9.Drug-Receptor Theories

Example of intracellular receptors

IP$_3$ binds to a specific intracellular receptor calcium channel on the endoplasmic reticulum, releasing sequestered Ca^{+2}

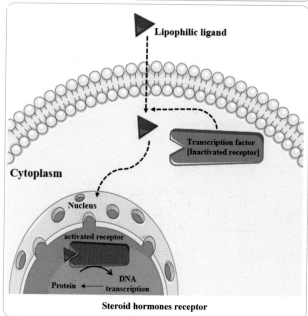

Lipophilic ligand

Transcription factor [Inactivated receptor]

Cytoplasm

Nucleus

activated receptor

Protein ← DNA transcription

Steroid hormones receptor

Lipophilic or hydrophobic ligands (steroid hormones) enter the cells by diffusion and bind to a receptor in cytoplasm or nucleus

The activator receptor complex regulates transcription and protein synthesis

Transduction of extracellular signals

The plasma membrane of all cells contain specific receptor allowing the cell to respond to external chemical stimuli that cannot cross membrane

Chemotaxis

Chemical signal via cell surface receptor to the flagella in bacteria causing the bacterium swim toward food or away from toxic chemicals

Hormones

Molecules that allow cells in one part of an organisms to communicate with cells in another part of the same organism

Neurotransmitters

Substances that transmit nerve messages at synapses

Growth factor

Proteins that regulate cell proliferation

General mechanism for signal transduction

A ligand binds to its specific receptor on the surface of the target cell

This generates a signal passed through a membrane protein transducer to a membrane bound effector enzyme

The action of the effector enzyme generates an intracellular second messenger which may be nuclear effectors and cellular response

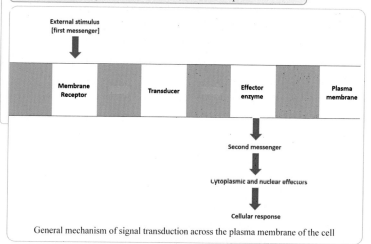

External stimulus [first messenger]

| Membrane Receptor | | Transducer | | Effector enzyme | | Plasma membrane |

Second messenger

Cytoplasmic and nuclear effectors

Cellular response

General mechanism of signal transduction across the plasma membrane of the cell

Cell-surface (extracellular) receptors: G-Protein as signal transducers:
1.The adenylyl cyclase signaling pathway
2.The Inositol-Phospholipid Signaling Pathway

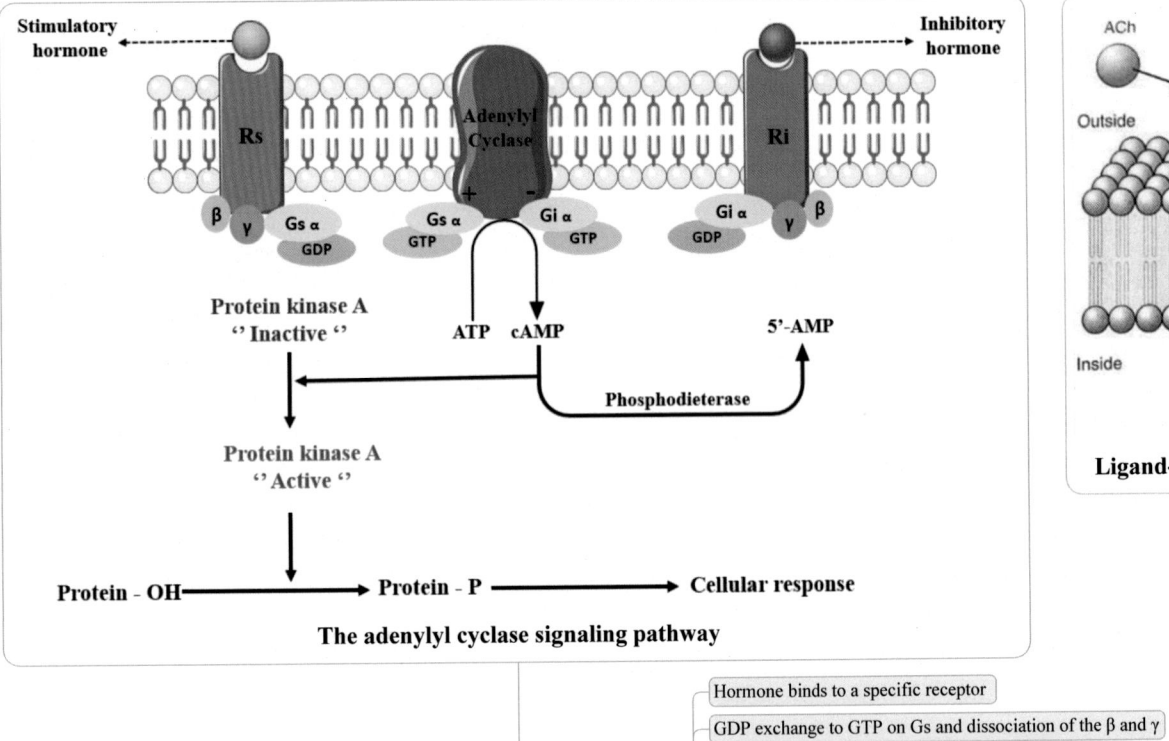

The adenylyl cyclase signaling pathway

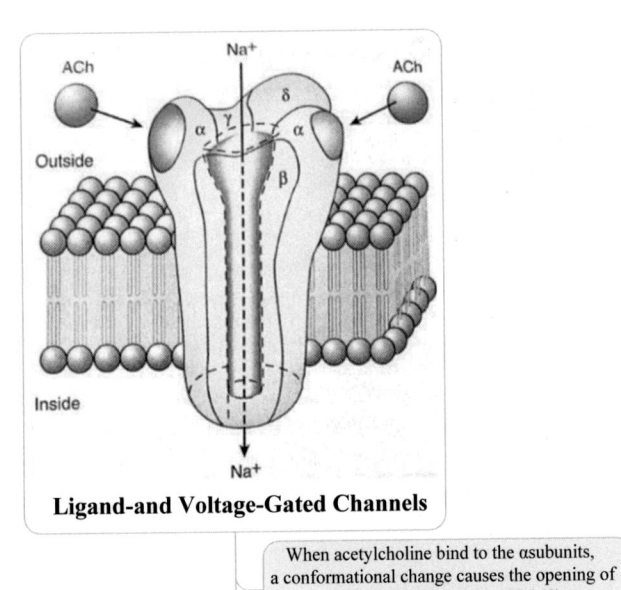

Ligand-and Voltage-Gated Channels

When acetylcholine bind to the αsubunits, a conformational change causes the opening of the ion in the nicotinic acetylcholine receptor (nAChR) also called ionotropc receptor

Which allows Na⁺ to follow downs its concentration gradients into cells, producing a localized excitatory postsynaptic potential a depolarization

Involved in fast synaptic transmission

Mechanism
- Hormone binds to a specific receptor
- GDP exchange to GTP on Gs and dissociation of the β and γ
- (GSα and GTP), moves to adenylyl cyclase (effector enzyme) and activates it
- Adenylyl cyclase cleaves ATP to cAMP and PPi
- cAMP (second messenger) activate protein kinase A at the cytosol
- Phosphorylation of cellular proteins to get cellular responses to the hormone

Regulation of The adenylyl cyclase signaling pathway
- Hormone that bind to inhibitory G protein (Gi) inhibit adenylyl cyclase activity
- cAMP concentration in the cytosol increases
  - cAMP phosphodieterase catalyzes the hydrolysis of cAMP to 5`AMP
- GTPase convert GTP to GDP, results inhibit adenylyl cyclase activity

Cell-surface (extracellular) receptors:

G-Protein as signal transducers:

1. The adenylyl cyclase signaling pathway

2. The Inositol-Phospholipid Signaling Pathway

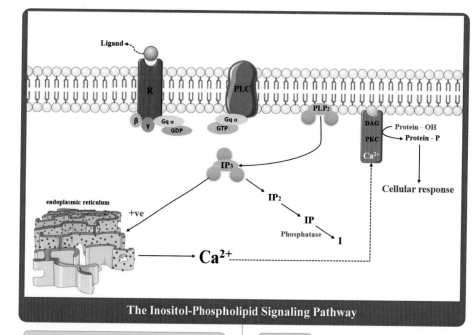

The Inositol-Phospholipid Signaling Pathway

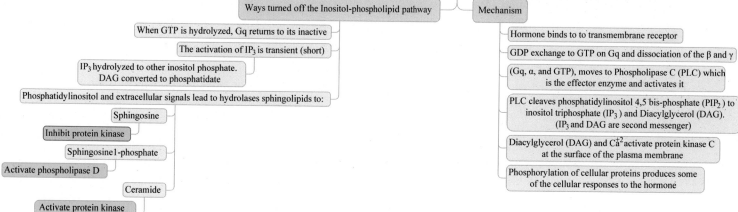

Ways turned off the Inositol-phospholipid pathway

When GTP is hydrolyzed, Gq returns to its inactive

The activation of IP$_3$ is transient (short)

IP$_3$ hydrolyzed to other inositol phosphate.
DAG converted to phosphatidate

Phosphatidylinositol and extracellular signals lead to hydrolases sphingolipids to:

Sphingosine

Inhibit protein kinase

Sphingosine1-phosphate

Activate phospholipase D

Ceramide

Activate protein kinase
and protein phosphatase

Mechanism

Hormone binds to to transmembrane receptor

GDP exchange to GTP on Gq and dissociation of the β and γ

(Gq, α, and GTP), moves to Phospholipase C (PLC) which
is the effector enzyme and activates it

PLC cleaves phosphatidylinositol 4,5 bis-phosphate (PIP$_2$) to
inositol triphosphate (IP$_3$) and Diacylglycerol (DAG).
(IP$_3$ and DAG are second messenger)

Diacylglycerol (DAG) and Ca^{+2} activate protein kinase C
at the surface of the plasma membrane

Phosphorylation of cellular proteins produces some
of the cellular responses to the hormone

Lipids and membrane : Exercises

Q 1: Circle the best correct answer:

1.Which of the following compound is responsible for cell surface recognition such as ABO blood group system?
a.Peripheral protein
b.Gangliosides
c.Ceramide
d.Integral protein

2.Which of the following statement about Lipid bilayer cell membrane is false?
a. Triacylglycerol is a major component of cell membrane.
b. stabilize by hydrophobic interaction
c. Consist of two sheet
d. flexible self-seal

3.In humans, a dietary essential fatty acid is:
a. Palmitic acid
b. Stearic acid
c. Oleic acid
d. Linoleic acid

4.Which one of the following is not a sphingolipids?
a. Ceramide
b. Plasmalogen
c. Cerebrosides
d. Gangliosides

5.Cerebrosides are a combination of:
a. Ceramide with galactose
b. Glycerol with galactose
c. Sphingosine with galactose
d. phospholipids with vinyl ether link

6.Ceramide is precursor for all of the following except:
a. Plasmalogens
b. Cerebrosides
c. Gangliosides
d. Sphingolipids

7.An enzyme which brings about lysis of bacterial cell wall by cleavage the glyosidic bond is:
a. Elastase
b. Lysozyme
c. Trypsin
d. Phospholipase A1

8.The function of Eicosanoids and Prostaglandins is:
a. storage fatty acids in human.
b. waterproof coating
c. Forming blood clot
d. Consist of cell membrane

9.Which of the following is not a fat-soluble vitamin?
a. A
b. C
c. D
d. E and K

10.The enzyme that is catalyze the hydrolysis of phospholipids and produce diacylglycerol is.
a. Phospholipase C
b. Phospholipase D
c. Phospholipase A1
d. Phospholipase A2

11.Fatty acids are generally stored as:
a. Plasmalogens
b. Phosphatidylserine
c. Triacylglycerol
d. Sphingomyelins

Lipids and membrane : Exercises

Q 1: Circle the best correct answer:

12. The enzyme that is included in venom and catalyze the hydrolysis of phospholipids and produce fatty acids is:
a. Phospholipase A1
b. Phospholipase A2
c. Phospholipase C
d. Phospholipase D

13. Movement of lipids in cell membrane from one face of the bilayer to the other is:
a. Lateral diffusion
b. Transverse diffusion or flip-flop
c. Uniport
d. Symport

14. Which of the following proteins is considered a transporter protein (channel)?
a. Integral membrane proteins.
b. Peripheral membrane proteins.
c. Lipid-anchored membrane proteins.
d. all of above

15. Which of the following statements about passive transport is true?
a. K^+ channel is example of active transport
b. need ATP
c. Transport from high concentration to low concentration
d. $Na^+ K^+$ ATPase is an example of passive transport

16. Which of the following statements about Tyrosine kinase receptors is true?
a. Autophosphorylation of tyrosine in IRSs
b. PLC is the effector enzyme
c. cAMP is a second messenger
d. Phospholipase C is the effector enzyme

17. The second messenger of Inositol-Phospholipid Signaling Pathway are:
a. Ca^{2+}
b. IP_3
c. Diacylglycerol (DAG)
d. all of these

18. Steroid hormones enter into the cells by:
a. Through the transport proteins
b. diffuse across the bilayer
c. Endocytosis
d. Pinocytosis

19. Which of the following is an example of G Protein receptor?
a. Receptor Tyrosine kinases
b. Ligand-and Voltage-Gated Channels
c. The Inositol-Phospholipid Signaling Pathway
d. Steroid hormones receptor

20. The adenylyl cyclase & Inositol-Phospholipid Signaling Pathway that is an example of a ...... signal transduction system:
a. Ligand-gated ion channel
b. G protein
c. receptor-enzyme
d. voltage-gated

21. Intracellular receptor Lipophilic or hydrophobic ligands (steroid hormones) enter the cells by:
a. Through the transport proteins
b. diffuse across the bilayer
c. Endocytosis
d. Pinocytosis

22. Protein associated with cell membranes by covalent bond called:
a. Integral membrane proteins
b. Peripheral membrane proteins
c. Lipid-anchored membrane proteins
d. all of these

Lipids and membrane : Exercises

Q 1: Circle the best correct answer:

23.The transducer of Inositol-Phospholipid signaling pathway is:
a. GTP-Gqα
b. Phospholipase C (PLC)
c. Phosphokinase C (PKC)
d. Calcium Channel

24.Which of the following statements about the adenylyl cyclase signaling pathway is false?
a. The adenylyl cyclase formation of cAMP from ATP
b. cAMP is a second messenger
c. Protein kinase A activated by cAMP
d. Gγ and β subunit activate adenylyl cyclase

25.Plasmalogens may also be classified as:
a. Sphingolipids
b. Sulpholipids
c. Glycerophospholipids
d. Glycolipids

Q 2. Circle the fatty acid in each pair that has the higher melting point :

a. 18:2 and 18:3
b. 16:0 and 18:0

Q 3. Write short note on:

1.Types of lipids in cell membrane.
2.Types of protein in cell membrane.
3.Types of transportation through the cell membrane.
4.The major function of triacylglycerol.
5.The functions of cholesterol in the cell membrane of mammals cells.
6.Explain. Phospholipase A_1, Phospholipase A_2, and Phospholipase C cause hemolysis in RBCs.
7.Inositol-Phospholipid signaling.
8.Adenylyl cyclase signaling pathway.
9.Insulin tyrosine kinase receptor.

Chapter 15 : Lipid Metabolism

Lipids play an important role in cell structure and metabolism. TAGs are the major storage form of energy. Cholesterol is a component of cell membranes and precursor of steroid hormones. Lipid digestion occurs at lipid water interfaces since TAG is insoluble in water and digestive enzymes are water soluble. Lipids are digested and absorbed with the help of bile salts. Products of lipid digestion aggregate to form mixed micelles and are absorbed into the small intestine. Lipids are transported in the form of lipoproteins.

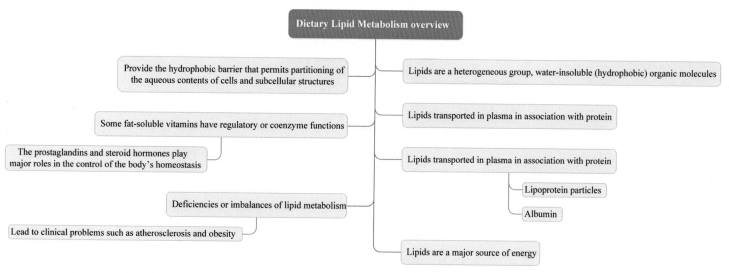

15.10. Digestion, Absorption, Secretion, and Utilization of Dietary Lipids

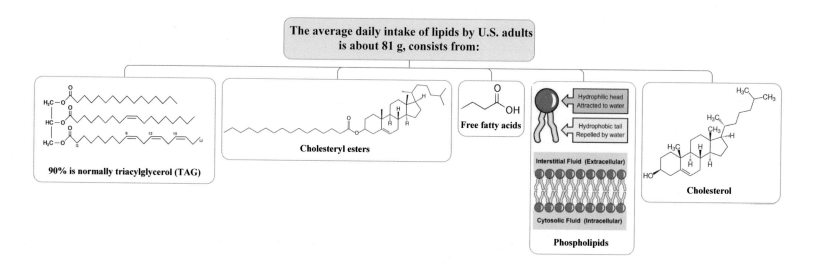

15.10.Digestion, Absorption, Secretion, and Utilization of Dietary Lipids

Processing of dietary lipid in the stomach

| The digestion of lipids begins in the stomach | Triacylglycerols (TAGs) from milk contain short- to medium-chain length fatty acids | That degraded in the stomach by two acid lipases: These are acid stable (pH 4-6) and important in neonates for milk fat digestion |

Lingual lipase   Gastric lipase

Cystic Fibrosis disease (CF)

Mutation in transmembrane conductance regulator (CFTR) protein

In pancreas cause thickened secretion that clog the pancreatic ducts

Function as chloride channel on epithelium

Defective CFTR results in decreased secretion of chloride and increased reabsorption of sodium and water

Emulsification of dietary lipid in the small intestine

Emulsification of dietary lipids occurs in the duodenum

Emulsification increases the surface area of the hydrophobic lipid droplets

The dietary lipids are emulsified in the small intestine via using

Mechanical peristaltic action   Bile salts as detergent

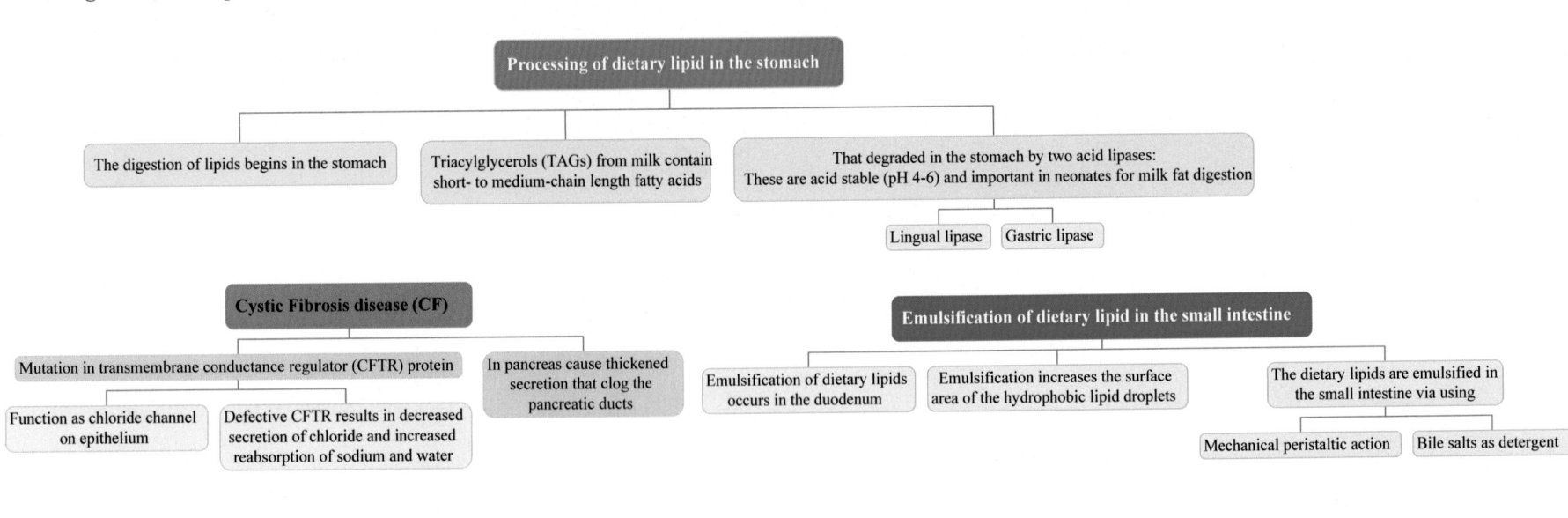

Removes the fatty acids at carbons 1 and 3 from TAG, forming fatty acid and 2-Monoacylglycerol

Consist 2%-3% of pancreatic secretion and colipase

Pancreatic secrete different enzymes

- Cholesteryl ester hydrolase (cholesterol esterase)
- Phospholipase A2
- Lysophospholipase
- Pancreatic lipase
- Colipase
  - restores activity to lipase in the presence of inhibitory substances like bile acids that bind the micelles
  - activated in the intestine by trypsin
  - Colipase binds the lipase at a ratio of 1:1, at the lipid-aqueous interface

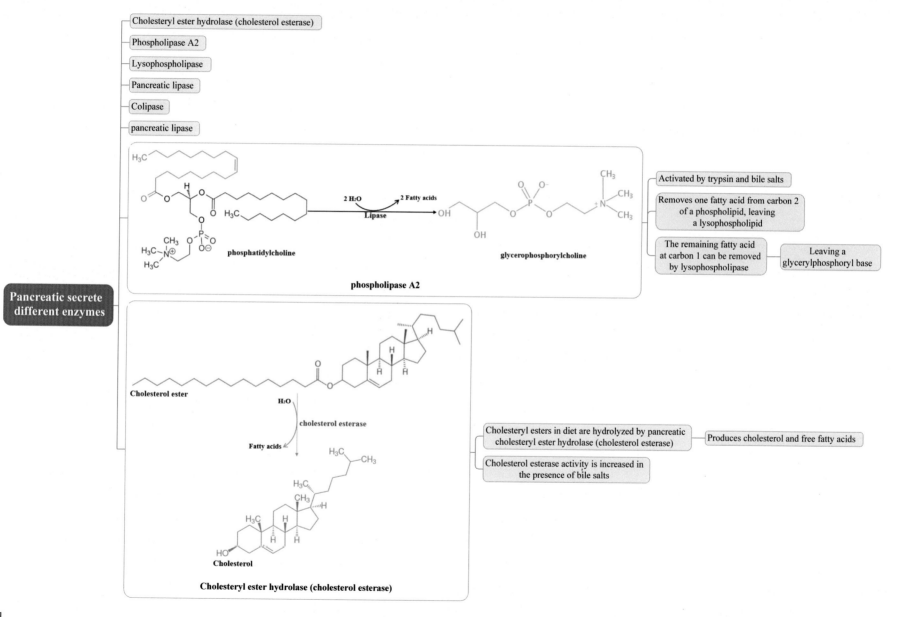

Cholesteryl ester hydrolase (cholesterol esterase)

Phospholipase A2

Lysophospholipase

Pancreatic lipase

Colipase

pancreatic lipase

Pancreatic secrete different enzymes

phosphatidylcholine

2 H₂O

2 Fatty acids

Lipase

glycerophosphorylcholine

phospholipase A2

Activated by trypsin and bile salts

Removes one fatty acid from carbon 2 of a phospholipid, leaving a lysophospholipid

The remaining fatty acid at carbon 1 can be removed by lysophospholipase

Leaving a glycerylphosphoryl base

Cholesterol ester

H₂O

cholesterol esterase

Fatty acids

Cholesterol

Cholesteryl ester hydrolase (cholesterol esterase)

Cholesteryl esters in diet are hydrolyzed by pancreatic cholesteryl ester hydrolase (cholesterol esterase)

Produces cholesterol and free fatty acids

Cholesterol esterase activity is increased in the presence of bile salts

Control of lipid digestion by two hormones

Cholecystokinin (CCK) — The effect of CCK
- Gallbladder release bile salts
- Exocrine cells of the pancreas (release digestive enzymes)
- Decrease gastric motility and contents

Secretin
- Released in low pH, causes:
  - Pancreas and liver release a solution rich in bicarbonate
    - Helps neutralize the pH of the intestinal contents

Absorption of lipids by intestinal mucosal cells (enterocytes)

mixed micelles
- facilitate the absorption of dietary lipids by intestinal mucosal cells (enterocytes)
- Consist from
  - 2-monoacylglycerol
  - cholesterol
  - free fatty acid
  - fat-soluble vitamins (A,D,E & K)

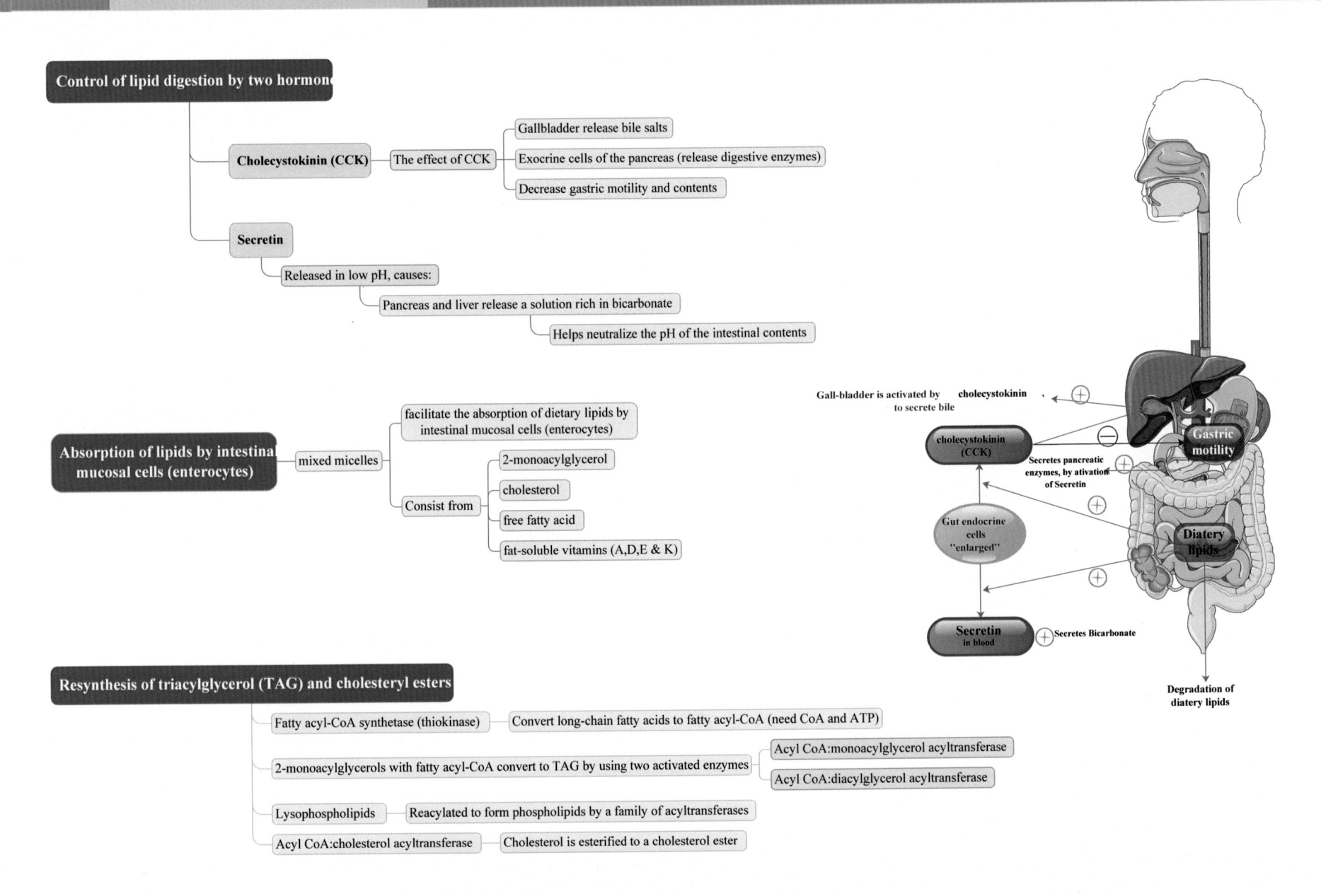

Gall-bladder is activated by cholecystokinin to secrete bile

cholecystokinin (CCK)

Secretes pancreatic enzymes, by ativation of Secretin

Gut endocrine cells "enlarged"

Gastric motility

Diatery lipids

Secretin in blood — Secretes Bicarbonate

Degradation of diatery lipids

Resynthesis of triacylglycerol (TAG) and cholesteryl esters

- Fatty acyl-CoA synthetase (thiokinase) — Convert long-chain fatty acids to fatty acyl-CoA (need CoA and ATP)
- 2-monoacylglycerols with fatty acyl-CoA convert to TAG by using two activated enzymes
  - Acyl CoA:monoacylglycerol acyltransferase
  - Acyl CoA:diacylglycerol acyltransferase
- Lysophospholipids — Reacylated to form phospholipids by a family of acyltransferases
- Acyl CoA:cholesterol acyltransferase — Cholesterol is esterified to a cholesterol ester

15.11.Fatty Acid, Ketone Body, and Triacylglycerol Metabolism

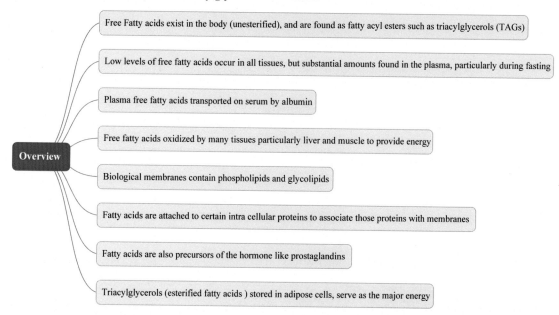

Overview
- Free Fatty acids exist in the body (unesterified), and are found as fatty acyl esters such as triacylglycerols (TAGs)
- Low levels of free fatty acids occur in all tissues, but substantial amounts found in the plasma, particularly during fasting
- Plasma free fatty acids transported on serum by albumin
- Free fatty acids oxidized by many tissues particularly liver and muscle to provide energy
- Biological membranes contain phospholipids and glycolipids
- Fatty acids are attached to certain intra cellular proteins to associate those proteins with membranes
- Fatty acids are also precursors of the hormone like prostaglandins
- Triacylglycerols (esterified fatty acids) stored in adipose cells, serve as the major energy

Essential fatty acid refers to fatty acids required for biological processes but does not include the fats that only act as fuel. Essential fatty acids should not be confused with essential oils, which are "essential" in the sense of being a concentrated essence. Only two fatty acids are known to be essential for humans: alpha-linolenic acid (an omega-3 fatty acid) and linoleic acid (an omega-6 fatty acid). Some other fatty acids are sometimes classified as "conditionally essential", meaning that they can become essential under some developmental or disease conditions; examples include docosahexaenoic acid (an omega-3 fatty acid) and gamma-linolenic acid (an omega-6 fatty acid).

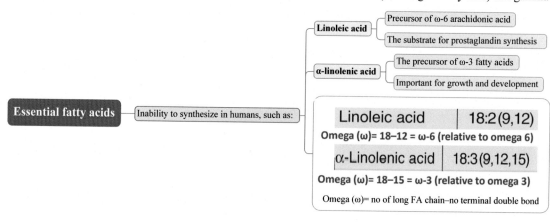

Essential fatty acids — Inability to synthesize in humans, such as:

- **Linoleic acid**
  - Precursor of ω-6 arachidonic acid
  - The substrate for prostaglandin synthesis
- **α-linolenic acid**
  - The precursor of ω-3 fatty acids
  - Important for growth and development

Linoleic acid	18:2 (9,12)

Omega (ω)= 18–12 = ω-6 (relative to omega 6)

α-Linolenic acid	18:3 (9,12,15)

Omega (ω)= 18–15 = ω-3 (relative to omega 3)

Omega (ω)= no of long FA chain–no terminal double bond

Saturation of fatty Acid a fatty acid in which all of the carbon atoms in the hydrocarbon chain are joined by single bonds. They exist mostly as components of fats (triglycerides) or other lipids of animal origin. Foods rich in saturated fatty acids include beef, lamb, pork, veal, whole-milk products, butter, most cheeses, and a few plant products such as cocoa butter, coconut oil, and palm oil. Ordinary oleomargarine and hydrogenated shortenings also contain saturated fatty acids. A diet high in saturated fatty acids may contribute to a high serum cholesterol level and appears to be associated with an increased incidence of coronary heart disease in some populations.

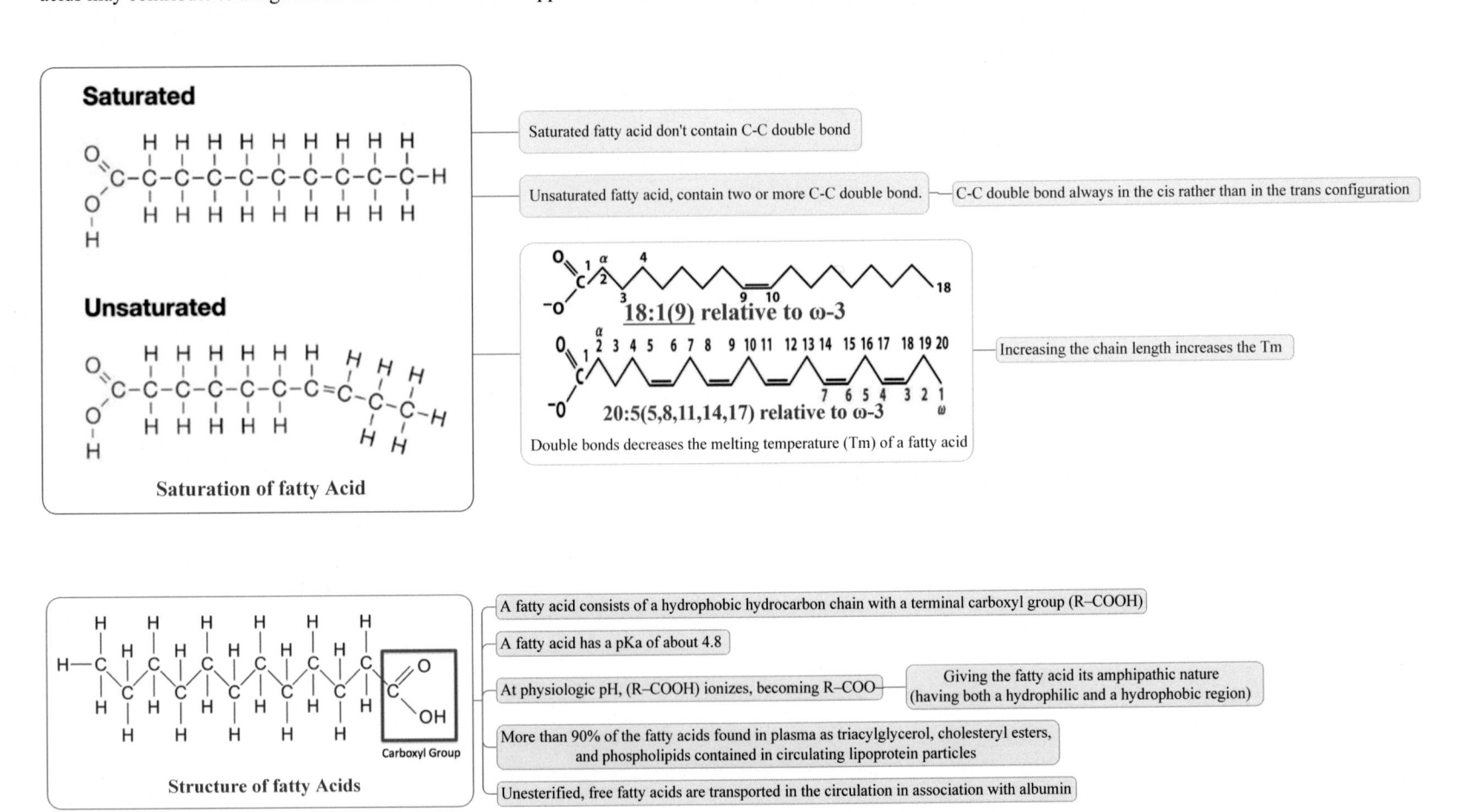

Saturated

Unsaturated

Saturation of fatty Acid

Saturated fatty acid don't contain C-C double bond

Unsaturated fatty acid, contain two or more C-C double bond. — C-C double bond always in the cis rather than in the trans configuration

18:1(9) relative to ω-3

20:5(5,8,11,14,17) relative to ω-3

Double bonds decreases the melting temperature (Tm) of a fatty acid

Increasing the chain length increases the Tm

Structure of fatty Acids

Carboxyl Group

A fatty acid consists of a hydrophobic hydrocarbon chain with a terminal carboxyl group (R–COOH)

A fatty acid has a pKa of about 4.8

At physiologic pH, (R–COOH) ionizes, becoming R–COO — Giving the fatty acid its amphipathic nature (having both a hydrophilic and a hydrophobic region)

More than 90% of the fatty acids found in plasma as triacylglycerol, cholesteryl esters, and phospholipids contained in circulating lipoprotein particles

Unesterified, free fatty acids are transported in the circulation in association with albumin

15.12.De novo synthesis of Fatty Acids : fatty acids stored as triacylglycerols.fatty acid synthesis occurs in cytosol of liver and lactating mammary glands and, to a lesser extent, in adipose tissue

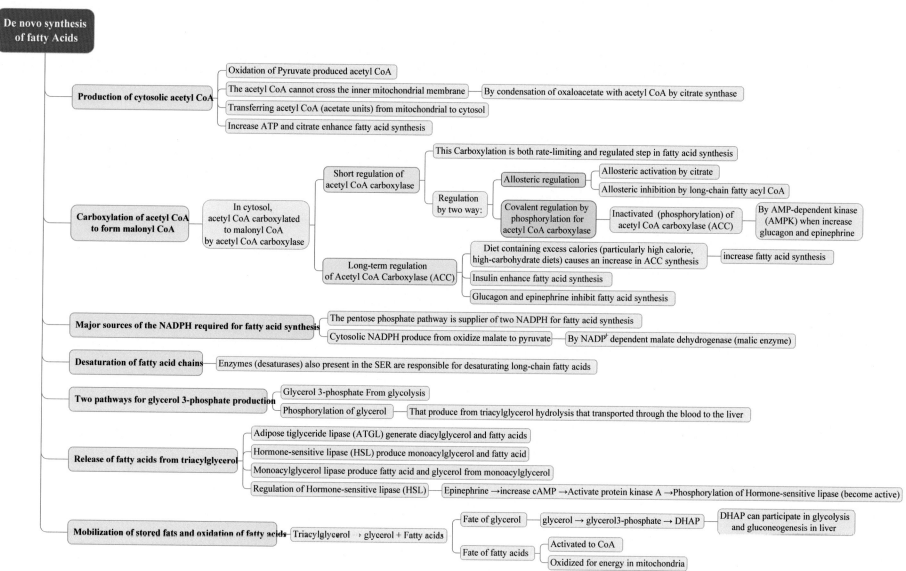

15.13.Fatty acid β-oxidation is a multistep process by which fatty acids are broken down by various tissues to produce energy. Fatty acids primarily enter a cell via fatty acid protein transporters on the cell surface

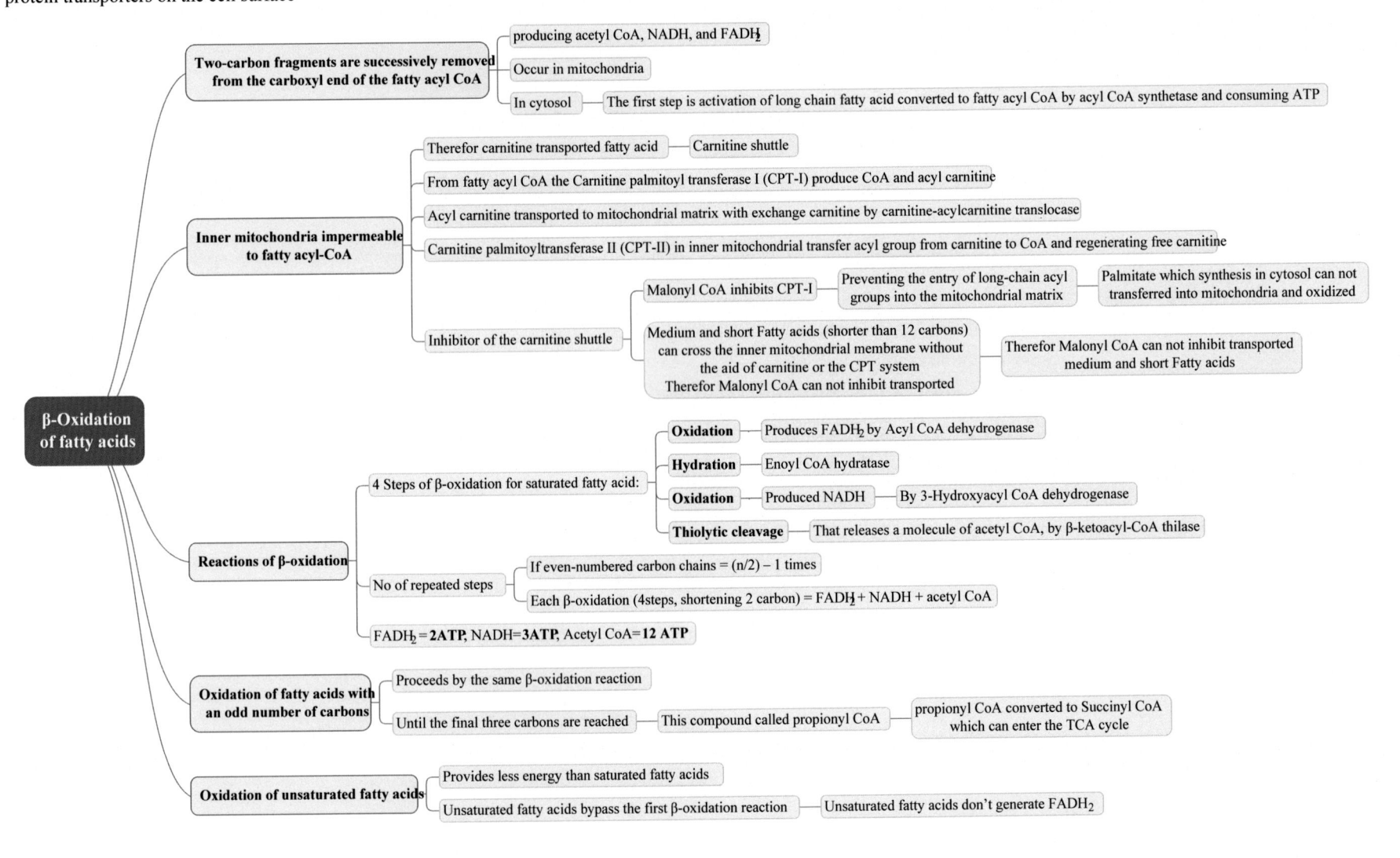

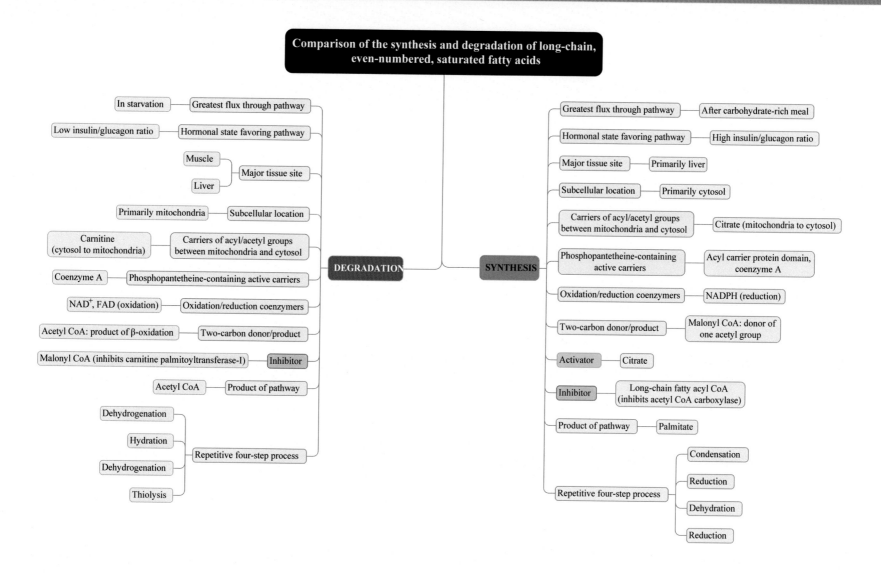

Comparison of the synthesis and degradation of long-chain, even-numbered, saturated fatty acids

DEGRADATION

In starvation	—	Greatest flux through pathway
Low insulin/glucagon ratio	—	Hormonal state favoring pathway
Muscle / Liver	—	Major tissue site
Primarily mitochondria	—	Subcellular location
Carnitine (cytosol to mitochondria)	—	Carriers of acyl/acetyl groups between mitochondria and cytosol
Coenzyme A	—	Phosphopantetheine-containing active carriers
NAD⁺, FAD (oxidation)	—	Oxidation/reduction coenzymers
Acetyl CoA: product of β-oxidation	—	Two-carbon donor/product
Malonyl CoA (inhibits carnitine palmitoyltransferase-I)	—	Inhibitor
Acetyl CoA	—	Product of pathway
Dehydrogenation / Hydration / Dehydrogenation / Thiolysis	—	Repetitive four-step process

SYNTHESIS

Greatest flux through pathway	—	After carbohydrate-rich meal
Hormonal state favoring pathway	—	High insulin/glucagon ratio
Major tissue site	—	Primarily liver
Subcellular location	—	Primarily cytosol
Carriers of acyl/acetyl groups between mitochondria and cytosol	—	Citrate (mitochondria to cytosol)
Phosphopantetheine-containing active carriers	—	Acyl carrier protein domain, coenzyme A
Oxidation/reduction coenzymers	—	NADPH (reduction)
Two-carbon donor/product	—	Malonyl CoA: donor of one acetyl group
Activator	—	Citrate
Inhibitor	—	Long-chain fatty acyl CoA (inhibits acetyl CoA carboxylase)
Product of pathway	—	Palmitate
Repetitive four-step process	—	Condensation / Reduction / Dehydration / Reduction

15.14.Eicosanoids: Prostaglandins and related compounds

Eicosanoid: A lipid mediator of inflammation derived from the 20-carbon atom arachidonic acid or a similar fatty acid. The eicosanoids include the prostaglandins, prostacyclin, thromboxane, and leukotrienes

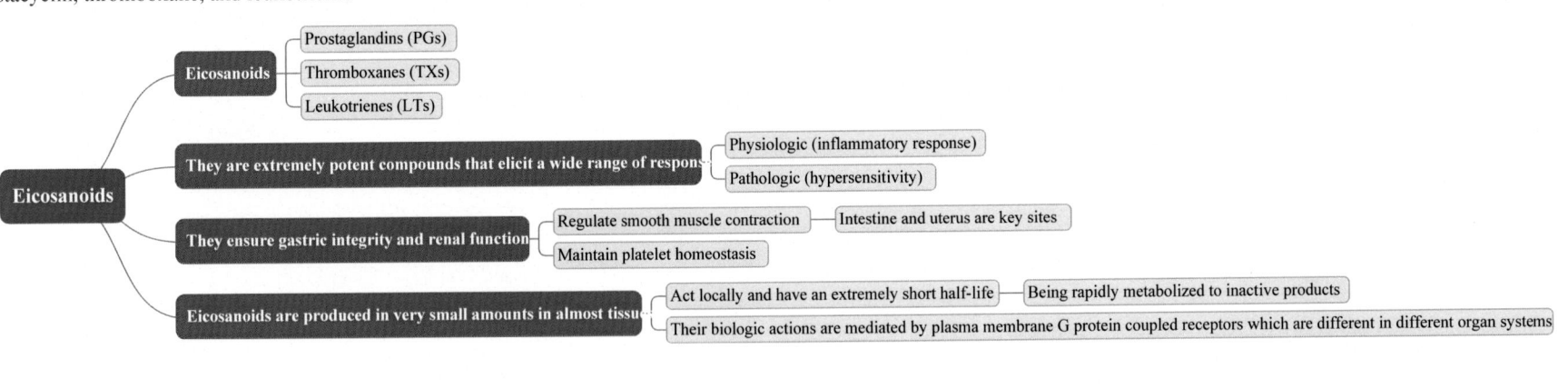

Eicosanoids

- Eicosanoids
  - Prostaglandins (PGs)
  - Thromboxanes (TXs)
  - Leukotrienes (LTs)
- They are extremely potent compounds that elicit a wide range of respons
  - Physiologic (inflammatory response)
  - Pathologic (hypersensitivity)
- They ensure gastric integrity and renal function
  - Regulate smooth muscle contraction — Intestine and uterus are key sites
  - Maintain platelet homeostasis
- Eicosanoids are produced in very small amounts in almost tissue
  - Act locally and have an extremely short half-life — Being rapidly metabolized to inactive products
  - Their biologic actions are mediated by plasma membrane G protein coupled receptors which are different in different organ systems

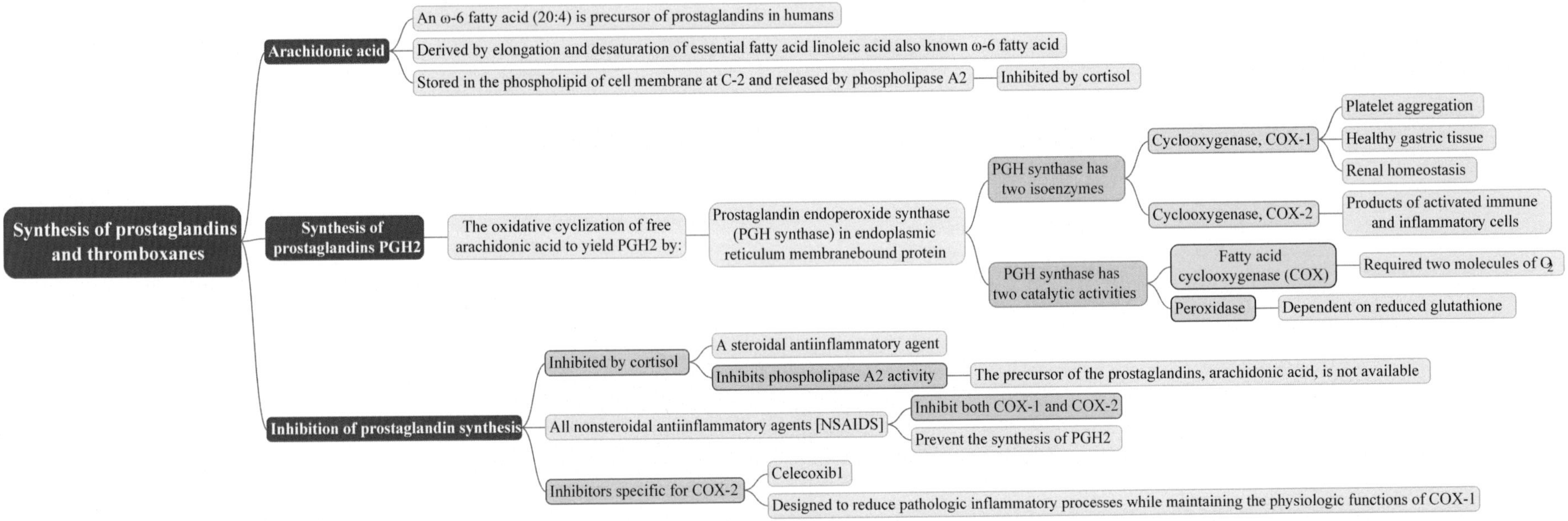

Synthesis of prostaglandins and thromboxanes

- Arachidonic acid
  - An ω-6 fatty acid (20:4) is precursor of prostaglandins in humans
  - Derived by elongation and desaturation of essential fatty acid linoleic acid also known ω-6 fatty acid
  - Stored in the phospholipid of cell membrane at C-2 and released by phospholipase A2 — Inhibited by cortisol
- Synthesis of prostaglandins PGH2
  - The oxidative cyclization of free arachidonic acid to yield PGH2 by:
    - Prostaglandin endoperoxide synthase (PGH synthase) in endoplasmic reticulum membranebound protein
      - PGH synthase has two isoenzymes
        - Cyclooxygenase, COX-1
          - Platelet aggregation
          - Healthy gastric tissue
          - Renal homeostasis
        - Cyclooxygenase, COX-2 — Products of activated immune and inflammatory cells
      - PGH synthase has two catalytic activities
        - Fatty acid cyclooxygenase (COX) — Required two molecules of O_2
        - Peroxidase — Dependent on reduced glutathione
- Inhibition of prostaglandin synthesis
  - Inhibited by cortisol
    - A steroidal antiinflammatory agent
    - Inhibits phospholipase A2 activity — The precursor of the prostaglandins, arachidonic acid, is not available
  - All nonsteroidal antiinflammatory agents [NSAIDS]
    - Inhibit both COX-1 and COX-2
    - Prevent the synthesis of PGH2
  - Inhibitors specific for COX-2
    - Celecoxib1
    - Designed to reduce pathologic inflammatory processes while maintaining the physiologic functions of COX-1

15.15.Ketone body metabolism

Ketone bodies are acetoacetate, β-hydroxy butyrate and acetone. Ketone bodies are synthesized in the liver but they are utilized by extra hepatic tissues as fuels. Ketone bodies are accumulated in the blood if the rate of synthesis exceeds the ability of extra hepatic tissues to utilize them. This leads to excess ketone bodies in blood, excretion of ketone bodies in urine and smell of acetone in breath. All these three together are known as ketosis. In uncontrolled diabetes mellitus and starvation, ketone bodies are formed

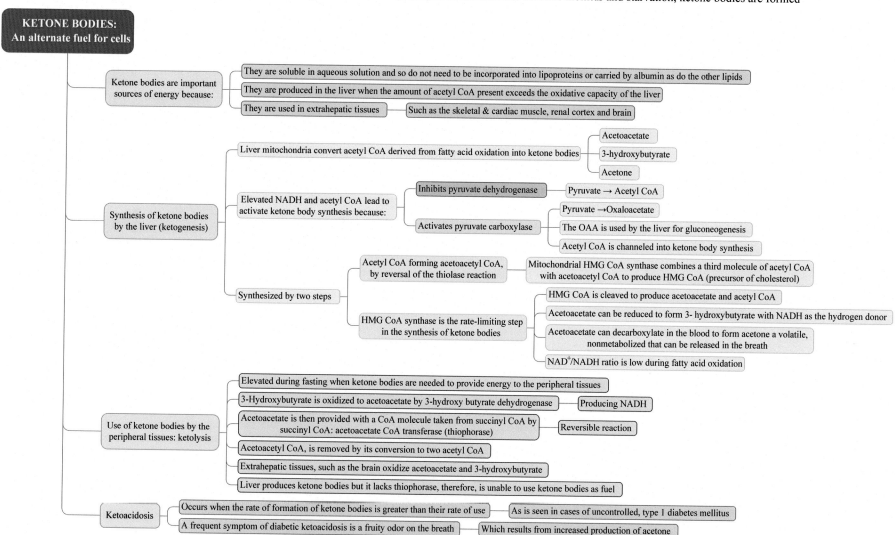

15.16.Cholesterol and steroids metabolism

Cholesterol, the characteristic steroid alcohol of animal tissues, performs a number of essential functions in the body. For example, cholesterol is a structural component of all cell membranes, modulating their fluidity, and, in specialized tissues, cholesterol is a precursor of bile acids, steroid hormones, and vitamin D. It is therefore of critical importance that the cells of the body be assured an appropriate supply of cholesterol. To meet this need, a complex series of transport, biosynthetic, and regulatory mechanisms has evolved. The liver plays a central role in the regulation of the body's cholesterol homeostasis. For example, cholesterol enters the liver's cholesterol pool from a number of sources including dietary cholesterol, as well as cholesterol synthesized de novo by extrahepatic tissues and by the liver itself. Cholesterol is eliminated from the liver as unmodified cholesterol in the bile, or it can be converted to bile salts that are secreted into the intestinal lumen. It can also serve as a component of plasma lipoproteins sent to the peripheral tissues. In humans, the balance between cholesterol influx and efflux is not precise, resulting in a gradual deposition of cholesterol in the tissues, particularly in the endothelial linings of blood vessels. This is a potentially life-threatening occurrence when the lipid deposition leads to plaque formation, causing the narrowing of blood vessels (atherosclerosis) and increased risk of cardio-, cerebro- and peripheral vascular disease.

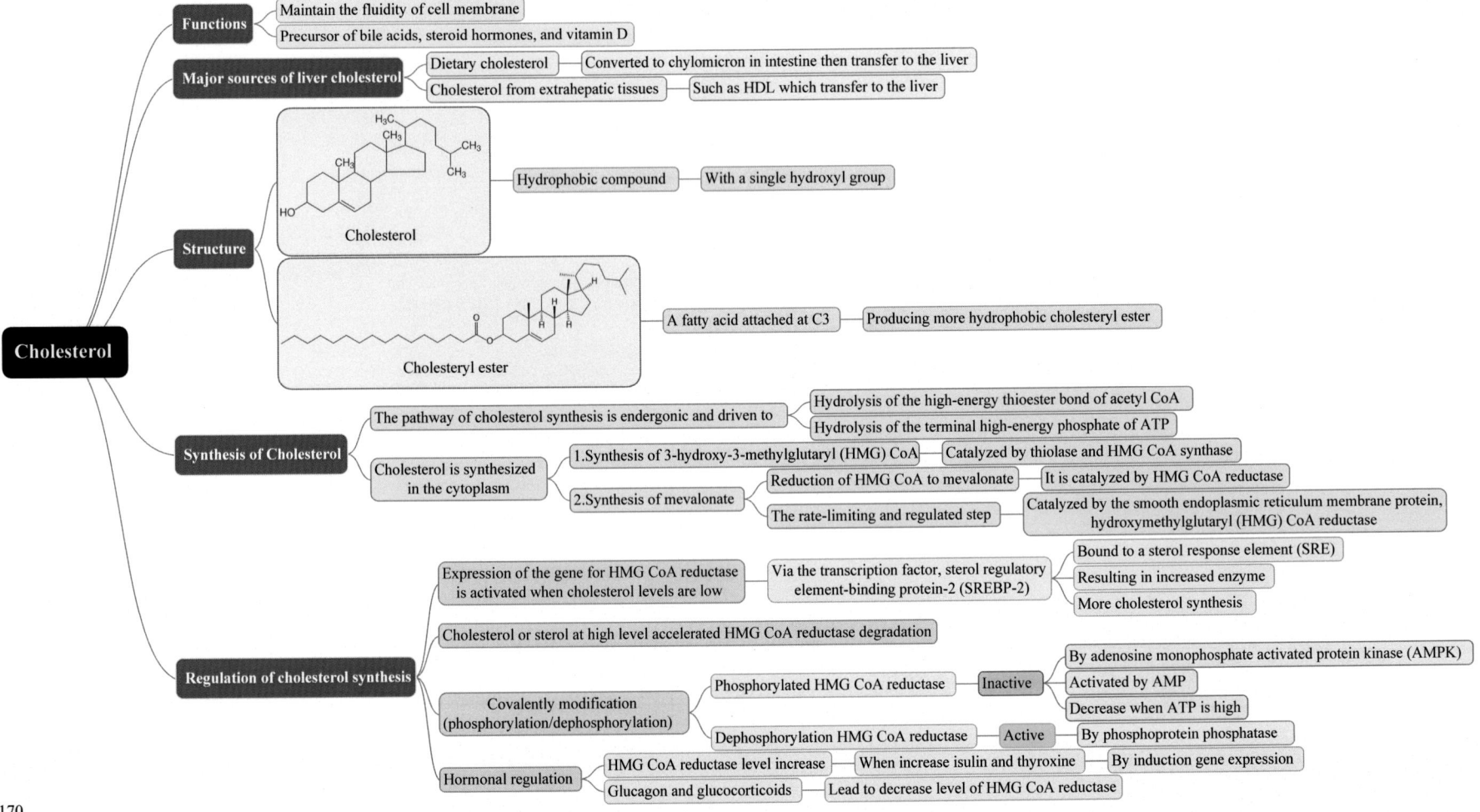

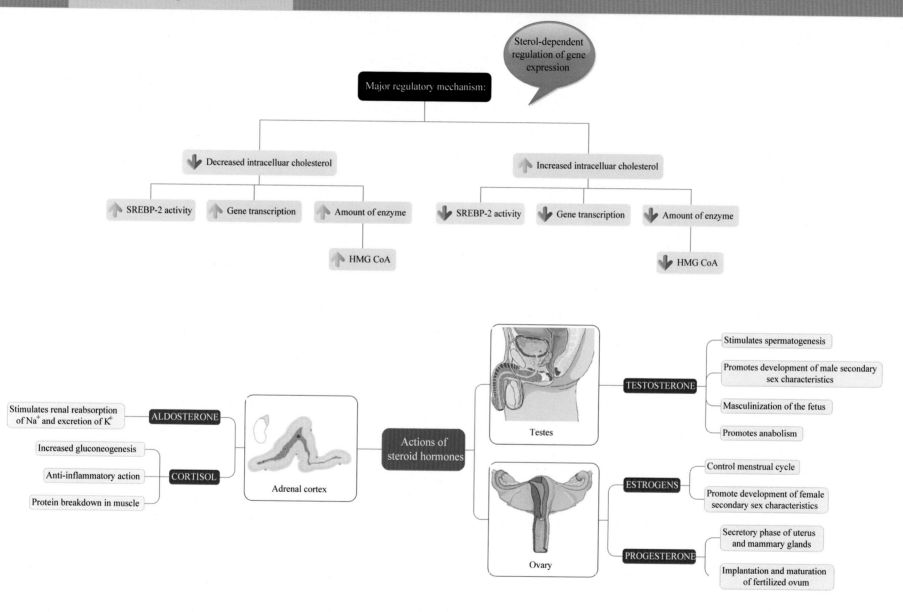

Sterol-dependent regulation of gene expression

Major regulatory mechanism:

↓ Decreased intracelluar cholesterol

↑ SREBP-2 activity ↑ Gene transcription ↑ Amount of enzyme

↑ HMG CoA

↑ Increased intracelluar cholesterol

↓ SREBP-2 activity ↓ Gene transcription ↓ Amount of enzyme

↓ HMG CoA

Stimulates renal reabsorption of Na⁺ and excretion of K⁺ — ALDOSTERONE

Increased gluconeogenesis
Anti-inflammatory action — CORTISOL
Protein breakdown in muscle

Adrenal cortex

Actions of steroid hormones

Testes — TESTOSTERONE
Stimulates spermatogenesis
Promotes development of male secondary sex characteristics
Masculinization of the fetus
Promotes anabolism

Ovary — ESTROGENS
Control menstrual cycle
Promote development of female secondary sex characteristics

PROGESTERONE
Secretory phase of uterus and mammary glands
Implantation and maturation of fertilized ovum

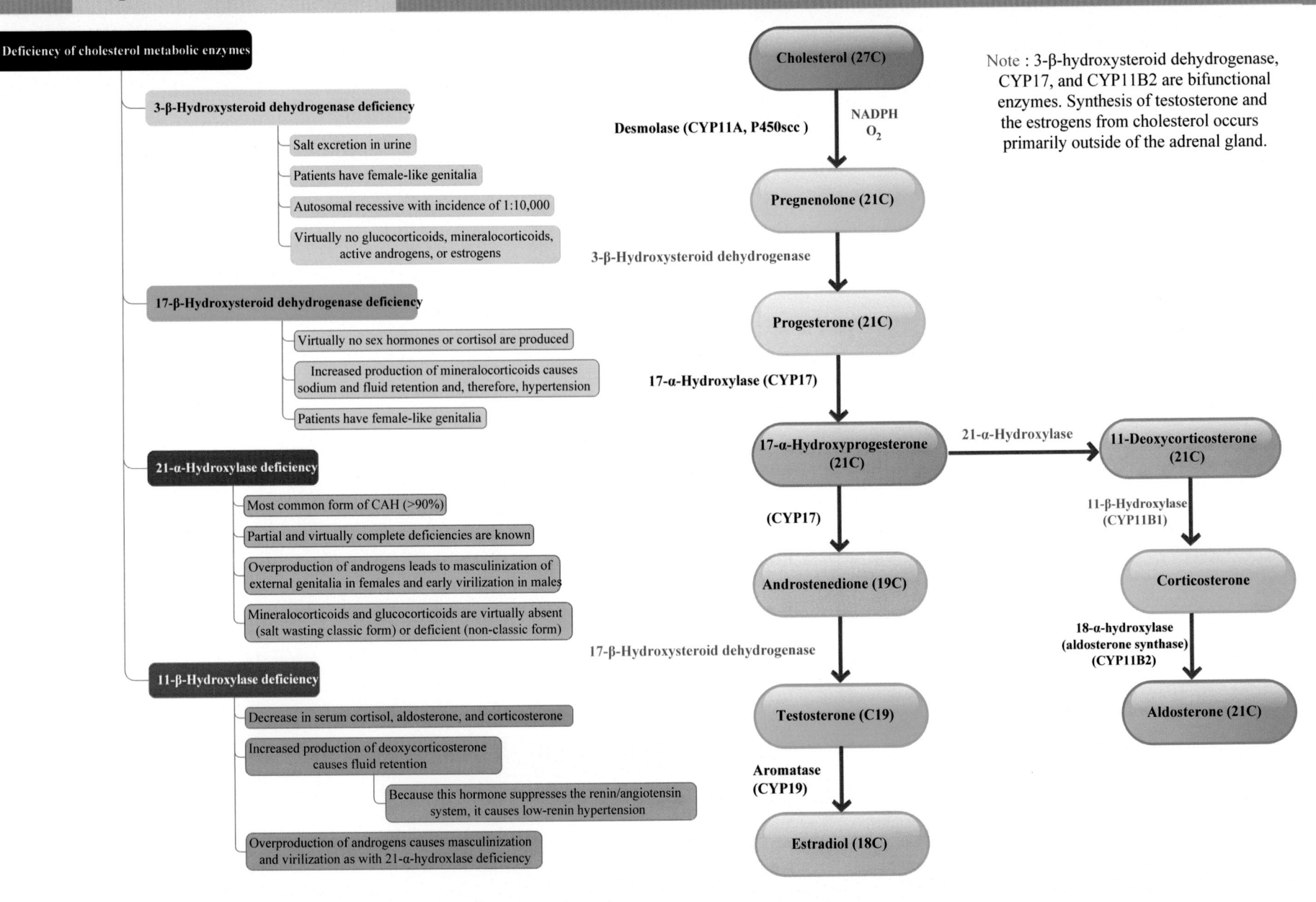

Deficiency of cholesterol metabolic enzymes

3-β-Hydroxysteroid dehydrogenase deficiency

- Salt excretion in urine
- Patients have female-like genitalia
- Autosomal recessive with incidence of 1:10,000
- Virtually no glucocorticoids, mineralocorticoids, active androgens, or estrogens

17-β-Hydroxysteroid dehydrogenase deficiency

- Virtually no sex hormones or cortisol are produced
- Increased production of mineralocorticoids causes sodium and fluid retention and, therefore, hypertension
- Patients have female-like genitalia

21-α-Hydroxylase deficiency

- Most common form of CAH (>90%)
- Partial and virtually complete deficiencies are known
- Overproduction of androgens leads to masculinization of external genitalia in females and early virilization in males
- Mineralocorticoids and glucocorticoids are virtually absent (salt wasting classic form) or deficient (non-classic form)

11-β-Hydroxylase deficiency

- Decrease in serum cortisol, aldosterone, and corticosterone
- Increased production of deoxycorticosterone causes fluid retention
- Because this hormone suppresses the renin/angiotensin system, it causes low-renin hypertension
- Overproduction of androgens causes masculinization and virilization as with 21-α-hydroxlase deficiency

Cholesterol (27C)

Desmolase (CYP11A, P450scc)   NADPH O₂

Pregnenolone (21C)

3-β-Hydroxysteroid dehydrogenase

Progesterone (21C)

17-α-Hydroxylase (CYP17)

17-α-Hydroxyprogesterone (21C)   →   21-α-Hydroxylase   →   **11-Deoxycorticosterone (21C)**

(CYP17)

11-β-Hydroxylase (CYP11B1)

Androstenedione (19C)

Corticosterone

17-β-Hydroxysteroid dehydrogenase

18-α-hydroxylase (aldosterone synthase) (CYP11B2)

Testosterone (C19)

Aromatase (CYP19)

Aldosterone (21C)

Estradiol (18C)

Note : 3-β-hydroxysteroid dehydrogenase, CYP17, and CYP11B2 are bifunctional enzymes. Synthesis of testosterone and the estrogens from cholesterol occurs primarily outside of the adrenal gland.

15.17.Lipoprotein : any member of a group of substances containing both lipid (fat) and protein. They occur in both soluble complexes as in egg yolk and mammalian blood plasma and insoluble ones, as in cell membranes. Lipoproteins in blood plasma have been intensively studied because they are the mode of transport for cholesterol through the bloodstream and lymphatic fluid.

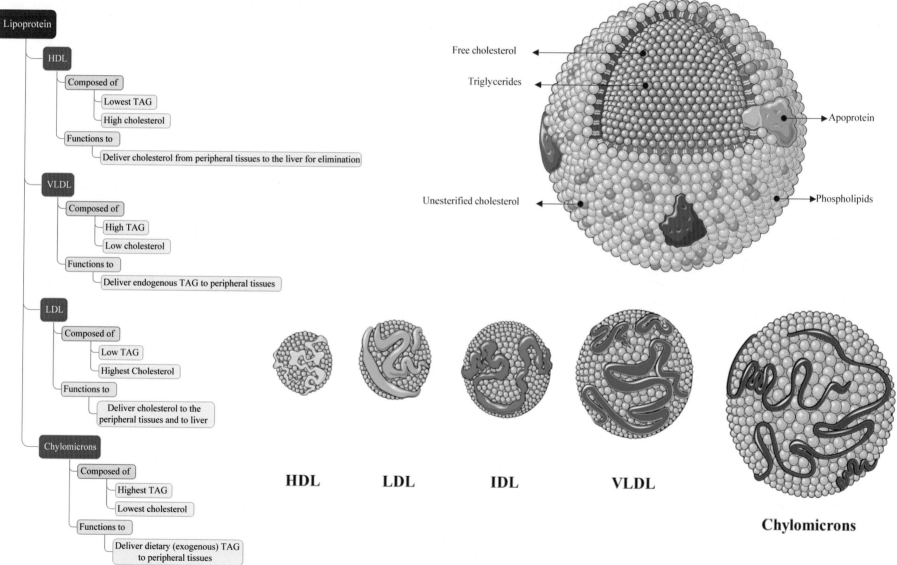

- Lipoprotein
  - HDL
    - Composed of
      - Lowest TAG
      - High cholesterol
    - Functions to
      - Deliver cholesterol from peripheral tissues to the liver for elimination
  - VLDL
    - Composed of
      - High TAG
      - Low cholesterol
    - Functions to
      - Deliver endogenous TAG to peripheral tissues
  - LDL
    - Composed of
      - Low TAG
      - Highest Cholesterol
    - Functions to
      - Deliver cholesterol to the peripheral tissues and to liver
  - Chylomicrons
    - Composed of
      - Highest TAG
      - Lowest cholesterol
    - Functions to
      - Deliver dietary (exogenous) TAG to peripheral tissues

Free cholesterol
Triglycerides
Apoprotein
Unesterified cholesterol
Phospholipids

HDL   **LDL**   **IDL**   **VLDL**

Chylomicrons

Q 1: Circle the best correct answer:

1.Which of the following is required as a reductant in fatty acid
synthesis?
a. NADH
b. NADPH
c. $FADH_2$
d. $FMNH_2$

2.The decarboxylation reaction in pentose phosphate pathway
(PPP) is catalyzed by:
a. Gluconolactone hydrolase
b. Glucose 6-phosphate dehydrogenase
c. 6-Phosphogluconate dehydrogenase
d. Transaldolase

3.The rate of PPP is increased by:
a. Insulin
b. Growth hormone
c. Glucagon
d. Epinephrine

4.Two important byproducts of PPP are:
a. $FADH_2$ and pentose sugars
b. Pentose sugars and $FADH_2$
c. Pentose sugars and sedoheptulose
d. NADPH and pentose sugars

5.The energy yield in TCA cycle are 3 NADH,
$FADH_2$, and GTP.
a. True
b. False

6.Reduced glutathione functions in R.B.Cs to:
a. Produce NADPH
b. Reduce methemoglobin to hemoglobin
c. Produce NADH
d. Reduce oxidizing agents such as H_2O_2

8.The mitochondrial cytochrome P450 monooxygenase system uses NADPH to:
a. Synthesis of steroid hormone, fatty acids, and regeneration of
reduced glutathione.
b. Produce 2 ATP
c. Drugs detoxification
d. Produce 3 ATP

9.All the following compounds are the fates of pyruvate
except:
a. Lactate
b. Acetyl CoA
c. Citrate
d. Ethanol

10.Which of the following compounds is the competitive
inhibitor for PPP?
a. NADH
b. NADPH
c. $FADH_2$
d. Glucose 6-phosphate

11.The importance of reversible non-oxidative reaction of
the pentose phosphate pathway is:
a. produce 3, 4, 5, and 6 carbon sugars, synthesis
intermediates for glycolysis
b. ATP synthesis
c. Produced NADPH and ribulose-5-phosphate.
d. Generate GTP, 3NADH and $FADH_2$

12.Transketolase has the coenzyme:
a. NAD^+
b. Riboflavin
c. Thiamin pyrophosphate (TPP)
d. Pyridoxol phosphate

13.The generation of reduced glutathione (G-SH) is needed to:
a. Catalase and superoxide dismutase
b. $NADP^+$ and glutathione peroxidase
c. NADH
d. NADPH and glutathione reductase

Q 1: Circle the best correct answer:

14. Transaldose catalyzes transfer…… from seven carbon sugars to glyceraldehyde 3-phosphate.
a. Two carbon
b. Three carbon
c. Four sugar
d. Six carbon

15. The oxidative deamination of glutamate to α-ketoglutarate is subjected by:
a. Pyruvate dehydrogenase complex
b. Glutamate dehydrogenase
c. Glutaminase
d. Pyruvate kinase

16. The apolipoprotein which forms the integral component of chylomicron is apo
a. B-48
b. B-100
c. C-II
d. D

17. The major storage form of fatty acids is:
a. Esterified cholesterol
b. Glycerophospholipids
c. Triglycerides
d. Sphingolipids

18. Exogenous triglycerides are transported from intestine to the liver by:
a. Chylomicrons
b. VLDL
c. HDL
d. LDL

19. Endogenous triglycerides are transported from liver to extrahepatic tissues by:
a. Chylomicrons
b. VLDL
c. HDL
d. LDL

20. Which of the following compounds is the precursor of eicosanoids?
a. Glycerol
b. Vitamin D
c. Cholesterol
d. Arachidonic acid

21. Which of the following compounds is the main catabolism substrate during starvation?
a. Glucose
b. Glycogen
c. Fatty acid
d. Protein

22. Which of the following compounds is the main catabolism substrate during prolong fast?
a. Glucose
b. Glycogen
c. Fatty acid
d. Protein

23. The fatty acid 18:1(9) is relative to ………
a. Omega 3
b. Omega6
c. Omega 9
d. Omega 2

24. The example of Essential fatty acids is………
a. Linoleic acid
b. Arachidonic acid
c. Prostaglandins (PGs)
d. Oleic acid

25. Long chain fatty acyl CoA transfer from cytosol to mitochondria by:
a. Palmitate
b. Carnitine shuttle
c. Sorbitol
d. DNP

Lipids metabolism : Exercises

Q 1: Circle the best correct answer:

26.The rate limiting step in fatty acid synthesis is:
a. Oxidative decarboxylated Pyruvate to acetyl CoA
b. Condensation of acetyl- CoA with malonyl CoA
c. Carboxylated acetyl CoA to malonyl CoA
d. Transfer the acetyl CoA from mitochondria to cytosol as citrate

27.The beta oxidation of odd fatty acid (15 C), will yield:
a. 7 NADH, 7 FADH$_2$, 8 acetyl CoA
b. 6 NADH, 6 FADH$_2$, 6 acetyl CoA, Popionyl CoA
c. 7 NADH, 7FADH$_2$, 7 acetyl CoA
d. 15 NADH, 15 FADH$_2$, 15 acetyl CoA, Popionyl CoA

28.The rate limiting step in beta oxidization of fatty acid is:
a. Acetyl CoA carboxylated to malonyl COA
b. Malonyl CoA inhibit carnitine palmitoyltransferaseII (CPT-II)
c. The reaction catalyzed by acetyl- CoA
d. Malonyl CoA inhibit carnitine palmitoyltransferase1 (CPT-I)

29.During fatty acid synthesis, Acetyl CoA condensation with oxaloacetate for transport from matrix to cytosol by converted to.........
a. Malate
b. Citrate
c. Succinate
d. Malonyl CoA

30.Acetyl CoA can be formed from the catabolism of pyruvate, fatty acid , and ketone bodies:
a. True
b. False

31.Which of the following fatty acids are synthesized by De novo synthesis of fatty acid?
a. Arachidonic acid
b. Linoleic acid
c. Palmitate
d. Oleic acid

32.The major sources of the NADPH is:
a. pentose phosphate pathway
b. Cytosolic NADPH produce from oxidize malate to pyruvate
c. Glycolysis and gluconeogenesis.
d. Both a and b

33.Which of the following statements about ketone bodies is FALSE:
a. Ketone bodies synthesis occurs in kidney
b. Ketone bodies are spare of glucose in the brain
c. Acetoacetate, and β-hydroxybutyrate, transport to other tissue for converted to acetyl CoA and generate energy
d. Acetone is present during diabetic ketoacidosis which is excrete in urine and breath

34.Which of the following compounds is not stored in the body?
a. Fatty acid
b. Amino acids
c. Glycogen
d. Cholesterol

35.Which of the following enzymes is the regulatory enzyme for cholesterol synthesis?
a. HMG-CoA synthase
b. Thiokinase
c. Acetyl-CoA carboxylase
d. HMG-CoA reductase

36.The integrator between the TCA cycle and urea cycle is:
a. Fumarate
b. Malate
c. Pyruvate
d. Citrate

37.Ubiquitin is a peptide used for labelling of...... for degradation:
a. Exogenous proteins (dietary protein)
b. Endogenous proteins (Cellular proteins)
c. Exo-and endogenous proteins
d. Digestive enzyme

Lipids metabolism : Exercises

Q 1: Circle the best correct answer:

38. Which of the following statements about urea cycle is true?
a. Converts ammonia to urea
b. Need 3 ATP
c. Takes places primarily in liver
d. All of these

39. The ammonia (NH_3) is transported from muscle to the liver as......
a. Alanine
b. Glutamine
c. Aspartate
d. Lysine

40. The urea cycle occurs in ....
a. Mitochondria only
b. Cytosol only
c. Mitochondria and Cytosol
d. Endoplasmic reticulum only

41. The integrator between the TCA cycle and fatty acid is......
a. Fumarate
b. Sccinyl CoA
c. Malate
d. Citrate

42. Which of the following statements about glutamate dehydrogenase is false?
a. Catalyzes forward and backward reaction
b. Need NADPH in reductive amination
c. Need NAD^+ in oxidative deamination
d. Need FAD in oxidative deamination

43. Non-steroidal anti-inflammatory drugs, such as aspirin act by inhibiting the activity of the enzyme:
a. Lipoxygenase
b. Cyclooxygenase (COX)
c. Phospholipase A2
d. Lipoprotein lipase

44. A steroidal anti-inflammatory drugs, such as cortisol act by inhibiting the activity of phosphollpase A2.
a. True
b. False

45. Which of the following compounds are NOT involve in the Key junction points?
a. Glucose-6-Phosphate
b. Pyruvate
c. Acetyl CoA
d. Oxaloacetate

46. Which of the following is the main function of Ghrelin?
a. Sensor of satiety
b. Sensor of thirsty
c. Enhances appetite
d. All of these

47. The transport of electrons from NADH to O_2 via the electron transport chain generates:
a. ATP
b. 2ATP
c. 3ATP
d. 2GTP

48. Pyruvate dehydrogenase complex (PDHC) is required for the production of:
a. Acetyl-CoA
b. Lactate
c. Phosphoenolpyruvate
d. Enolpyruvate

49. All the following compounds are activated glycogen degradation except:
a. Glucagon and adrenalin
b. Ca^{2+}
c. AMP
d. ATP

Q 1: Circle the best correct answer:

50. Glycogen stores in:
a. Muscle only
b. Liver only
c. Liver and muscle
d. Brain and Kidney

51. The breakdown of glucose to pyruvate is termed:
a. Glycolysis
b. Oxidative decarboxylation
c. Specific dynamic action
d. Gluconeogenesis

52. Which of the following enzymes is important in reciprocal regulation of glycolysis and gluconeogenesis?
a. PEP Carboxykinas
b. PFK2-FBP2
c. Aldolase
d. Hexokinase

53. Phosphofructokinase1 (PFK1) is allosterically activated by………
a. AMP, Fructose 2,6 bisphosphate
b. Citrate, ATP
c. Pyruvate, PEP
d. G6-P, F6-P

54. The first step of glycolysis is………
a. Decarboxylation
b. Dehydration
c. phosphorylation
d. Oxidation

55. All the following compounds are members of the electron transport chain except:
a. Ubiquinone
b. Carnitine
c. NADH dehydrogenase
d. Succinate dehydrogenase

56. Urea is produced by the action of the enzyme:
a. Ornithine transcarbamoylase
b. Glutaminase
c. Arginase
d. Aldolase

57. Control of urea cycle involves the enzyme:
a. Carbamoyl phosphate synthetase I
b. Ornithine transcarbamoylase
c. Argininosuccinase
d. Arginase

58. Substrate level phosphorylation in TCA cycle is in step:
a. Isocitrate dehydrogenase
b. Malate dehydrogenase
c. Aconitase
d. Succinate thiokinase

Q 2: Write short notes on:

1. The importance of Pentose phosphate pathway (PPP).
2. The importance of microsomal (ER) cytochrome P450 monooxygenase system.
3. Describe the regulation of pentose phosphate pathway (PPP).
4. Explain glucose 6-phosphate dehydrogenase deficiency led to hemolysis of RBCs and favism.
5. How the Lipids are transported in blood?
6. What is the major function of glutathione? and How the oxidized glutathione is reduced?
7. What are the uses of NADPH?
8. Functions of chylomicron and VLDL.
9. Glucogenic amino acids.
10. Ketogenic amino acids.
11. Non-shivering thermogenesis theory.
12. Describe the regulation of beta oxidation of fatty acids.
13. Functions of ketone bodies.
14. What is the regulatory enzyme for De novo synthesis of Fatty Acids?
15. Describe the regulation of De novo synthesis of fatty acids.
16. The role of carnitine-shuttle in the β-oxidation of fatty acids.
17. Describe the regulation of cholesterol synthesis.
18. Amino acid pool.
19. protein turnover.
20. Explain, If NADH transported from cytosol into mitochondrial matrix by Malate-Aspartate shuttle produce 3 ATP.
21. Functions of COX-1 and COX-2.

Q 3. Indicate the effect of insulin (increases or decreases) for each of the following pathways:

PATHWAY	EFFECT OF INSULIN
1.Glycolysis	
2.Gluconeogenesis	
3.Glycogen degradation	
4.Glycogen synthesis	
5.Pentose phosphate pathway	
6.De novo synthesis of fatty acids	
7.β-oxidation of fatty acids	
8.Ketolysis (ketone bodies degradation)	
9.ketone bodies synthesis	

OVERVIEW

Unlike fats and carbohydrates, amino acids are not stored by the body, that is, no protein exists whose sole function is to maintain a supply of amino acids for future use. Therefore, amino acids must be obtained from the diet, synthesized de novo, or produced from normal protein degradation. Any amino acids in excess of the biosynthetic needs of the cell are rapidly degraded. The first phase of catabolism involves the removal of the a-amino groups (usually by transamination and subsequent oxidative deamination), forming ammonia and the corresponding a-keto acid the "carbon skeletons" of amino acids. A portion of the free ammonia is excreted in the urine, but most is used in the synthesis of urea. These compounds can be metabolized to CO_2 and water, glucose, fatty acids, or ketone bodies by the central pathways of metabolism

16.1.Nitrogen:

Human needs amino acids and for that nitrogen is important sources which further help to synthesize human proteins. A metabolic process in our body depends upon enzymes, which contains various kinds of proteins. The nucleic acid DNA makes up your genes and RNA is involved in protein synthesis which needs nitrogen for it. We all know that without DNA we would not be alive. For proper digestion of food and growth human body needs nitrogen. It is extremely important in the development of the human fetus.

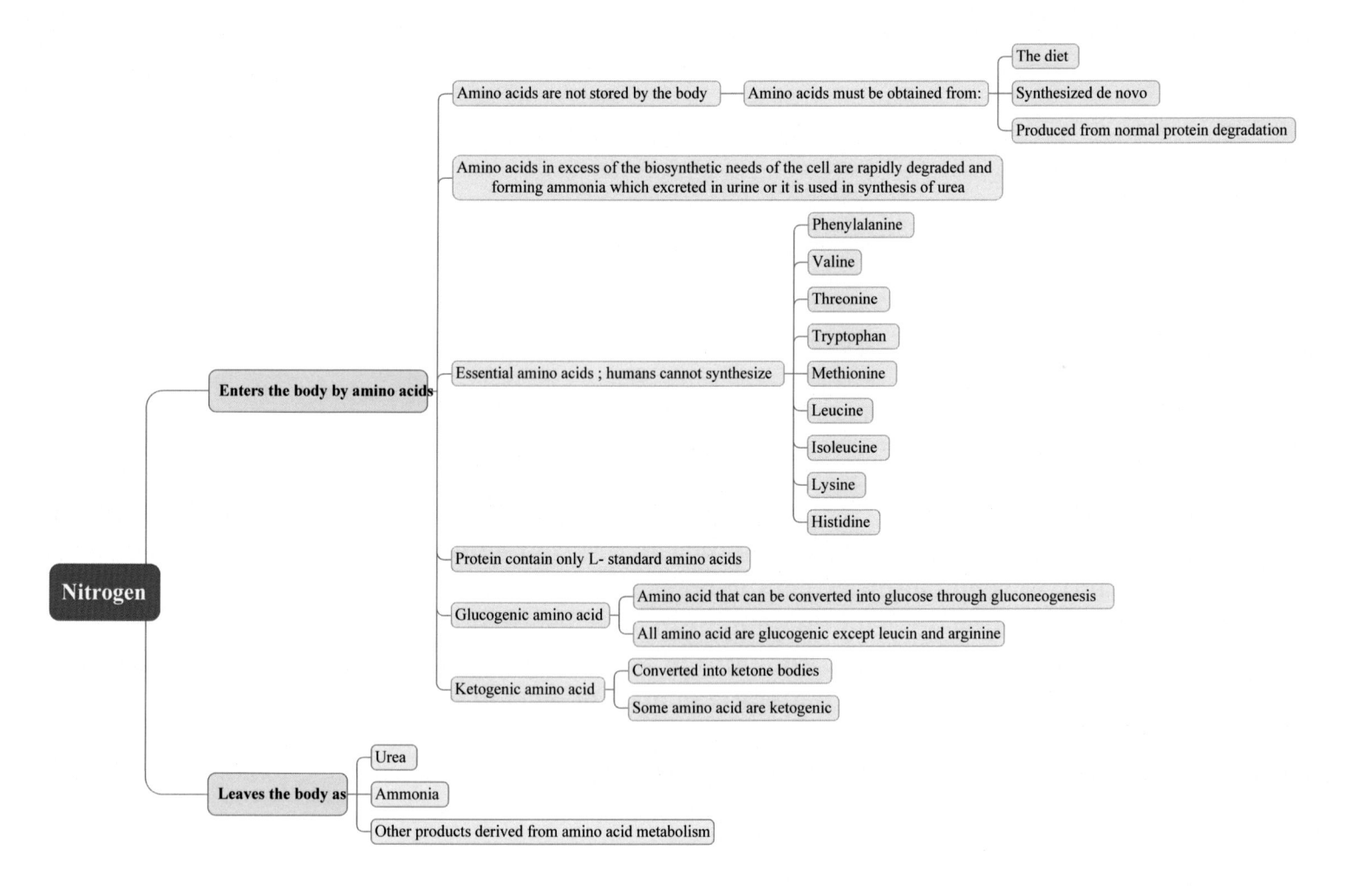

16.2.Nitrogen metabolism : it is the polymeric nitrogen containing compounds proteins and nucleic acids that define the major attributes of organism such as function and structure. Operation and mechanism of metabolic pathways is provided by proteins. Genetic information is stored in nucleic acid polymers. Each of the monomer of these macromolecules has an individual metabolic pathway. In addition, the monomeric nucleotides are essential for energy turnover as key intermediates in all metabolic pathways and also as second messenger molecules, often in form of cyclic nucleotides.Amino acids contribute to carbohydrate synthesis via gluconeogenesis, to fat synthesis or energy production via acetyl-CoA, and special nitrogen compounds such as catecholamines (neurotransmitters), thyroid hormones, creatine(-phosphate), the protoporphyrin ring (heme), and contribute to nucleic acid and phospholipid synthesis as nitrogen group donor.

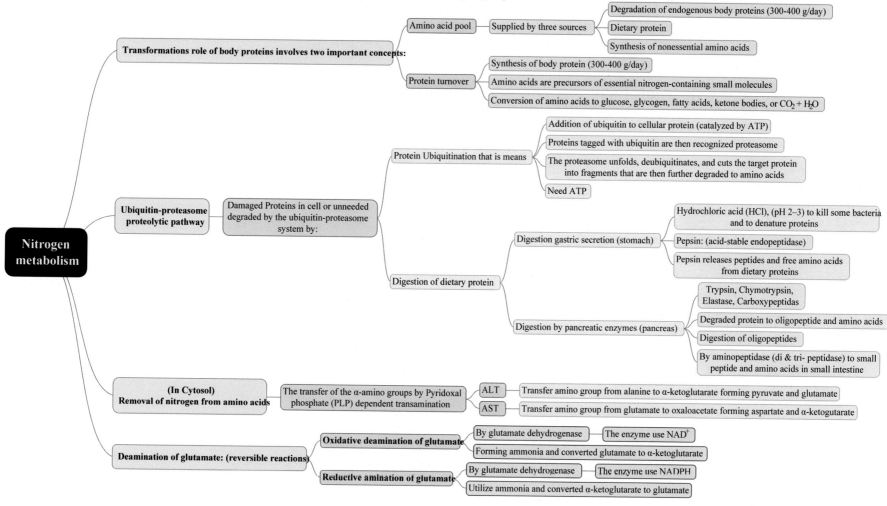

16.2. Urea cycle

Ammonia is converted to urea in the hepatocytes of the liver in five steps via urea cycle- in the mitochondria (first 2 steps) and cytosol (last 3 steps). The urea then travels through the blood stream to the kidney and is excreted in the urine. The urea cycle was discovered by Hans Krebs (who also discovered Citric acid or Krebs cycle) and his student associate Kurt Henseleit in 1932.

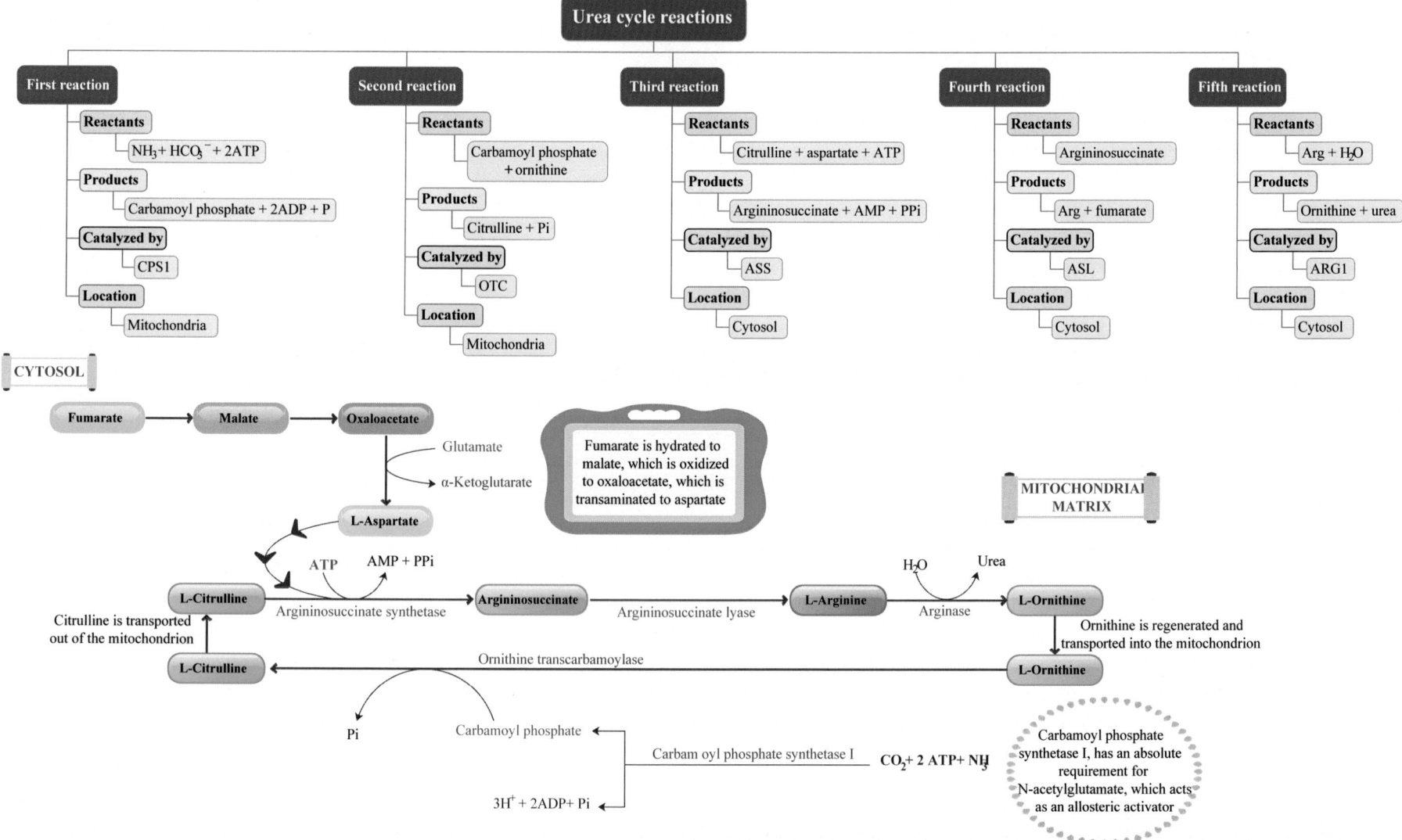

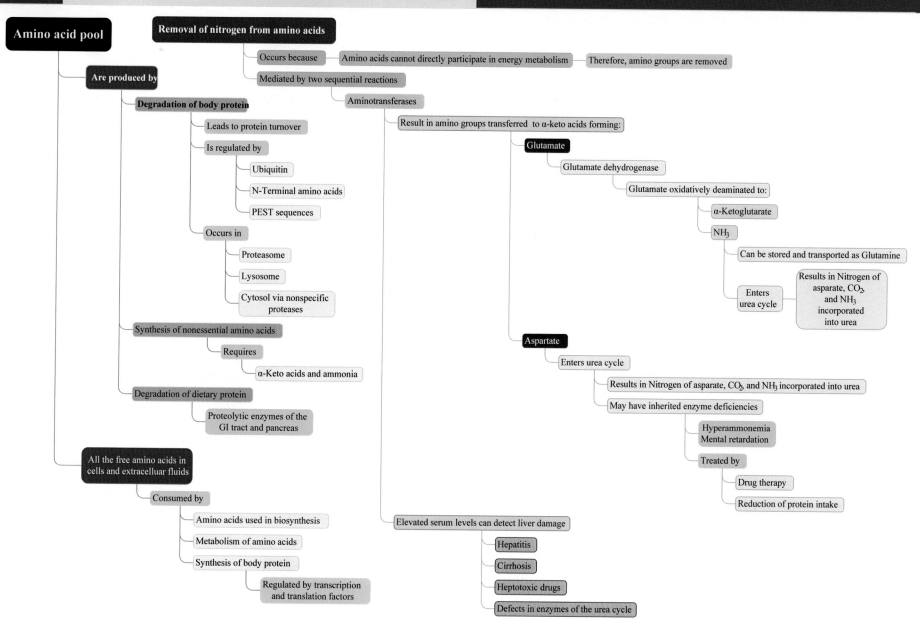

Amino acid pool

Are produced by

Degradation of body protein
- Leads to protein turnover
- Is regulated by
  - Ubiquitin
  - N-Terminal amino acids
  - PEST sequences
- Occurs in
  - Proteasome
  - Lysosome
  - Cytosol via nonspecific proteases

Synthesis of nonessential amino acids
- Requires
  - α-Keto acids and ammonia

Degradation of dietary protein
- Proteolytic enzymes of the GI tract and pancreas

All the free amino acids in cells and extracelluar fluids

Consumed by
- Amino acids used in biosynthesis
- Metabolism of amino acids
- Synthesis of body protein
  - Regulated by transcription and translation factors

Removal of nitrogen from amino acids

Occurs because — Amino acids cannot directly participate in energy metabolism — Therefore, amino groups are removed

Mediated by two sequential reactions

Aminotransferases

Result in amino groups transferred to α-keto acids forming:

Glutamate
- Glutamate dehydrogenase
  - Glutamate oxidatively deaminated to:
    - α-Ketoglutarate
    - NH_3
      - Can be stored and transported as Glutamine
      - Enters urea cycle — Results in Nitrogen of asparate, CO_2, and NH_3 incorporated into urea

Aspartate
- Enters urea cycle
- Results in Nitrogen of asparate, CO_2, and NH_3 incorporated into urea
- May have inherited enzyme deficiencies
  - Hyperammonemia Mental retardation
  - Treated by
    - Drug therapy
    - Reduction of protein intake

Elevated serum levels can detect liver damage
- Hepatitis
- Cirrhosis
- Heptotoxic drugs
- Defects in enzymes of the urea cycle

OVERVIEW

Nucleic acids are required for the storage and expression of genetic information. There are two chemically distinct types of nucleic acids: deoxyribonucleic acid (DNA) and ribonucleic acid (RNA). DNA, the repository of genetic information, is present not only in chromosomes in the nucleus of eukaryotic organisms, but also in mitochondria and the chloroplasts of plants. Prokaryotic cells, which lack nuclei, have a single chromosome, but may also contain nonchromosomal DNA in the form of plasmids. The genetic information found in DNA is copied and transmitted to daughter cells through DNA replication. The DNA contained in a fertilized egg encodes the information that directs the development of an organism. This development may involve the production of billions of cells. Each cell is specialized, expressing only those functions that are required for it to perform its role in maintaining the organism. Therefore, DNA must be able to not only replicate precisely each time a cell divides, but also to have the information that it contains be selectively expressed. Transcription (RNA synthesis) is the first stage in the expression of genetic information.

17.1. DNA Structure: Deoxyribonucleic acid or DNA is a molecule that contains the instructions an organism needs to develop, live and reproduce. These instructions are found inside every cell, and are passed down from parents to their children. DNA is made up of molecules called nucleotides. Each nucleotide contains a phosphate group, a sugar group and a nitrogen base. The four types of nitrogen bases are adenine (A), thymine (T), guanine (G) and cytosine (C). The order of these bases is what determines DNA's instructions, or genetic code. Human DNA has around 3 billion bases, and more than 99 percent of those bases are the same in all people, according to the U.S. National Library of Medicine (NLM)

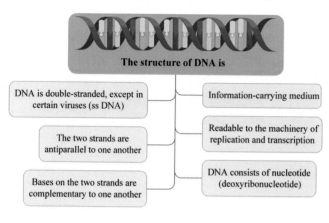

The structure of DNA is

- DNA is double-stranded, except in certain viruses (ss DNA)
- The two strands are antiparallel to one another
- Bases on the two strands are complementary to one another
- Information-carrying medium
- Readable to the machinery of replication and transcription
- DNA consists of nucleotide (deoxyribonucleotide)

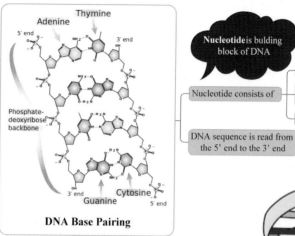

DNA Base Pairing

Nucleotide is bulding block of DNA

Nucleotide consists of
- Nitrogenous base
- Five-Carbon sugar ribose [in RNA] and deoxyribose [in DNA]
- Phosphate group

DNA sequence is read from the 5' end to the 3' end — (5'-ACGT-3') is read "adenine, cytosine, guanine, thymine"

Attached to each sugar ring is a nucleotide base, one of the four bases Adenine (A), Guanine (G), Cytosine (C), and Thymine (T). The first two (A, G) are examples of a purine which contains a six atom ring and five atom ring sharing two atoms. The second two (C, T) are examples of a pyrimidine which is composed of a single six atom ring. A base pair is one of the pairs A-T or C-G. Notice that each base pair consists of a purine and a pyrimidine. The nucleotides in a base pair are complementary which means their shape allows them to bond together with hydrogen bonds. The A-T pair forms two hydrogen bonds. The C-G pair forms three. The hydrogen bonding between complementary bases holds the two strands of DNA together. Hydrogen bonds are not chemical bonds. They can be easily disrupted. This permits the DNA strands to separate for transcription (copying DNA to RNA) and replication (copying DNA to DNA). In our simple model, the entire base pair structure is represented by the single blue rod. Various more elaborate models can be constructed to represent base pairs, including the one above which shows individual atoms and bonds.

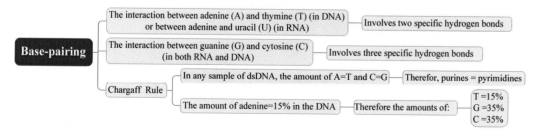

Base-pairing
- The interaction between adenine (A) and thymine (T) (in DNA) or between adenine and uracil (U) (in RNA) — Involves two specific hydrogen bonds
- The interaction between guanine (G) and cytosine (C) (in both RNA and DNA) — Involves three specific hydrogen bonds
- Chargaff Rule
  - In any sample of dsDNA, the amount of A=T and C=G — Therefor, purines = pyrimidines
  - The amount of adenine=15% in the DNA — Therefore the amounts of: — T =15% / G =35% / C =35%

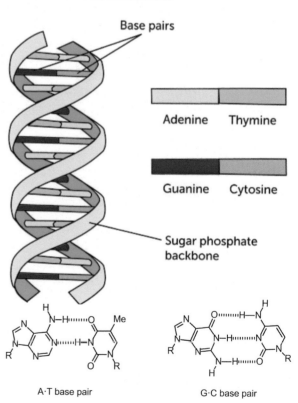

Base pairs

Adenine — Thymine

Guanine — Cytosine

Sugar phosphate backbone

A·T base pair

G·C base pair

17.2. DNA replication

Steps in prokaryotic DNA synthesis

1. Separation of ds DNA or "melt" a origin of replication (rich in A=T)
- Origin of replication (rich in A=T) is a site in a DNA molecules at which helicase unwinds the double helix
  - Allowing DNA replication to commence
  - A prokaryotic chromosome has a single origin of replication
- DNA replication occurs in the S phase of the cell cycle
- The strands are separated locally, forming two replication forks.
- Replication of dsDNA is bidirectional
- Because the polymerases use only ssDNA as a template by DNA helicase

2. DNA replication requires a proteins
- For separation and maintaining the separation of the parental strands and formation of the replication fork
- These proteins include the following:
  - DnaA protein
    - Binds at origin of replication
    - Results in strand separation with the formation of localized regions of ssDNA
  - DNA helicases — Require energy (ATP)
    - For unwinding DNA
    - That is causes supercoiling in other region of DNA
  - Single-stranded DNA-binding (SSB) proteins — Bind to the ssDNA generated by helicases For
    - Keep the two strands of DNA separated
    - Protect the DNA from nucleases that degrade ssDNA

3. Solving the problem of supercoils
- When ds DNA are separated, a problem is encountered are positive supercoils in the region of DNA ahead of the replication fork as result of overwinding and negative supercoils in the region behind the fork
- Type I DNA topoisomerases
  - Cut one strand of the DNA duplex
  - Relax negative supercoiled DNA
- Type II DNA topoisomerases
  - Cut both strands of a DNA duplex
  - Relax either negatively or positively supercoild DNA molecules

4. Formation of RNA primer by primas
- primase
  - A specific RNA polymerase, called primase (DnaG)
  - Responsible for synthesis of RNA primer
- Primer
  - Is a short, single-stranded segment of DNA or RNA
  - Provide a 3-OH group for DNA synthesis
  - Results serves as the essential starting material for a new DNA strand

Steps in prokaryotic DNA synthesis

5.Elongation of the leading and lagging strands

DNA elongation (DNA pol III) is catalyzed by DNA polymerase III

Properties of DNA polymerase III
- Synthesis of DNA in 5'→3' direction using templet (ssDNA) — Antiparallel to the parental strand
- "proofreading" and erorr correction activity (3'→5') exonuclease — 3'→5' exonuclease remove the misplaced nucleotide the 5' →3 polymerase activity then replaces it with the correct nucleotide

Leading strand — One strand is leading strand, grows continuously and uninterruptedly from its 5 `→3` in the same direction of movement of the replication fork

Lagging strand
- Direction of DNA on away from the replication fork is synthesized discontinuously from their 5 `→3 until it is blocked by proximity to an RNA primer
- The strand growing in opposite direction to unwinding = lagging strand

6.Excision of RNA primers and their replacement by DN

The RNA is excised and the gap filled by DNA polymerase I

Properties of DNA polymerase I:
- DNA polymerase I remove the RNA primer
  - 5'→3' exonuclease activity
  - 3'→5' Exonuclease activity
- Replaces it with deoxyribonucleotides
  - Synthesizing DNA in the 5'→3' direction
  - 5'→3' polymerase activity

7.DNA ligase

Joined (ligated) the fragment DNA (Need energy from ATP convert to AMP + PPi) — By phosphodiester linkage between the 5'-phosphate group on the DNA chain synthesized by DNA polymerase III and the 3'-hydroxyl group on the chain made by DNA polymerase I is catalyzed by DNA ligase

8.Termination
- Sequence-specific binding of the protein, to replication sites on the DNA
- Stopping the movement of DNA polymerase

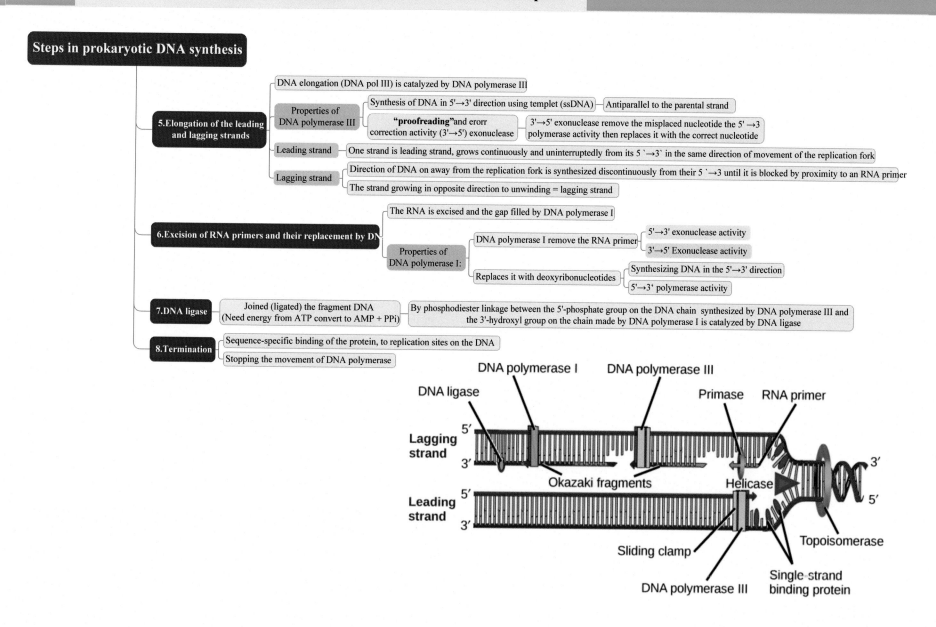

Chapter 17 : DNA Structure, Replication, Repair and RNA Transcription

DNA Synthesis: The discovery of the double-helical nature of DNA by Watson & Crick explained how genetic information could be duplicated and passed on to succeeding generations. The strands of the double helix can separate and serve as templates for the synthesis of daughter strands. In conservative replication the two daughter strands would go to one daughter cell and the two parental strands would go to the other daughter cell. In semiconservative replication one parental and one daughter strand would go to each of the daughter cells

What is the different between DNA replication in eukaryotic and prokaryotic

- Multiple origins of replication in eukaryotic cells versus single origins of replication in prokaryotes

- RNA primers are removed by RNase H rather than by a DNA polymeras

- Nucleoside analogs
  - Containing modified sugars can be used to block DNA chain growth
  - They are useful in anticancer and antiviral chemotherapy

- Telomeres
  - Are repetitive non coding DNA sequences plus protein at the end of linear chromosomes
  - Function of telomeres:
    - Preventing attack by nucleases
    - As most cells divide and age, these sequences are shortened, contributing to senescence — In cells that do not senesce — (For example, germ line and cancer cells)

- Some of the enzymes involved in eukaryotic replication are different — These include 5 enzymes and their functions
  - Polymerases α
    - Contain primase
    - Initiate DNA synthesis
  - Polymerases β — Repair
  - Polymerases γ — Replicates mitochondrial DNA
  - Polymerases δ — Thought to elongate okazaki fragments of the lagging strand
  - Polymerases ε — Thought to elongate the leading strand

- Telomerase — Are complex contains (1. protein + 2. short RNA)
  - Protein acts as a reverse transcriptase
  - Short piece of RNA RNA as a template for the 5'→3synthesis 5'→3 of DNA

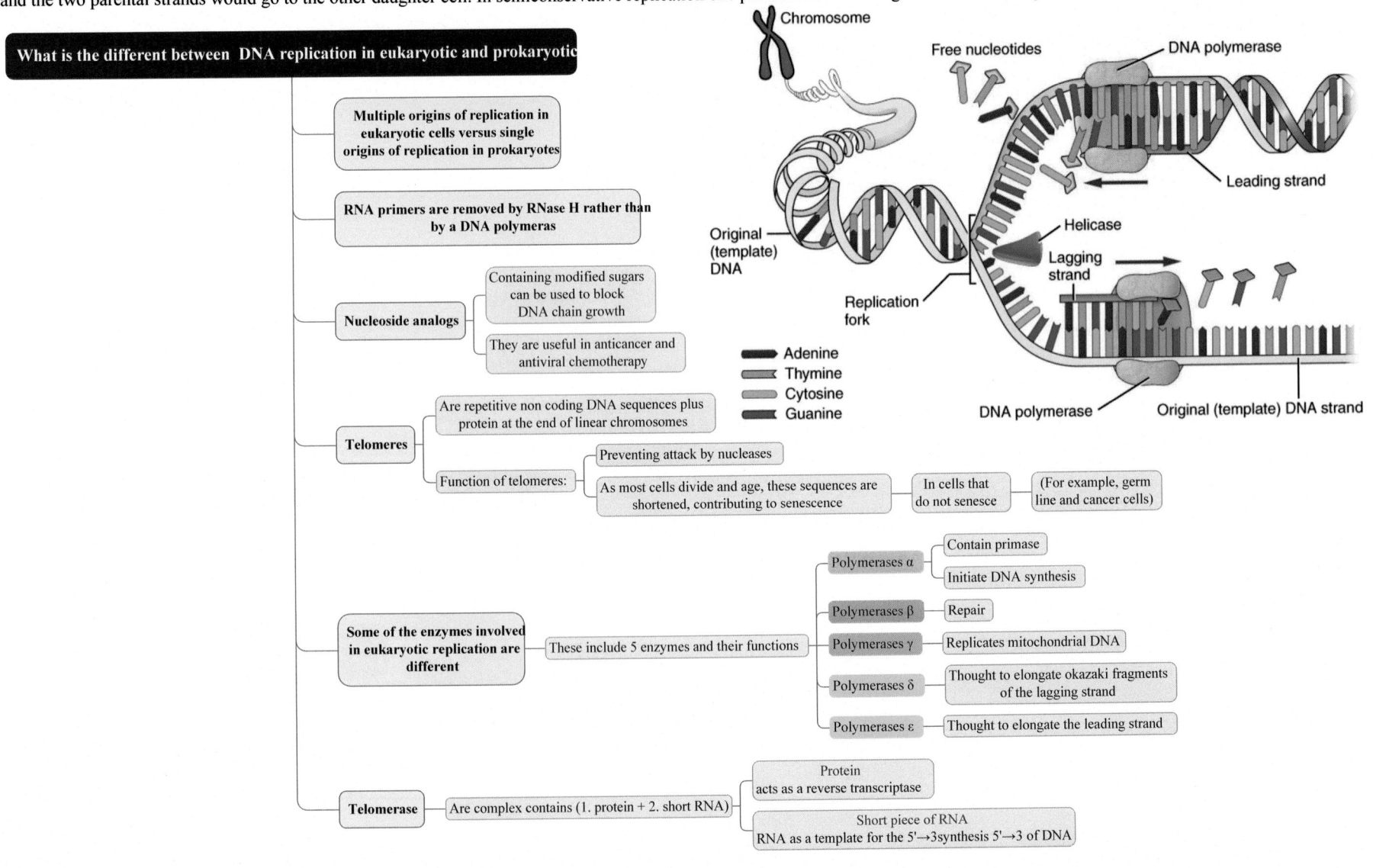

Chromosome

Free nucleotides

DNA polymerase

Leading strand

Original (template) DNA

Helicase

Lagging strand

Replication fork

- Adenine
- Thymine
- Cytosine
- Guanine

DNA polymerase

Original (template) DNA strand

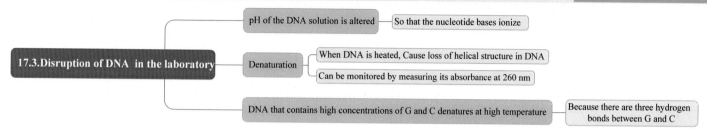

17.3.Disruption of DNA in the laboratory
- pH of the DNA solution is altered — So that the nucleotide bases ionize
- Denaturation
  - When DNA is heated, Cause loss of helical structure in DNA
  - Can be monitored by measuring its absorbance at 260 nm
- DNA that contains high concentrations of G and C denatures at high temperature — Because there are three hydrogen bonds between G and C

17.4.DNA repair: is a collection of processes by which a cell identifies and corrects damage to the DNA molecules that encode its genome. In human cells, both normal metabolic activities and environmental factors such as radiation can cause DNA damage, resulting in as many as 1 million individual molecular lesions per cell per day. Many of these lesions cause structural damage to the DNA molecule and can alter or eliminate the cell's ability to transcribe the gene that the affected DNA encodes. Other lesions induce potentially harmful mutations in the cell's genome, which affect the survival of its daughter cells after it undergoes mitosis. As a consequence, the DNA repair process is constantly active as it responds to damage in the DNA structure. When normal repair processes fail, and when cellular apoptosis does not occur, irreparable DNA damage may occur, including double-strand breaks and DNA cross linkages (. This can eventually lead to malignant tumors, or cancer as per the two hit hypothesis

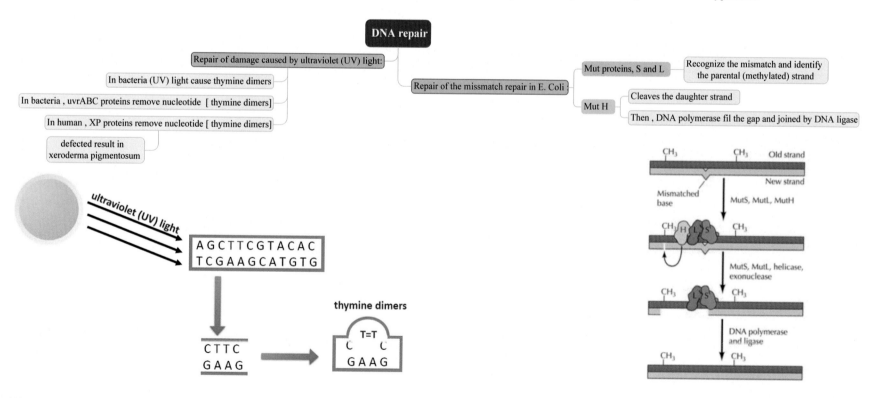

DNA repair

Repair of damage caused by ultraviolet (UV) light:
- In bacteria (UV) light cause thymine dimers
- In bacteria , uvrABC proteins remove nucleotide [thymine dimers]
- In human , XP proteins remove nucleotide [thymine dimers]
  - defected result in xeroderma pigmentosum

Repair of the missmatch repair in E. Coli :
- Mut proteins, S and L — Recognize the mismatch and identify the parental (methylated) strand
- Mut H
  - Cleaves the daughter strand
  - Then , DNA polymerase fil the gap and joined by DNA ligase

ultraviolet (UV) light

AGCTTCGTACAC
TCGAAGCATGTG

thymine dimers

T=T
C   C
CTTC   →   GAAG
GAAG

CH₃   CH₃   Old strand
                   New strand
Mismatched
base   MutS, MutL, MutH

CH₃ H L S CH₃

MutS, MutL, helicase,
exonuclease

CH₃ L S   CH₃

DNA polymerase
and ligase

CH₃   CH₃

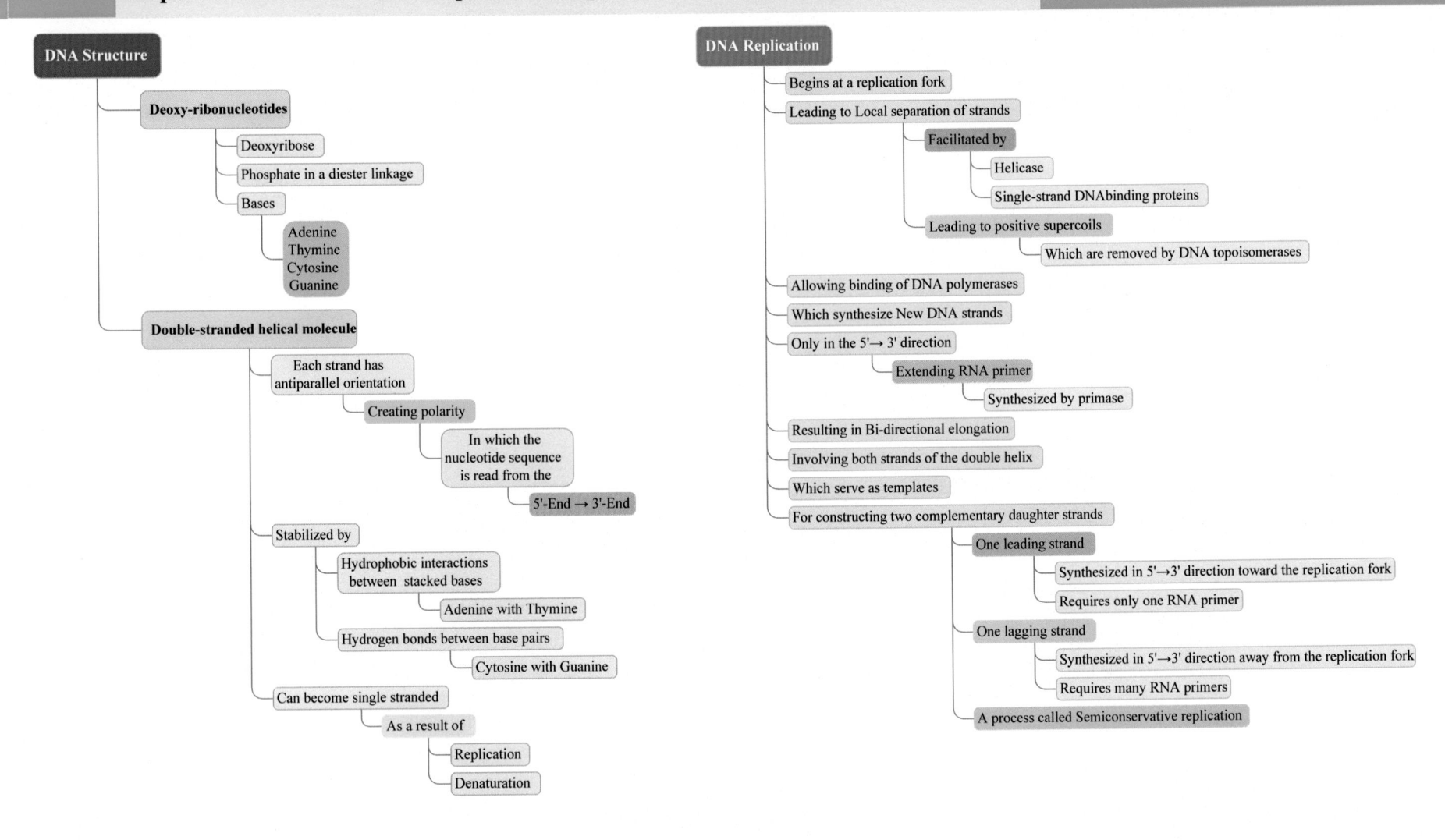

DNA Structure

- **Deoxy-ribonucleotides**
  - Deoxyribose
  - Phosphate in a diester linkage
  - Bases
    - Adenine
    - Thymine
    - Cytosine
    - Guanine
- **Double-stranded helical molecule**
  - Each strand has antiparallel orientation
    - Creating polarity
      - In which the nucleotide sequence is read from the
        - 5'-End → 3'-End
  - Stabilized by
    - Hydrophobic interactions between stacked bases
      - Adenine with Thymine
    - Hydrogen bonds between base pairs
      - Cytosine with Guanine
  - Can become single stranded
    - As a result of
      - Replication
      - Denaturation

DNA Replication

- Begins at a replication fork
- Leading to Local separation of strands
  - Facilitated by
    - Helicase
    - Single-strand DNAbinding proteins
  - Leading to positive supercoils
    - Which are removed by DNA topoisomerases
- Allowing binding of DNA polymerases
- Which synthesize New DNA strands
- Only in the 5'→ 3' direction
  - Extending RNA primer
    - Synthesized by primase
- Resulting in Bi-directional elongation
- Involving both strands of the double helix
- Which serve as templates
- For constructing two complementary daughter strands
  - One leading strand
    - Synthesized in 5'→3' direction toward the replication fork
    - Requires only one RNA primer
  - One lagging strand
    - Synthesized in 5'→3' direction away from the replication fork
    - Requires many RNA primers
  - A process called Semiconservative replication

OVERVIEW

Genetic information, stored in the chromosomes and transmitted to daughter cells through DNA replication, is expressed through transcription to RNA and, in the case of messenger RNA (mRNA), subsequent translation into proteins (polypeptide chains). The pathway of protein synthesis is called translation because the "language" of the nucleotide sequence on the mRNA is translated into the "language" of an amino acid sequence. The process of translation requires a genetic code, through which the information contained in the nucleic acid sequence is expressed to produce a specific sequence of amino acids. Any alteration in the nucleic acid sequence may result in an incorrect amino acid being inserted into the polypeptide chain, potentially causing disease or even death of the organism. Newly made proteins undergo a number of processes to achieve their functional form. They must fold properly, and misfolding can result in degradation of the protein. Many proteins are covalently modified to activate them or alter their activities. Finally, proteins are targeted to their final intra- or extracellular destinations by signals present in the proteins themselves.

18.1. Structure of RNA. RNA is typically single stranded and is made of ribonucleotides that are linked by phosphodiester bonds. A ribonucleotide in the RNA chain contains ribose (the pentose sugar), one of the four nitrogenous bases (A, U, G, and C), and a phosphate group. The subtle structural difference between the sugars gives DNA added stability, making DNA more suitable for storage of genetic information, whereas the relative instability of RNA makes it more suitable for its more short-term functions. The RNA-specific pyrimidine uracil forms a complementary base pair with adenine and is used instead of the thymine used in DNA. Even though RNA is single stranded, most types of RNA molecules show extensive intramolecular base pairing between complementary sequences within the RNA strand, creating a predictable three-dimensional structure essential for their function.

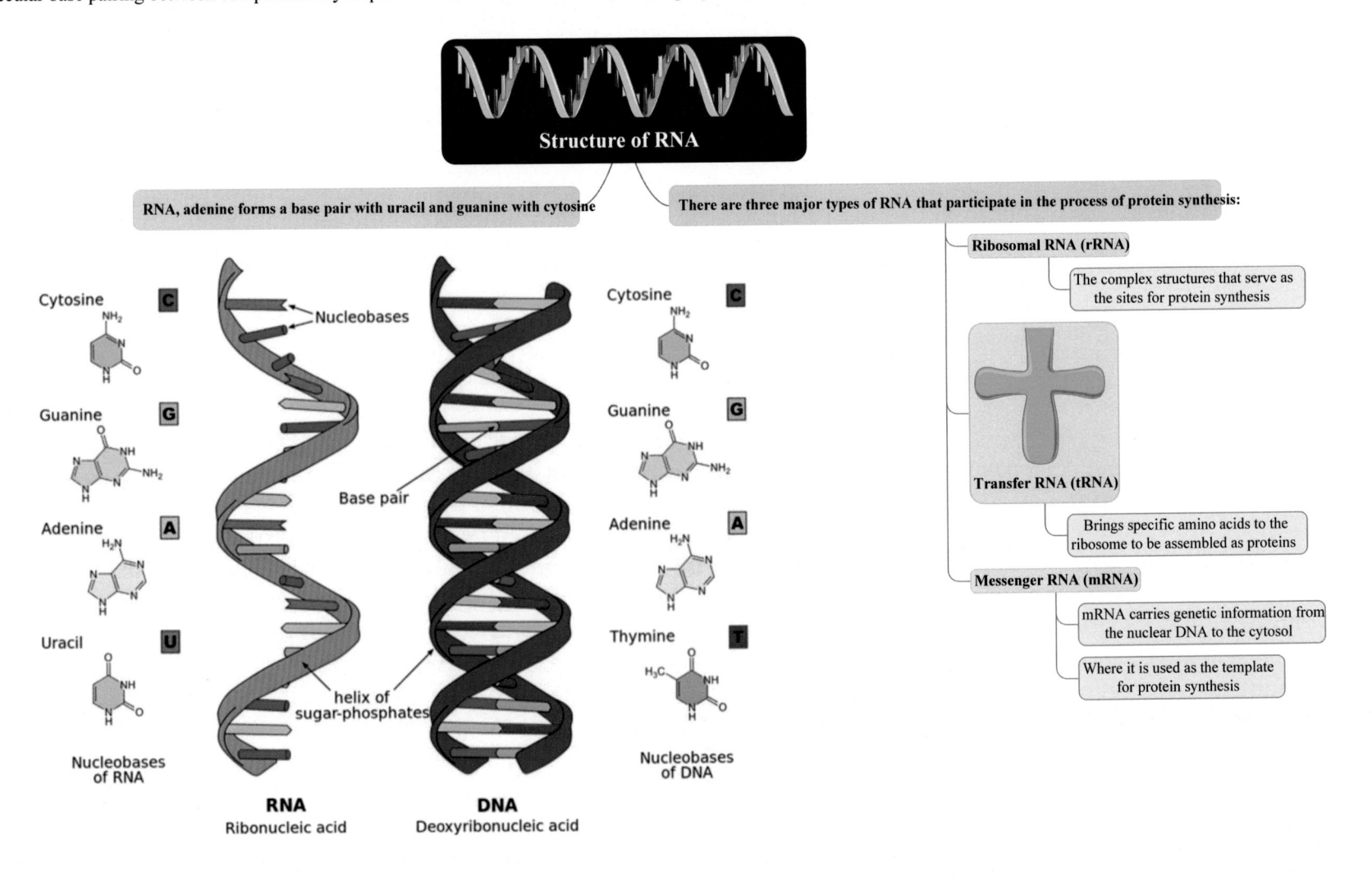

18.2. The central dogma of molecular biology describes the two-step process, transcription and translation, by which the information in genes flows into proteins: DNA → RNA → protein.

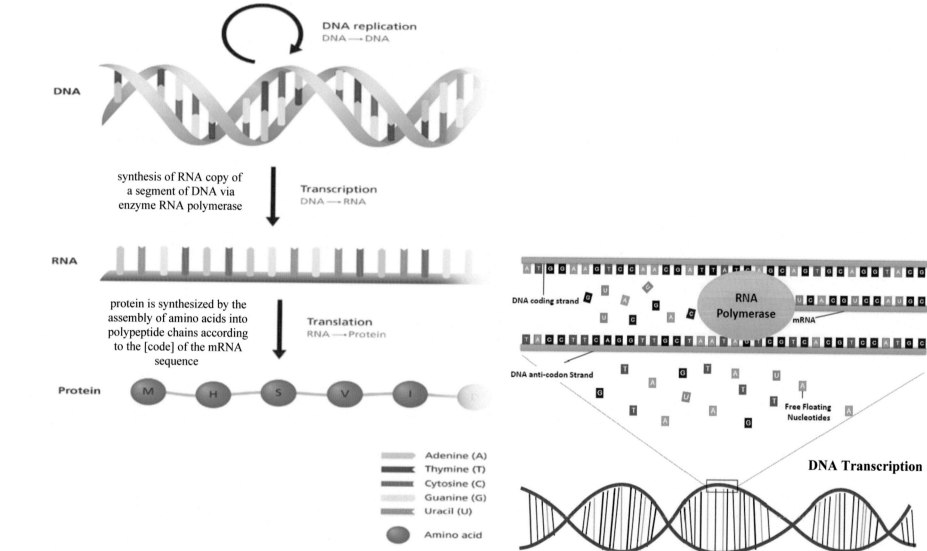

DNA replication
DNA ⟶ DNA

DNA

synthesis of RNA copy of
a segment of DNA via
enzyme RNA polymerase

Transcription
DNA ⟶ RNA

RNA

protein is synthesized by the
assembly of amino acids into
polypeptide chains according
to the [code] of the mRNA
sequence

Translation
RNA ⟶ Protein

Protein

M H S V I D

Adenine (A)
Thymine (T)
Cytosine (C)
Guanine (G)
Uracil (U)

Amino acid

DNA coding strand

RNA
Polymerase

mRNA

DNA anti-codon Strand

Free Floating
Nucleotides

DNA Transcription

Chapter 18 : Protein Synthesis

Transcription is the synthesis of RNA from DNA. Genetic information flows from DNA into protein, the substance that gives an organism its form. This flow of information occurs through the sequential processes of transcription (DNA to RNA) and translation (RNA to protein).During transcription, only one strand of DNA is usually copied. This is called the template strand, and the RNA molecules produced are single-stranded messenger RNAs (mRNAs). The DNA strand that would correspond to the mRNA is called the coding or sense strand. In eukaryotes (organisms that possess a nucleus) the initial product of transcription is called a pre-mRNA. Pre-mRNA is extensively edited through splicing before the mature mRNA is produced and ready for translation by the ribosome, the cellular organelle that serves as the site of protein synthesis. Transcription of any one gene takes place at the chromosomal location of that gene, which is a relatively short segment of the chromosome. The active transcription of a gene depends on the need for the activity of that particular gene in a specific cell or tissue or at a given time.

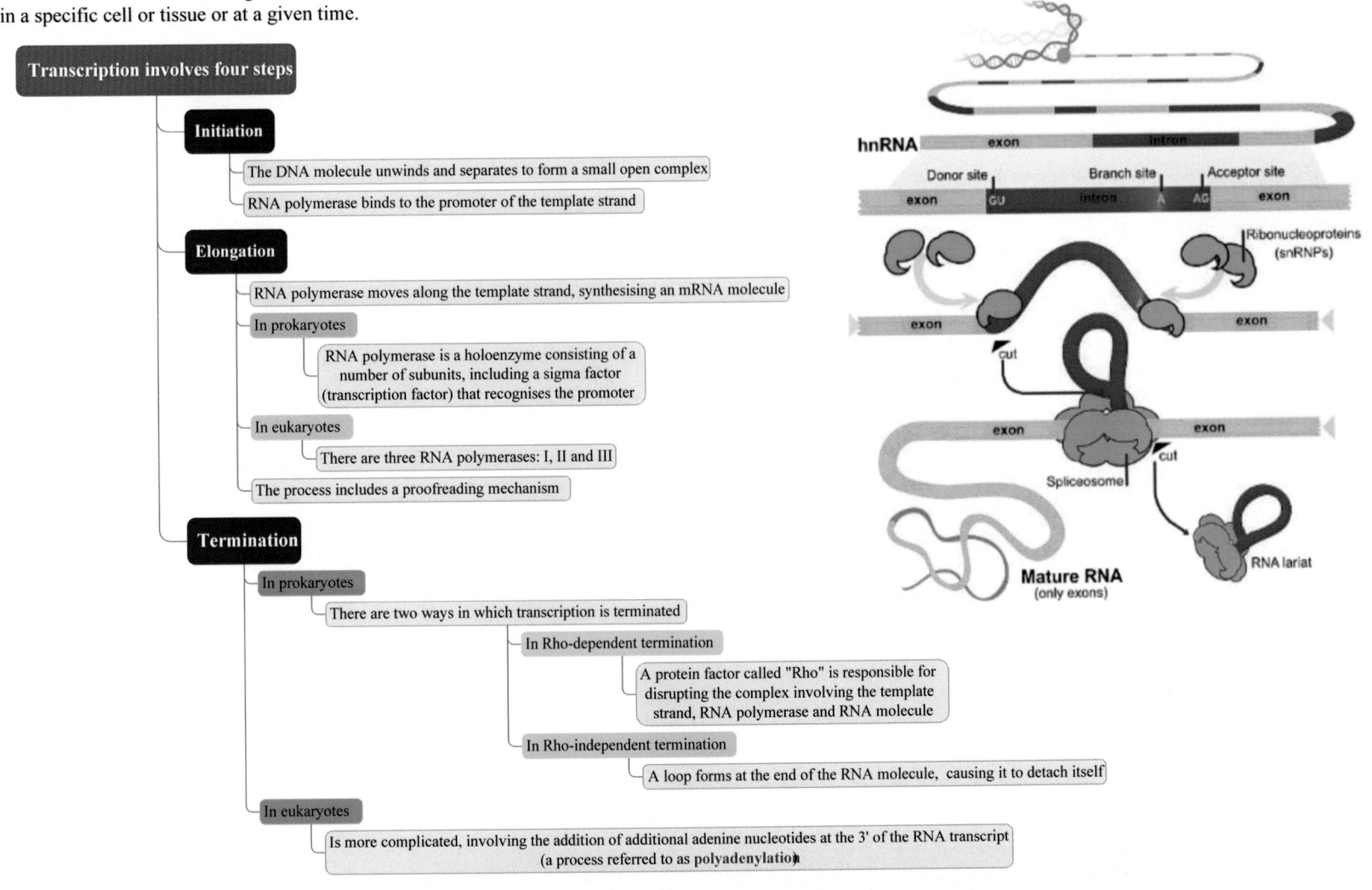

Transcription involves four steps

- **Initiation**
  - The DNA molecule unwinds and separates to form a small open complex
  - RNA polymerase binds to the promoter of the template strand

- **Elongation**
  - RNA polymerase moves along the template strand, synthesising an mRNA molecule
  - In prokaryotes
    - RNA polymerase is a holoenzyme consisting of a number of subunits, including a sigma factor (transcription factor) that recognises the promoter
  - In eukaryotes
    - There are three RNA polymerases: I, II and III
  - The process includes a proofreading mechanism

- **Termination**
  - In prokaryotes
    - There are two ways in which transcription is terminated
      - In Rho-dependent termination
        - A protein factor called "Rho" is responsible for disrupting the complex involving the template strand, RNA polymerase and RNA molecule
      - In Rho-independent termination
        - A loop forms at the end of the RNA molecule, causing it to detach itself
  - In eukaryotes
    - Is more complicated, involving the addition of additional adenine nucleotides at the 3' of the RNA transcript (a process referred to as polyadenylation)

18.3.Processing of mRNA

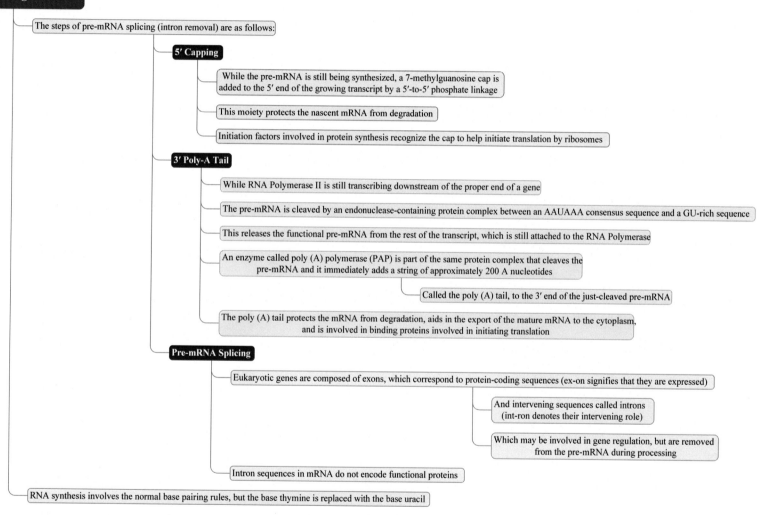

The steps of pre-mRNA splicing (intron removal) are as follows:

5′ Capping

While the pre-mRNA is still being synthesized, a 7-methylguanosine cap is added to the 5′ end of the growing transcript by a 5′-to-5′ phosphate linkage

This moiety protects the nascent mRNA from degradation

Initiation factors involved in protein synthesis recognize the cap to help initiate translation by ribosomes

3′ Poly-A Tail

While RNA Polymerase II is still transcribing downstream of the proper end of a gene

The pre-mRNA is cleaved by an endonuclease-containing protein complex between an AAUAAA consensus sequence and a GU-rich sequence

This releases the functional pre-mRNA from the rest of the transcript, which is still attached to the RNA Polymerase

An enzyme called poly (A) polymerase (PAP) is part of the same protein complex that cleaves the pre-mRNA and it immediately adds a string of approximately 200 A nucleotides

Called the poly (A) tail, to the 3′ end of the just-cleaved pre-mRNA

The poly (A) tail protects the mRNA from degradation, aids in the export of the mature mRNA to the cytoplasm, and is involved in binding proteins involved in initiating translation

Pre-mRNA Splicing

Eukaryotic genes are composed of exons, which correspond to protein-coding sequences (ex-on signifies that they are expressed)

And intervening sequences called introns (int-ron denotes their intervening role)

Which may be involved in gene regulation, but are removed from the pre-mRNA during processing

Intron sequences in mRNA do not encode functional proteins

RNA synthesis involves the normal base pairing rules, but the base thymine is replaced with the base uracil

18.4. The Genetic Code : specifically, the code defines a mapping between tri-nucleotide sequences called codons and amino acids; every triplet of nucleotides in a nucleic acid sequence specifies a single amino acid. Because the vast majority of genes are encoded with exactly the same code, this particular code is often referred to as the canonical or standard genetic code, or simply the genetic code, though in fact there are many variant codes; thus, the canonical genetic code is not universal. For example, in humans, protein synthesis in mitochondria relies on a genetic code that varies from the canonical code

The Genetic Code

Each 3 consecutive bases on RNA is a coded word (the codon) (triplets) that specifies an amino acid

Leads to the 'open reading frame' (ORF)

The genetic code consists of 64 codons, (4x4x4 resulting from a combination of 4 possible ribonucleotides)

But only 61 code amino acids

One codon, AUG, codes for methionine, and is also the start signal for the initiation of translation

Three codons act as signal terminators of translation called stop codon or non sensecodon

UAA
UAG
UGA

by binding release factors (RF), which cause the ribosomal subunits to disassociate, releasing the amino acid sequence

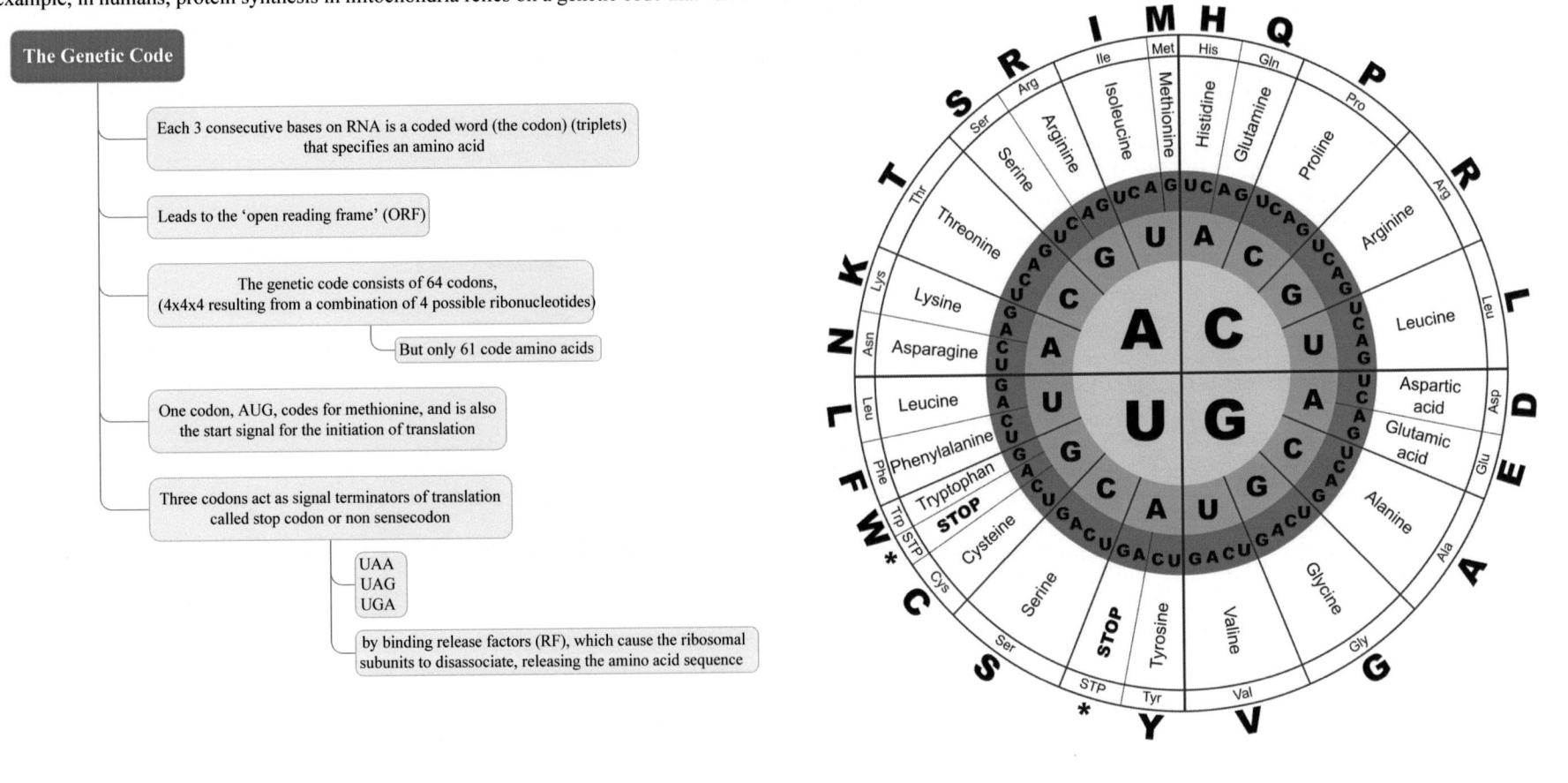

Components required for translation

Messenger RNA

Carries genetic information from the nuclear DNA to the cytosol

Functionally competent ribosomes

A ribosome consists of rRNA with proteins

Ribosomes consist of a large subunit and a small subunit

mRNA binds to the small subunit

Whose relative sizes are given in terms of their sedimentation coefficients, or S (Svedberg) values

Ribosomal RNA (rRNA)

The complex structures that serve as the sites for protein synthesis

rRNA has three binding sites for tRNA molecules

A-site (aminoacyl t RNA site)

Holds tRNA carrying next amino acid

P-site (peptidyl tRNA site)

Carrying growing polypeptide chain

E- site (exite site)

Empty tRNA leaves ribosome from exit site

Transfer RNA

Brings specific amino acids to the ribosome to be assembled as proteins

Amino acid attachment site:

Anticodon contains 3 bases that are specific for the attached amino acid base pairs to the complementary triplet code on mRNA (the codon)

When a tRNA has a covalently attached amino acid, it is said to be charged; when it does not, it is said to be uncharged

Anticodon:

Each tRNA molecule also contains a three-base nucleotide sequence

The anticodon, that pairs with a specific codon on the mRNA

Aminoacyl-tRNA synthetases

Aminoacyl-tRNA synthetases is required for attachment of amino acids to the 3' end of a tRNAs

Aminoacyl-tRNA synthetases catalyze the covalent attachment of the carboxyl group of an amino acid to the 3'-end of its corresponding (cognate) tRNA

Need energy, the enzyme splits ATP to AMP + PPi

The Aminoacyl-tRNA synthetases have a "proofreading" or "editing" activity

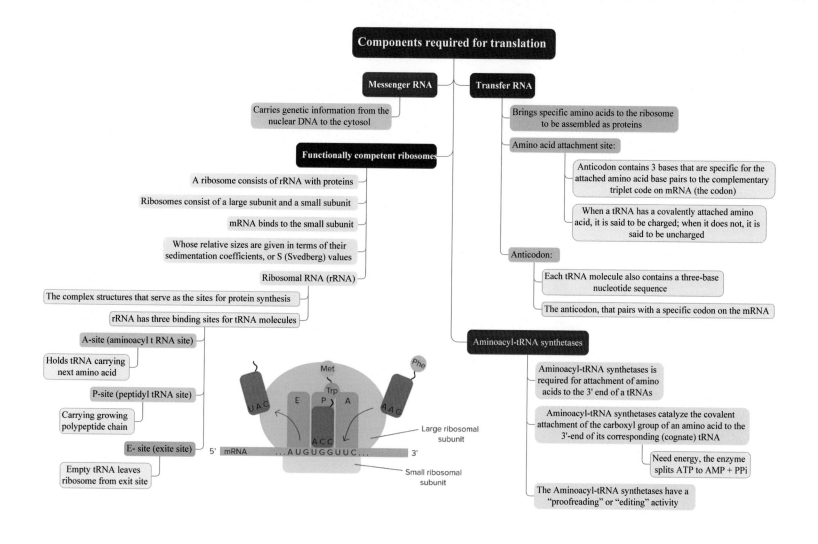

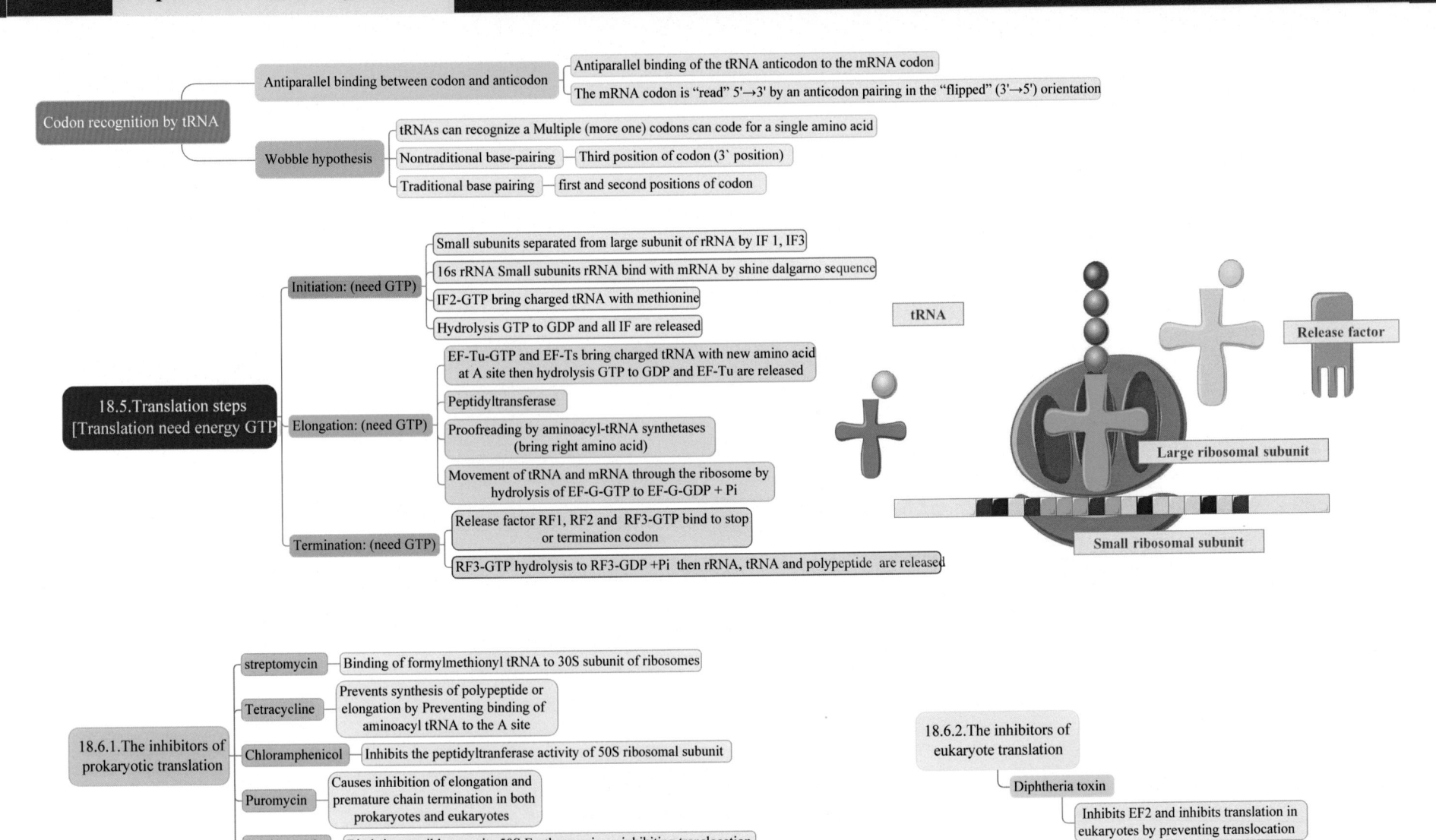

Codon recognition by tRNA

- Antiparallel binding between codon and anticodon
  - Antiparallel binding of the tRNA anticodon to the mRNA codon
  - The mRNA codon is "read" 5'→3' by an anticodon pairing in the "flipped" (3'→5') orientation
- Wobble hypothesis
  - tRNAs can recognize a Multiple (more one) codons can code for a single amino acid
  - Nontraditional base-pairing — Third position of codon (3` position)
  - Traditional base pairing — first and second positions of codon

18.5.Translation steps [Translation need energy GTP]

- Initiation: (need GTP)
  - Small subunits separated from large subunit of rRNA by IF 1, IF3
  - 16s rRNA Small subunits rRNA bind with mRNA by shine dalgarno sequence
  - IF2-GTP bring charged tRNA with methionine
  - Hydrolysis GTP to GDP and all IF are released
- Elongation: (need GTP)
  - EF-Tu-GTP and EF-Ts bring charged tRNA with new amino acid at A site then hydrolysis GTP to GDP and EF-Tu are released
  - Peptidyltransferase
  - Proofreading by aminoacyl-tRNA synthetases (bring right amino acid)
  - Movement of tRNA and mRNA through the ribosome by hydrolysis of EF-G-GTP to EF-G-GDP + Pi
- Termination: (need GTP)
  - Release factor RF1, RF2 and RF3-GTP bind to stop or termination codon
  - RF3-GTP hydrolysis to RF3-GDP +Pi then rRNA, tRNA and polypeptide are released

tRNA

Release factor

Large ribosomal subunit

Small ribosomal subunit

18.6.1.The inhibitors of prokaryotic translation

- streptomycin — Binding of formylmethionyl tRNA to 30S subunit of ribosomes
- Tetracycline — Prevents synthesis of polypeptide or elongation by Preventing binding of aminoacyl tRNA to the A site
- Chloramphenicol — Inhibits the peptidyltranferase activity of 50S ribosomal subunit
- Puromycin — Causes inhibition of elongation and premature chain termination in both prokaryotes and eukaryotes
- Erythromycin — Binds irreversibly to a site 50S Erythromycin so inhibiting translocation

18.6.2.The inhibitors of eukaryote translation

- Diphtheria toxin
  - Inhibits EF2 and inhibits translation in eukaryotes by preventing translocation

Translation steps

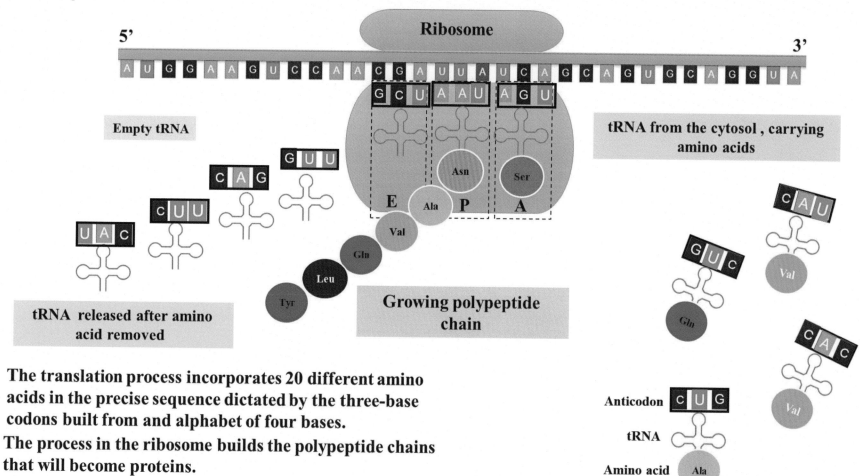

The translation process incorporates 20 different amino acids in the precise sequence dictated by the three-base codons built from and alphabet of four bases.

The process in the ribosome builds the polypeptide chains that will become proteins.

18.7. Mutation: is a change inDNA, the hereditary material of life. An organism's DNA affects how it looks, how it behaves, and its physiology. So a change in an organism's DNA can cause changes in all aspects of its life.

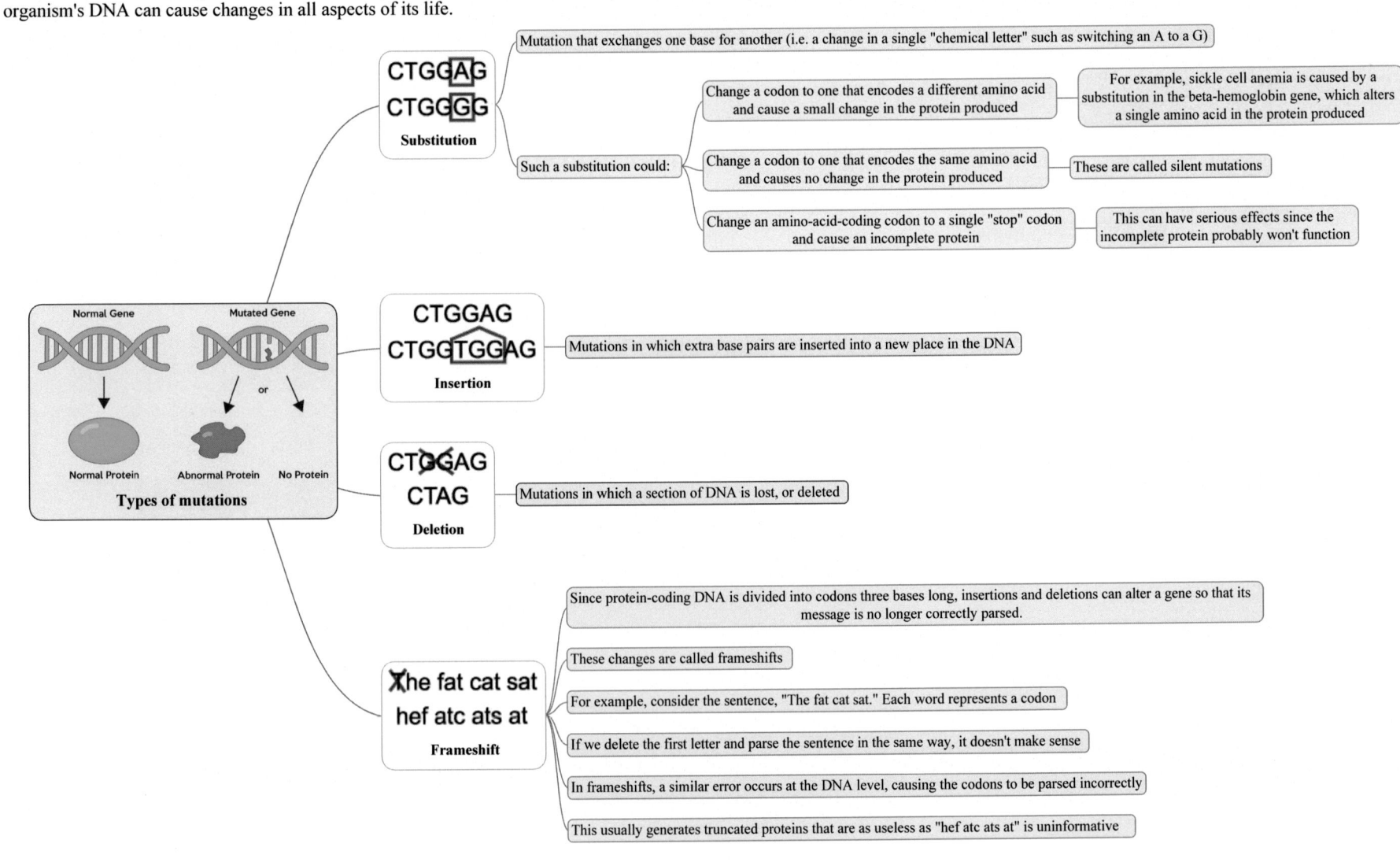

Mutation that exchanges one base for another (i.e. a change in a single "chemical letter" such as switching an A to a G)

CTGGAG
CTGGGG
Substitution

Such a substitution could:

Change a codon to one that encodes a different amino acid and cause a small change in the protein produced

For example, sickle cell anemia is caused by a substitution in the beta-hemoglobin gene, which alters a single amino acid in the protein produced

Change a codon to one that encodes the same amino acid and causes no change in the protein produced

These are called silent mutations

Change an amino-acid-coding codon to a single "stop" codon and cause an incomplete protein

This can have serious effects since the incomplete protein probably won't function

Normal Gene   Mutated Gene

or

Normal Protein   Abnormal Protein   No Protein

Types of mutations

CTGGAG
CTGGTGGAG
Insertion

Mutations in which extra base pairs are inserted into a new place in the DNA

CTGGAG
CTAG
Deletion

Mutations in which a section of DNA is lost, or deleted

The fat cat sat hef atc ats at
Frameshift

Since protein-coding DNA is divided into codons three bases long, insertions and deletions can alter a gene so that its message is no longer correctly parsed.

These changes are called frameshifts

For example, consider the sentence, "The fat cat sat." Each word represents a codon

If we delete the first letter and parse the sentence in the same way, it doesn't make sense

In frameshifts, a similar error occurs at the DNA level, causing the codons to be parsed incorrectly

This usually generates truncated proteins that are as useless as "hef atc ats at" is uninformative

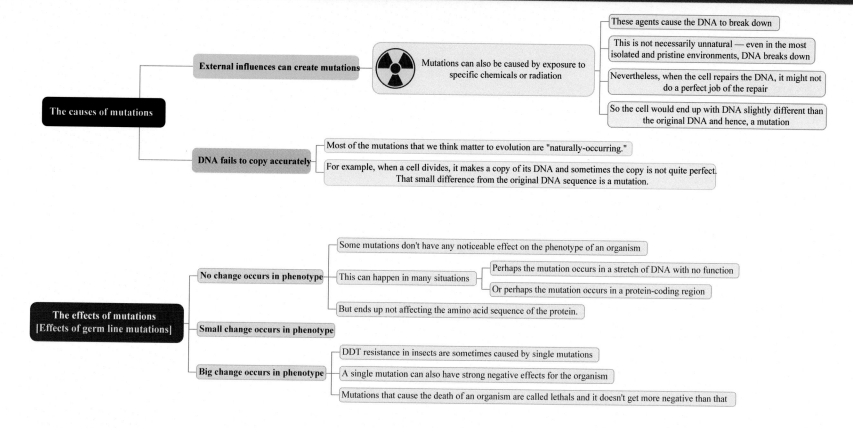

18.8.Genetic disorders

A genetic disease is any disease caused by an abnormality in the genetic makeup of an individual. The genetic abnormality can range from minuscule to major from a discrete mutation in a single base in the DNA of a single gene to a gross chromosomal abnormality involving the addition or subtraction of an entire chromosome or set of chromosomes. Some people inherit genetic disorders from the parents, while acquired changes or mutations in a preexisting gene or group of genes cause other genetic diseases. Genetic mutations can occur either randomly or due to some environmental exposure.

In an autosomal dominant disorder, the mutated gene is a dominant gene located on one of the non sex chromosomes (autosomes)

You need only one mutated gene to be affected by this type of disorder

A person with an autosomal dominant disorder — in this case, the father — has a 50 percent chance of having an affected child with one mutated gene (dominant gene) and a 50 percent chance of having an unaffected child with two normal genes (recessive genes)

18.8.1.Autosomal Dominant inheritance

Female with Huntington's disease

Well female

Male with Huntington's disease

Well male

Family pedigree showing autosomal dominant inheritance

To have an autosomal recessive disorder, you inherit two mutated genes, one from each parent

These disorders are usually passed on by two carriers

Their health is rarely affected, but they have one mutated gene (recessive gene) and one normal gene (dominant gene) for the condition

18.8.2.Autosomal Recessive Inheritance

Carrier Male

Well Male

Well Female

Male with disease

Female with disease

Carrier Female

With each pregnancy, two carriers have a 25 percent chance of having an unaffected child with two normal genes (left), a 50 percent chance of having an unaffected child who is also a carrier (middle), and a 25 percent chance of having an affected child with two recessive genes (right)

Family pedigree showing autosomal recessive inheritance

18.8.3.The Chromosomal Basis of Down Syndrome

The human body is made of cells; all cells contain chromosomes, structures that transmit genetic information

Most cells of the human body contain 23 pairs of chromosomes, half of which are inherited from each parent

Only the human reproductive cells, the sperm cells in males and the ovum in females, have 23 individual chromosomes, not pairs

Scientists identify these chromosome pairs as the XX pair, present in females, and the XY pair, present in males, and number them 1 through 22

When the reproductive cells, the sperm and ovum, combine at fertilization, the fertilized egg that results contains 23 chromosome pairs

A fertilized egg that will develop into a female contains chromosome pairs 1 through 22, and the XX pair

When the fertilized egg contains extra material from chromosome number 21, this results in Down syndrome

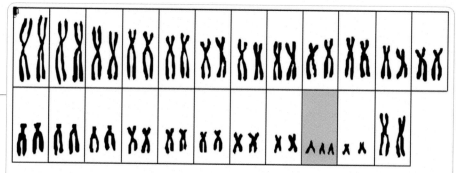

Karyotype of a person with Down syndrome

18.8.4.Fragile X Syndrome

Is the most common inherited form of mental retardation

It results from a change, or mutation, in a single gene, which can be passed from one generation to the next

Fragile X appears in families of every ethnic group and income level

The gene's chemical code for a protein has two parts:

- The introduction area (promoter)

- The instructions for creating the protein

Are inside the cell's nucleus, but the parts that actually make the protein are outside the nucleus

To send the instructions to the protein-producing areas of the cell, the gene "reads" the chemical code and rewrites it into a new form (called messenger RNA)

The new form is then sent out of the cell's nucleus to make proteins

But, if either the original code or the new form of the code is incorrect or has missing parts, the cell can't make the correct protein

Without the protein, the body may not develop or function normally

The FMR1 gene contains too many repeats of one specific sequence, CGG, which is an important part of the promoter region for making FMRP

18.8.5.Genetics of Huntington's Disease

Huntington's disease (HD) is a familial disease, passed from parent to child through a mutation in the normal gene. The genetic defect responsible for HD is a small sequence of DNA on chromosome 4 in which several base pairs are repeated many, many times

Each parent has two copies of every chromosome but gives only one copy to each child. Each child of an HD parent has a 50-50 chance of inheriting the HD gene

If a child does not inherit the HD gene, he or she will not develop the disease and cannot pass it to subsequent generations. A person who inherits the HD gene will sooner or later develop the disease

Whether one child inherits the gene has no bearing on whether others will or will not inherit the gene. In some families, all the children may inherit the HD gene; in others, none do

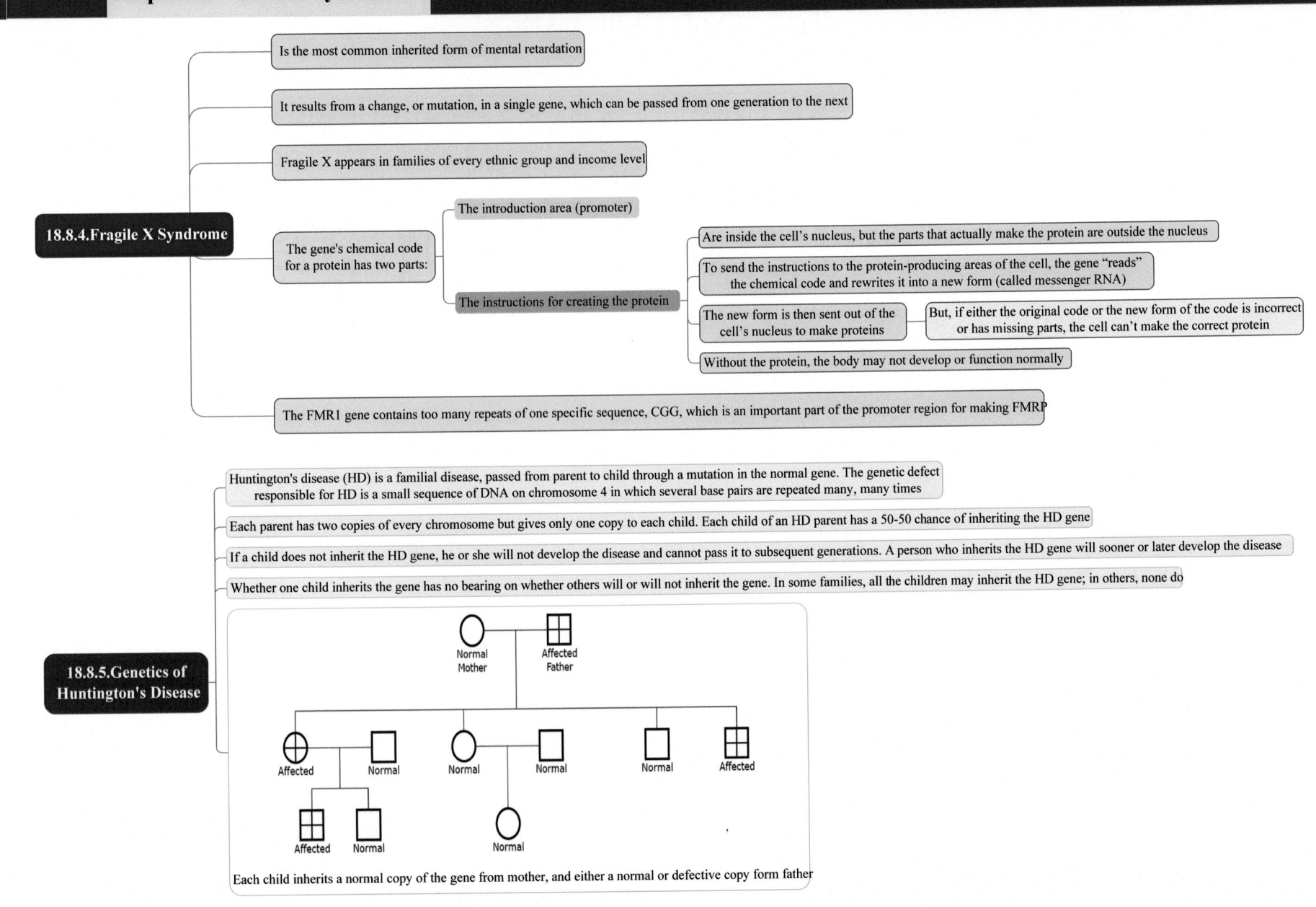

Each child inherits a normal copy of the gene from mother, and either a normal or defective copy form father

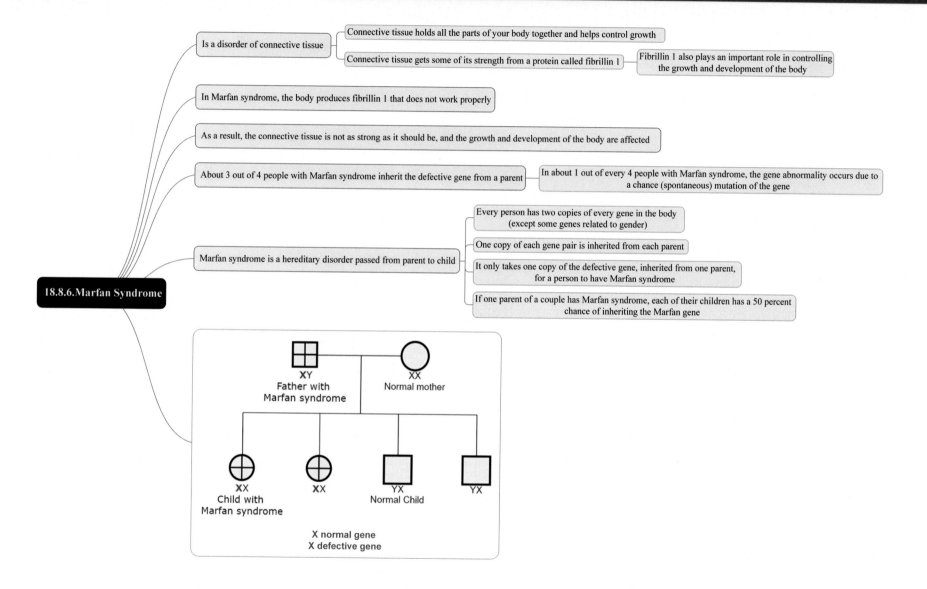

18.8.7.X-linked Dominant Inheritance

Is a mode of genetic inheritance by which a dominant gene is carried on the X chromosome.

As an inheritance pattern, it is less common than the Xlinked recessive type

In medicine, X-linked dominant inheritance indicates that a gene responsible for a genetic disorder is located on the X chromosome

And only one copy of the allele is sufficient to cause the disorder when inherited from a parent who has the disorder

In this case, someone who expresses an X-linked dominant allele will exhibit the disorder and be considered affected

Family pedigree showing X-linked dominant inheritance

18.8.7.X-linked Recessive Inheritance

Is a mode of inheritance which a mutation in a gene on the X chromosome causes the phenotype to be expressed in males

Who are necessarily hemizygous for the gene mutation because they have one X and one Y chromosome

And in females who are homozygous for the gene mutation

Females have two X chromosomes, while males have one X and one Y chromosome

Carrier females who have only one copy of the mutation do not usually express the phenotype

Although differences in X chromosome inactivation can lead to varying degrees of clinical expression in carrier females since some cells will express one X allele

Some scholars have suggested discontinuing the terms dominant and recessive when referring to X-linked inheritance

Due to the multiple mechanisms that can result in the expression of X-linked traits in females, which include cell autonomous expression, skewed X-inactivation, clonal expansion, and somatic mosaicism

Family pedigree showing X-linked recessive inheritance

Protein Synthesis : Exercises

Q 1: Circle the best correct answer:

1.In DNA, the amount of A=20%, therefore the amount of G is:
a. 20%
b. 30%
c. 40%
d. 60%

2.In prokaryotic mRNA 'Shine-Dalgarno' sequence is:
a. Allow tRNA to be processed
b. Are unique to eukaryotic mRNA
c. Occur at the 3' end of tRNA
d. binding site of 16s rRNA in prokaryotic mRNA helps to initiate protein synthesis

3.Direction of DNA synthesis and reading is:
a. 3'→5'
b. 5'→3'
c. Both A and B
d. None of these

4.The Wobble Hypothesis explains:
a. A Multiple (more one) codons can code for a single amino acid
b. Nonsense codons not code for amino acids
c. Solving the problem of supercoils
d. One codon can code for a single amino acid

5.Actinomycin D act as anticancer drugs due to:
a. Binding to β subunit of RNA polymerase
b. Inhibit translation
c. intercalating into the narrow groove so inhibit transcription
d. inhibit cell wall synthesis

6.Transcription is the formation of:
a. DNA from DNA
b. RNA from DNA
c. Protein through mRNA
d. mRNA from pre mRNA

7.An Okazaki fragment is a :
a. Fragment of DNA resulting from endonuclease action
b. Fragment of RNA that is a subunit of the 30S ribosome
c. Piece of DNA that is synthesized in the 3' → 5' direction
d. Segment of RNA primer and short fragment DNA that is an intermediate in the synthesis of lagging strand

8.Which one of the following statements about DNA polymerase I is not correct?
a. Synthesis of DNA in 5'→3' direction
b. Has a "proofreading" and error correction activity (3'→5' exonuclease)
c. Synthesis of RNA primer
d. Remove the RNA primer (5'→3' exonuclease activity)

9.protein synthesis (translation) required:
a. ATP
b. GTP
c. CTP
d. TTP

10.In eukaryotic, DNA wrapped around a set of eight proteins called:
a. Nucleotides
b. Histones
c. Nucleosome
d. Chromosome

11.In repair of the mismatch for double-stranded DNA, the Mut S and L proteins in methyl-directed repair system:
a. Recognize the mismatch and identify the parental (methylated) strand
b. Changes both the template strand and the newly replicated strand.
c. Cleaves mismatch on the daughter strand
d. Corrects the DNA strand that is methylated.

12.The function of nonsense or stop codons is.
a. Termination of translation
b. Termination of transcription
c. No function
d. Recognizes the amino acid

Protein Synthesis : Exercises

Q 1: Circle the best correct answer:

13.The XP protein and uvrABC protein is essential in:
a. base-excision repair
b. methyl-directed repair
c. Mismatch repair
d. Thymine dimer repair

14.Which of the following statements about aminoacyl-tRNA synthetases is false?
a. Have an editing/proofreading capability.
b. The enzyme attaches an amino acid to the 3' end of a tRNA.
c. Transferring the peptide chain from p site on to amino acid at the A site.
d. Need energy, the enzyme splits ATP to AMP^+ PPi.

15.Termination of protein synthesis (translation) does not require:
a. Release factor RF1, RF2 and RF3-GTP
b. GTP
c. stop or termination codon
d. p(rho) factor

16.The antibiotics with can be inhibited the transcription is:
a. Chloramphenicol
b. Penicillin
c. Puromycin
d. Rifampin

17.Which of the following statements about rRNA is true?
a. A ribosome is the complex that serves as the sites for protein synthesis.
b. Ribosomes contain one single protein.
c. rRNA are distributed in three separate, large ribosomal subunits.
d. There are four binding sites for aminoacyl-tRNAs on a ribosome.

18.The function of peptidyltransferase activity is:
a. bring charged tRNA with new amino acid at A site
b. Translocation, movement of tRNA and mRNA through the ribosome
c. forming peptide bond by transferring the amino acids (f methionine) or peptide chain from the P site onto the amino acid at the A site
d. Termination the protein synthesis

19.DNA fragments are sealed and joined by:
a. DNA polymerase II
b. DNA ligase
c. DNA gyrase
d. DNA topoisomerase II

20.Reverse transcriptase activity is present in the eukaryotic in:
a. DNA polymerase α
b. DNA polymerase γ
c. Telomerase
d. DNA polymerase II

21.The termination site for transcription is recognized by:
a. p (rho) factor
b. β−Subunit of RNA polymerase
c. X factor
d. α−Subunit o RNA polymerase

22.DNA topoisomerase II of Eukaryotic cells catalyses:
a. Relaxation of negatively supercoiled DNA
b. Relaxation of positively supercoiled DNA
c. Conversion of negatively supercoiled DNA into positively supercoiled DNA
d. Relaxation of both negative and positive supercoils.

23.Primase activity in eukaryotic cells is present in:
a. DNA polymerase I
b. DNA polymerase α
c. DNA polymerase III
d. DNA polymerase δ

Protein Synthesis : Exercises

Q 1: Circle the best correct answer:

24.Protein binds at origin of replication to start separation to form localized regions of ssDNA is:
a. DnaA protein
b. DNA polymerase III
c. Single-stranded DNA-binding (SSB) proteins
d. DNA polymerase I

25.Anticodons are presented on:
a. mRNA
b. tRNA
c. rRNA
d. DNA

26.The type of point mutation in HbSC anemia is:
a. Silent mutation
b. missense mutation
c. Nonsense mutation
d. Frame shift mutation

27.In the following partial sequence of mRNA, a mutation of the template DNA results in a change in codon 91 to UAA:

88   89   90   91   92   93   94
GUC GAC CAG CCU GGC UAA CCG

The type of mutation is:
a. Silent mutation
b. missense mutation
c. Nonsense mutation
d. Frame shift mutation

28.In eukaryotic, the modifications of Pre-mRNA are included:
a. Addition poly-A tail at 3`.
b. 7-methylguanosine cap at 5` at pre-mRNA.
c. Splicing of pre-mRNA to remove non-coding introns and join exons.
d. All of these

29.Nucleotide is building blocks of DNA that is binding together by:
a. Phosphodiester bond
b. Ester bond
c. Peptide bond
d. Hydrogen bond

30.The reason of the major β-thalasemia is:
a. absent on one β-globin gene
b. absent one α-globin gene
c. absent on two β-globin gene
d. absent on four α-globin gene

Q 2: Write short notes on:

1.The properties of DNA polymerase III.
2.The properties of DNA polymerase I.
3.The effect of UV on DNA.
4.Repair of damage caused by ultraviolet.
5.Repair of the mismatch mutation.
6.The functions of the major groove and the minor groove.
7.Types of RNA.
8.Describe the process of protein synthesis.
9.Describe the process of transcription.
10.Genetic code.
11.Frameshift mutation.
12.'Shine-Dalgarno' sequence.
13.Point mutation.
14.Solving the problem of supercoils.
15.Separation of ds DNA during process of DNA replication.
16.RNA primer.
17.Primase.
18.Eukaryotic mRNA processing.
19.DNA that contains high concentrations of G and C denatures at high temperature.
20.During eukaryotic mRNA processing, the intron is removed.

OVERVIEW

In the past, efforts to understand genes and their expression have been confounded by the immense size and complexity of human deoxyribonucleic acid (DNA). It is now possible to determine the nucleotide sequence of long stretches of DNA, and the entire sequence of the human genome has been determined. This effort (called the Human Genome Project) was made possible by several techniques that have already contributed to our understanding of many genetic diseases. These include, first, the discovery of restriction endonucleases that permit the dissection of huge DNA molecules into defined fragments. Second, the development of cloning techniques, providing a mechanism for amplification of specific nucleotide sequences. Finally, the ability to synthesize specific probes, which has allowed the identification and manipulation of nucleotide sequences of interest. These and other experimental approaches have permitted the identification of both normal and mutant nucleotide sequences in DNA.This knowledge has led to the development of methods for the diagnosis of genetic diseases, and initial successes in the treatment of patients by gene therapy.

Chapter 19 : Recombinant DNA Technology

19.1. What is gene cloning?

It is the isolation of a gene and its easy propagation within cells via a plasmid or virus (The plasmid or virus is said to be the vector).

Gene cloning

- A DNA fragment carrying the gene is inserted into the plasmid or viral DNA molecule to produce a recombinant DNA mol which is a hybrid molecule

- The technology of how this is done is known as recombinant DNA technology or genetic engineering

- Cloning allows genes and their gene products (proteins) to be easily characterized and easily isolate or purified and also cloning allows defined genetic experiments — e.g transgenic mice

Steps in gene cloning with pBR322

1. Purify chromosomal DNA from the specific organism, then cut the chromosomal DNA with restriction enzymes. (example, Bam H1)

2. Purifying vector or plasmid and cut with Bam H1.
E. coli host cell carries around 3000 plasmid per cell that is important for ease of propagation. (use the same restriction enzyme that is used in cutting of chromosomal DNA)

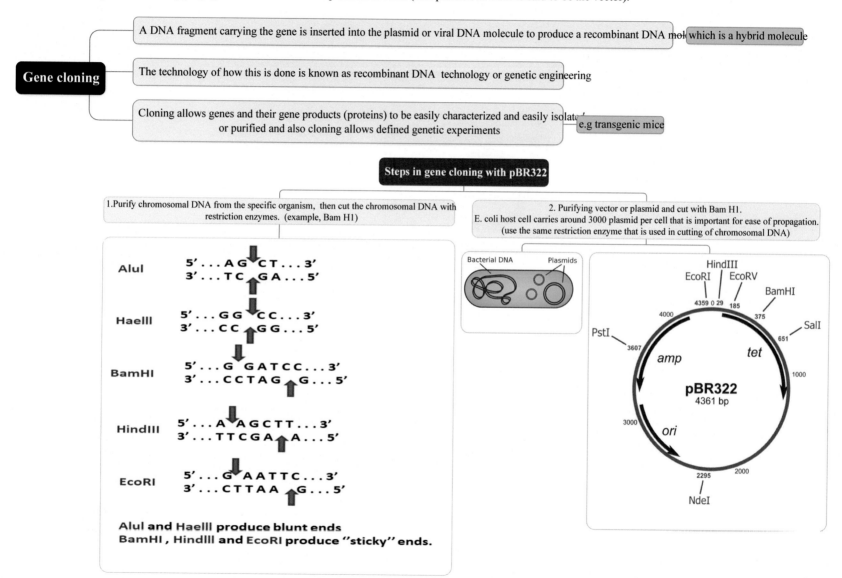

AluI
5'...AG CT...3'
3'...TC GA...5'

HaeIII
5'...GG CC...3'
3'...CC GG...5'

BamHI
5'...G GATCC...3'
3'...CCTAG G...5'

HindIII
5'...A AGCTT...3'
3'...TTCGA A...5'

EcoRI
5'...G AATTC...3'
3'...CTTAA G...5'

AluI and HaeIII produce blunt ends
BamHI , HindIII and EcoRI produce "sticky" ends.

Steps in gene cloning with pBR322

3. Ligation vector or plasmid and gene cut with BamH1 and the gene cut with BamH1. After ligation, insert can be cloned in either of 2 orientations.

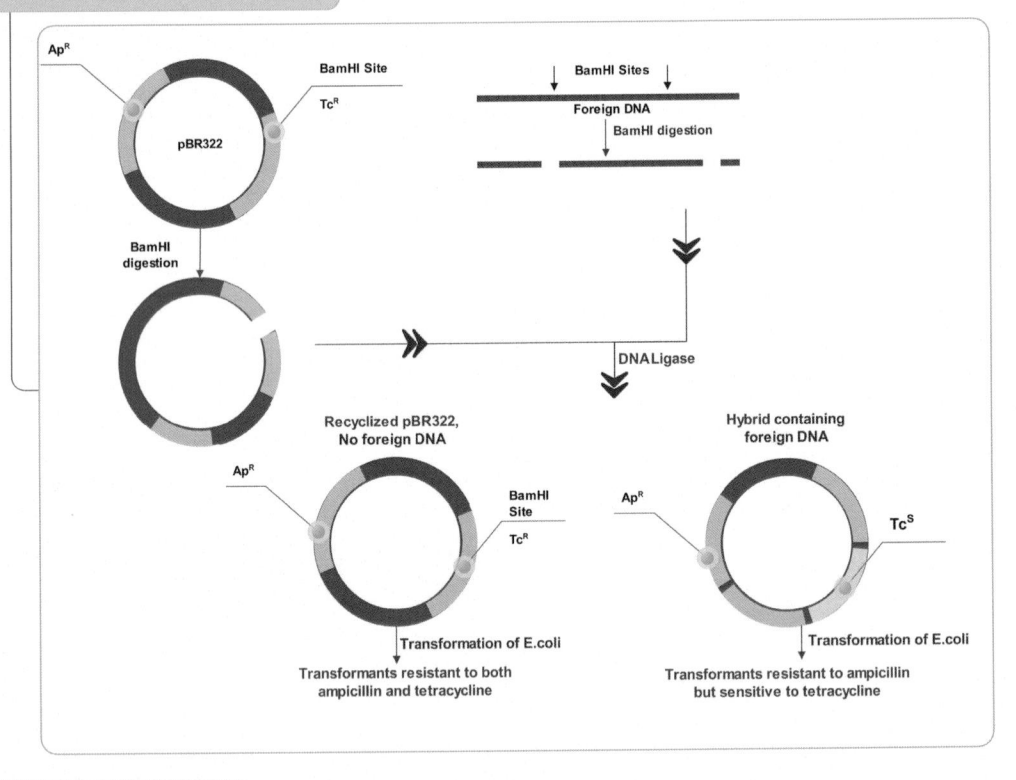

Ap^R

BamHI Site

Tc^R

pBR322

BamHI
digestion

BamHI Sites

Foreign DNA

BamHI digestion

DNALigase

Recyclized pBR322,
No foreign DNA

Hybrid containing
foreign DNA

Ap^R

BamHI
Site

Tc^R

Ap^R

Tc^S

Transformation of E.coli

Transformation of E.coli

Transformants resistant to both
ampicillin and tetracycline

Transformants resistant to ampicillin
but sensitive to tetracycline

4.Transformation of bacterial host cells with recombinant DNA molecules

Steps in gene cloning with pBR322

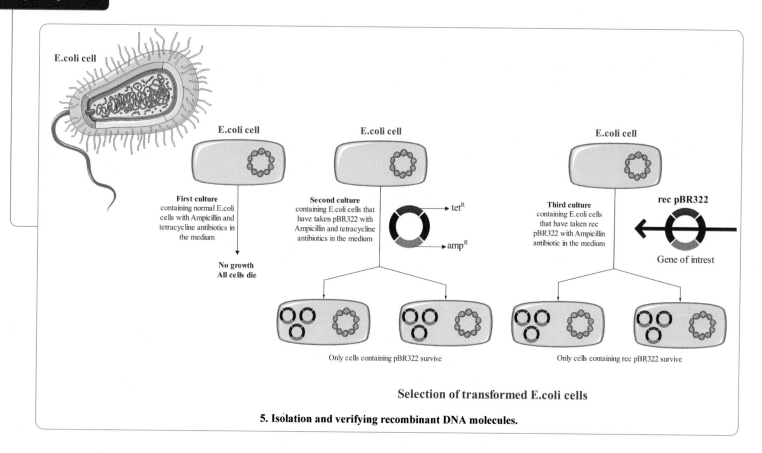

E.coli cell

E.coli cell

First culture
containing normal E.coli
cells with Ampicillin and
tetracycline antibiotics in
the medium

**No growth
All cells die**

E.coli cell

Second culture
containing E.coli cells that
have taken pBR322 with
Ampicillin and tetracycline
antibiotics in the medium

→ tet^R

→ amp^R

E.coli cell

Third culture
containing E.coli cells
that have taken rec
pBR322 with Ampicillin
antibiotic in the medium

rec pBR322

Gene of intrest

Only cells containing pBR322 survive

Only cells containing rec pBR322 survive

Selection of transformed E.coli cells

5. Isolation and verifying recombinant DNA molecules.

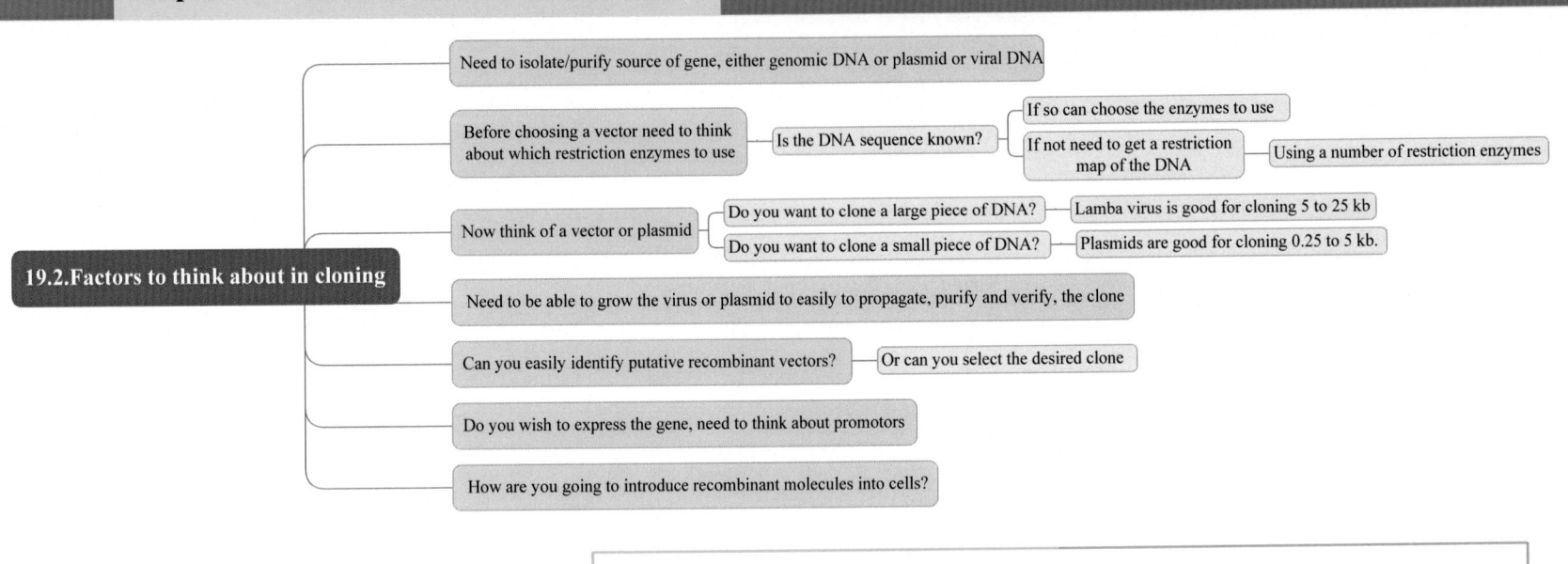

Need to isolate/purify source of gene, either genomic DNA or plasmid or viral DNA

Before choosing a vector need to think about which restriction enzymes to use — Is the DNA sequence known?
- If so can choose the enzymes to use
- If not need to get a restriction map of the DNA — Using a number of restriction enzymes

Now think of a vector or plasmid
- Do you want to clone a large piece of DNA? — Lamba virus is good for cloning 5 to 25 kb
- Do you want to clone a small piece of DNA? — Plasmids are good for cloning 0.25 to 5 kb.

19.2.Factors to think about in cloning

Need to be able to grow the virus or plasmid to easily to propagate, purify and verify, the clone

Can you easily identify putative recombinant vectors? — Or can you select the desired clone

Do you wish to express the gene, need to think about promotors

How are you going to introduce recombinant molecules into cells?

19.3.Gene cloning approaches:

19.3.1. Simple cloning of DNA

Often there is a need to clone a DNA fragment for as an intermediate step (in cloning, sequencing DNA analysis etc.). since the DNA is not to be expressed as protein. It would normally be cloned into a plasmid such as pBR322 or pUC 19. Particularly if the DNA fragment is small (<10 kb).

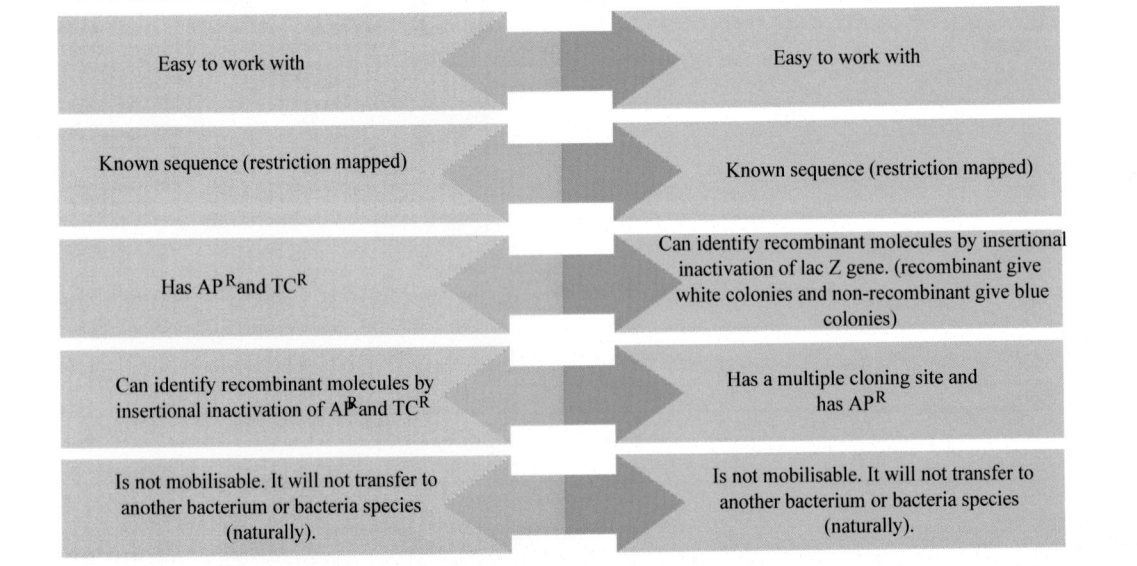

Advantage of pBR322:	Advantage of pUC119:
Easy to work with	Easy to work with
Known sequence (restriction mapped)	Known sequence (restriction mapped)
Has AP^R and TC^R	Can identify recombinant molecules by insertional inactivation of lac Z gene. (recombinant give white colonies and non-recombinant give blue colonies)
Can identify recombinant molecules by insertional inactivation of AP^R and TC^R	Has a multiple cloning site and has AP^R
Is not mobilisable. It will not transfer to another bacterium or bacteria species (naturally).	Is not mobilisable. It will not transfer to another bacterium or bacteria species (naturally).

LacZ (β-galactosidase) Alpha complementation

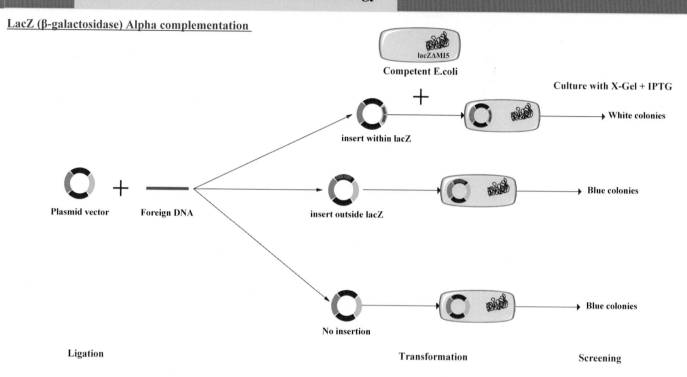

Competent E.coli

Culture with X-Gel + IPTG

Plasmid vector

Foreign DNA

insert within lacZ → White colonies

insert outside lacZ → Blue colonies

No insertion → Blue colonies

Ligation

Transformation

Screening

19.3.2.Cloning to express a gene in bacteria *(E. Coli)*

To express a gene in *E. Coli* it is important to place the start site of the gene (prockaryote or eukaryote) adjacent to a strong *E. Coli* viral promotor such as the T7 promotor. The T7 promotor is present on the host chromosome and is inducible. a gene expressed by this promotor can account for 20% of total protein expressed

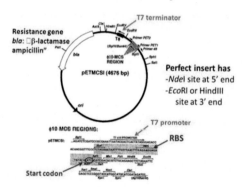

Resistance gene
bla: □β-lactamase
ampicillin"

pETMCSI (4676 bp)

T7 terminator

Perfect insert has
-*Nde*I site at 5' end
-*Eco*RI or HindIII
 site at 3' end

T7 promotor

RBS

Start codon

19.3.3. Simple cloning of large DNA fragments in lambda phage

Often there is a need to clone a large DNA fragment >10 kb for further analysis or to generate a library of large fragments. Generally used lambda DNA to clone fragments 5 to 25kb. Cut λ EMBL3 vector with Bam H1. Purify long and short arms and ligate with approximately 20 kb insert DNA. package λ virus using in vitro packaging extracts then infect E. Coli and isolate recombinant phage from plaques.

19.3.4. Cloning of very large DNA fragments

Very large fragments of DNA 300 to 1000kb can now be cloned into bacterial artificial chromosomes (BACs) based on the F sex factor and yeast artificial chromosomes based on 2 μm plasmid of Saccharomyces cerevisiae.

19.3.5. Cloning eukaryotic or human genes

Cloning of eukaryotic genes directly in form of DNA is rarely done. Gene are very large typically 5-20 kb and the genome is very large. Consequently, the mRNA is isolated instead from tissue in the form of cDNA (DNA that is complementary sequence to the mRNA. This is process is known as reverse transcriptase.

The mRNA has a poly A tail (150-200 residues). This is used to initiate reverse transcription using a complementary oligonucleotide p(dT) 12-15 which anneals (base-pairs) to the poly A site and primers the synthesis of the reverse strand.

OVERVIEW

Biochemistry also called as biological chemistry which is the study of chemical processes relating to living organisms. Much of biochemistry deals with the functions, structures and interactions of biological macromolecules which include nucleic acids, proteins, lipids and carbohydrates, which will provide structure of cells and help to perform many of the functions which are associated with life. Article is sometimes called a Scientific Article, a Peer-Reviewed Article, or a Scholarly Research Article. Together, journal articles in a particular field are often referred to as The Literature. Journal articles are most often Primary Research Articles. However, they can also be Review Articles. These types of articles have different aims and requirements. Sometimes, an article describes a new tool or method. Because articles in scientific journals are specific, meticulously cited and peer-reviewed, journal databases are the best place to look for information on previous research on your species. Without a background in the field, journal articles may be hard to understand - however, you do not need to understand an entire article to be able to get valuable information from it.

20.1.Scientists Have Confirmed a New DNA Structure Inside Human Cells

It's not just the double helix!

- For the first time, scientists have identified the existence of a new DNA structure never before seen in living cells

- The discovery of a 'twisted knot' of DNA in living cells
  - Confirms our complex genetic code is crafted with more intricate symmetry than just the double helix structure everybody associates with DNA
  - And the forms these molecular variants take affect how our biology functions

- "When most of us think of DNA, we think of the double helix," says antibody therapeutics researcher Daniel Christ from the Garvan Institute of Medical Research in Australia
  - This new research reminds us that totally different DNA structures exist and could well be important for our cells

- Called the intercalated motif (i-motif) structure, first discovered by researchers in the 1990s. but up until now had only ever been witnessed in vitro, not in living cells

- Now, thanks to Christ's team, we know the i-motif occurs naturally in human cells
  - Meaning the structure's significance to cell biology demands new attention from researchers
    - Which has previously been called into question, given it had only been demonstrated in the lab

- "The dual helical spirals shape of DNA made famous by Watson and Crick" explains genomicist Marcel Dinger, who co-led the research'

- The i-motif is a four-stranded 'knot' of DNA
  - In the knot structure, C [cytosine] letters on the same strand of DNA bind to each other
    - So this is very different from a double helix
      - Where 'letters' on opposite strands recognise each other, and where Cs bind to Gs [guanines]

- the i-motif is only one of a number of DNA structures that don't take the double helix form "According to Garvan's Mahdi Zeraati, the first author of the new study"
  - Including A-DNA, Z-DNA, triplex DNA and Cruciform DNA
    - And which could also exist in our cells

Watson and Crick Duplex

i-Motif C-Quadruplex

The new DNA structures

- G-quadruplex (G4) DNA
  - Was first visualised by researchers in human cells in 2013
  - Who made use of an engineered antibody to reveal the G4 within cells
    - Zeraati and fellow researchers employed the same kind of technique, developing an antibody fragment (called iMab)
      - That could specifically recognise and bind to i-motifs
      - In doing so, it highlighted their location in the cell with an immunofluorescent glow

- The transient i-motifs generally form late in a cell's 'life cycle'
  - Specifically called the late G1 phase, when DNA is being actively 'read'
  - Tend to appear in
    - Promoter regions — Areas of DNA that control whether genes are switched on or off
    - Telomeres — Genetic markers associated with ageing

Reference: Mahdi Zeraati, David B. Langley, Peter Schofield, Aaron L. Moye, Romain Rouet, William E. Hughes, Tracy M. Bryan, Marcel E. Dinger & Daniel Christ.I-motif DNA structures are formed in the nuclei of human cells.

Nature Chemistry volume 10, pages631–637 (2018)

Chapter 20 : The latest biochemical research articles

20.1.Scientists Have Confirmed a New DNA Structure Inside Human Cells

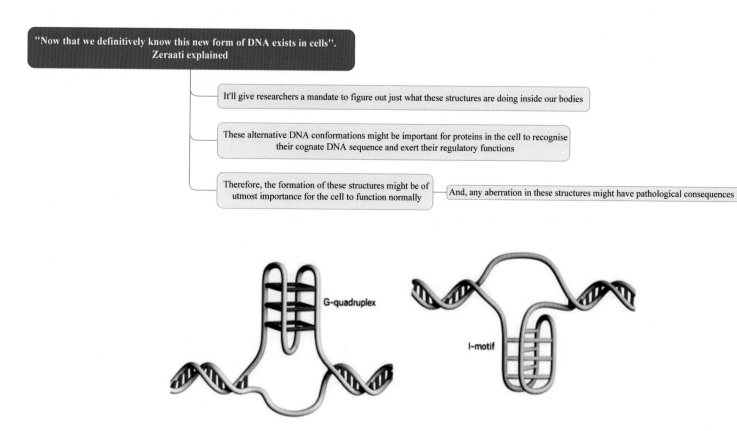

"Now that we definitively know this new form of DNA exists in cells".
Zeraati explained

It'll give researchers a mandate to figure out just what these structures are doing inside our bodies

These alternative DNA conformations might be important for proteins in the cell to recognise their cognate DNA sequence and exert their regulatory functions

Therefore, the formation of these structures might be of utmost importance for the cell to function normally

And, any aberration in these structures might have pathological consequences

G-quadruplex

I-motif

In DNA, guanine-guanine links (red) form G-quadruplexes, and connections between cytosines and protonated cytosines (green) form i-motifs.

Reference: Mahdi Zeraati, David B. Langley, Peter Schofield, Aaron L. Moye, Romain Rouet, William E. Hughes, Tracy M. Bryan, Marcel E. Dinger & Daniel Christ.I-motif DNA structures are formed in the nuclei of humaNature Chemistry volume 10, pages631–637 (2018)

20.2.Elephants Are Strangely Resistant to Cancer - And We May Finally Know Why

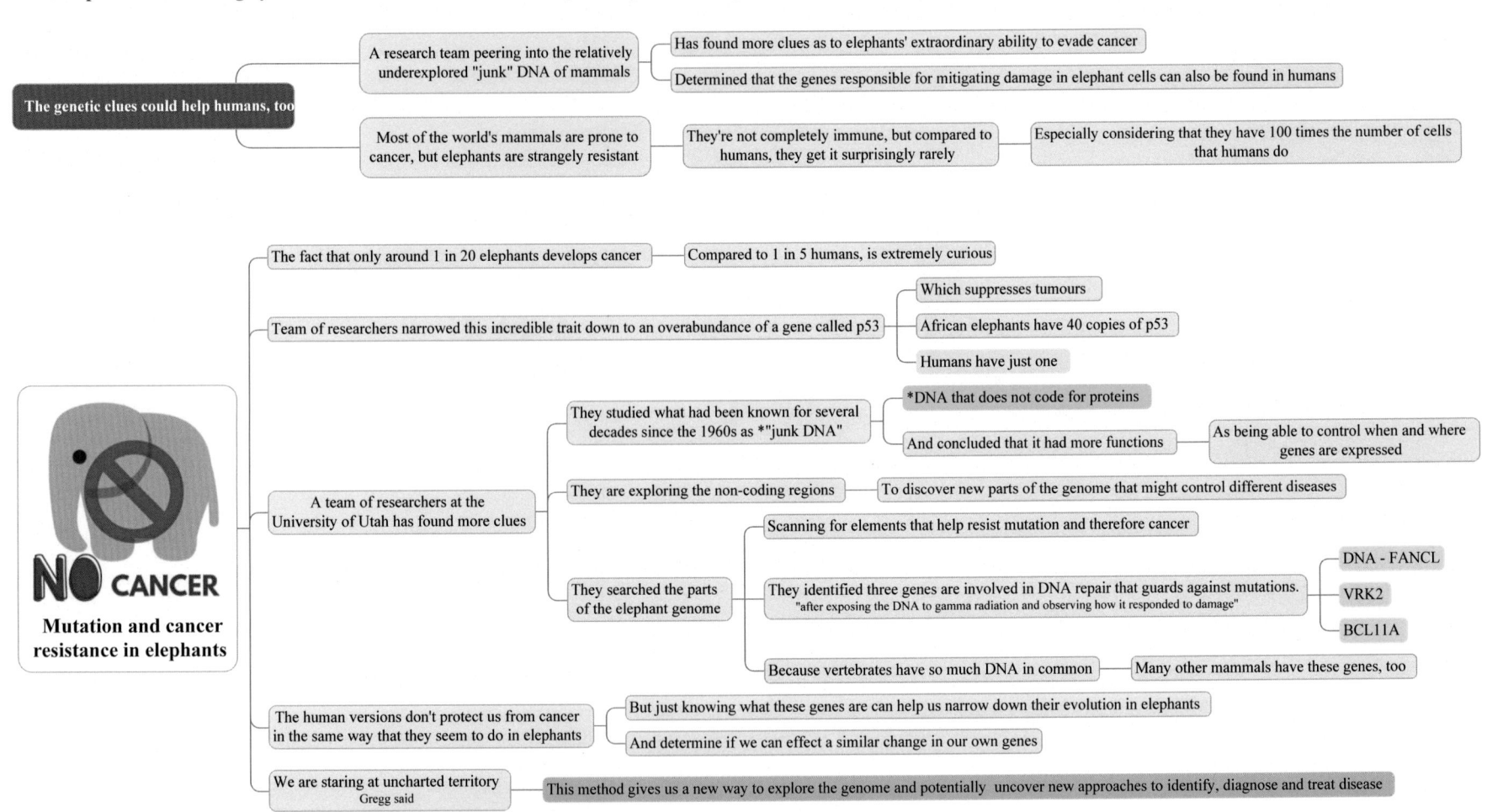

The genetic clues could help humans, too

- A research team peering into the relatively underexplored "junk" DNA of mammals
  - Has found more clues as to elephants' extraordinary ability to evade cancer
  - Determined that the genes responsible for mitigating damage in elephant cells can also be found in humans
- Most of the world's mammals are prone to cancer, but elephants are strangely resistant
  - They're not completely immune, but compared to humans, they get it surprisingly rarely
    - Especially considering that they have 100 times the number of cells that humans do

Mutation and cancer resistance in elephants

- The fact that only around 1 in 20 elephants develops cancer
  - Compared to 1 in 5 humans, is extremely curious
- Team of researchers narrowed this incredible trait down to an overabundance of a gene called p53
  - Which suppresses tumours
  - African elephants have 40 copies of p53
  - Humans have just one
- A team of researchers at the University of Utah has found more clues
  - They studied what had been known for several decades since the 1960s as *"junk DNA"
    - *DNA that does not code for proteins
    - And concluded that it had more functions
      - As being able to control when and where genes are expressed
  - They are exploring the non-coding regions
    - To discover new parts of the genome that might control different diseases
  - They searched the parts of the elephant genome
    - Scanning for elements that help resist mutation and therefore cancer
    - They identified three genes are involved in DNA repair that guards against mutations. "after exposing the DNA to gamma radiation and observing how it responded to damage"
      - DNA - FANCL
      - VRK2
      - BCL11A
    - Because vertebrates have so much DNA in common
      - Many other mammals have these genes, too
- The human versions don't protect us from cancer in the same way that they seem to do in elephants
  - But just knowing what these genes are can help us narrow down their evolution in elephants
  - And determine if we can effect a similar change in our own genes
- We are staring at uncharted territory
  Gregg said
  - This method gives us a new way to explore the genome and potentially uncover new approaches to identify, diagnose and treat disease

Reference: Elliott Ferris, Lisa M. Abegglen, Joshua D. Schiffman and Christopher Gregg. Accelerated Evolution in Distinctive Species Reveals Candidate Elements for Clinically Relevant Traits, Including Mutation and Cancer Resistance. Cell reports. Published: March 6, 2018.

Chapter 20 : The latest biochemical research articles

20.3.Site-specific phosphorylation of tau inhibits amyloid-β toxicity in Alzheimer's mice

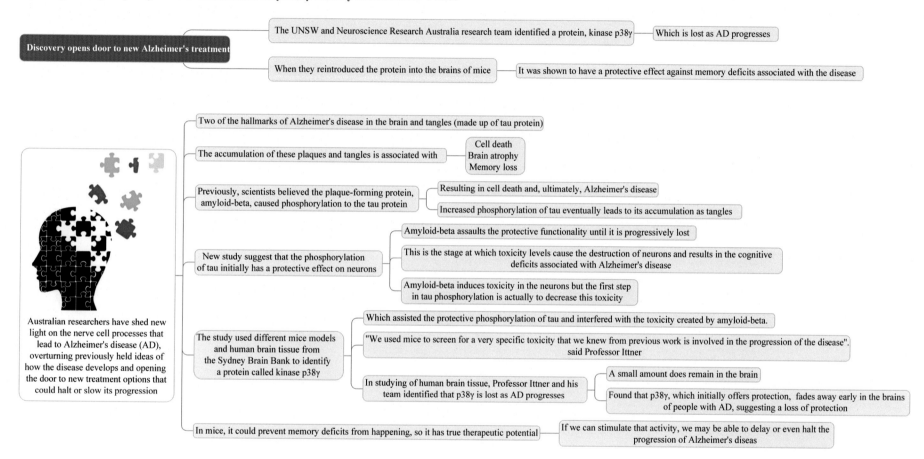

Discovery opens door to new Alzheimer's treatment

The UNSW and Neuroscience Research Australia research team identified a protein, kinase p38γ — Which is lost as AD progresses

When they reintroduced the protein into the brains of mice — It was shown to have a protective effect against memory deficits associated with the disease

Australian researchers have shed new light on the nerve cell processes that lead to Alzheimer's disease (AD), overturning previously held ideas of how the disease develops and opening the door to new treatment options that could halt or slow its progression

Two of the hallmarks of Alzheimer's disease in the brain and tangles (made up of tau protein)

The accumulation of these plaques and tangles is associated with
- Cell death
- Brain atrophy
- Memory loss

Previously, scientists believed the plaque-forming protein, amyloid-beta, caused phosphorylation to the tau protein
- Resulting in cell death and, ultimately, Alzheimer's disease
- Increased phosphorylation of tau eventually leads to its accumulation as tangles

New study suggest that the phosphorylation of tau initially has a protective effect on neurons
- Amyloid-beta assaults the protective functionality until it is progressively lost
- This is the stage at which toxicity levels cause the destruction of neurons and results in the cognitive deficits associated with Alzheimer's disease
- Amyloid-beta induces toxicity in the neurons but the first step in tau phosphorylation is actually to decrease this toxicity

The study used different mice models and human brain tissue from the Sydney Brain Bank to identify a protein called kinase p38γ
- Which assisted the protective phosphorylation of tau and interfered with the toxicity created by amyloid-beta.
- "We used mice to screen for a very specific toxicity that we knew from previous work is involved in the progression of the disease". said Professor Ittner
- In studying of human brain tissue, Professor Ittner and his team identified that p38γ is lost as AD progresses
  - A small amount does remain in the brain
  - Found that p38γ, which initially offers protection, fades away early in the brains of people with AD, suggesting a loss of protection

In mice, it could prevent memory deficits from happening, so it has true therapeutic potential — If we can stimulate that activity, we may be able to delay or even halt the progression of Alzheimer's diseas

Reference: Arne Ittner, Sook Wern Chua, Josefine Bertz, Alexander Volkerling, Julia van der Hoven, Amadeus Gladbach, Magdalena Przybyla, Mian Bi, Annika van Hummel, Claire H. Stevens, Stefania Ippati, Lisa S. Suh, Alexander Macmillan, Greg Sutherland, Jillian J. Kril, Ana P. G. Silva, Joel P. Mackay, Anne Poljak, Fabien Delerue, Yazi D. Ke, Lars M. Ittner. Site-specific phosphorylation of tau inhibits amyloid-β toxicity in Alzheimer's mice. Science 18 Nov 2016

20.4.This Newly Discovered Gene Variant Reduces The Risk of Severe Malaria by 40%

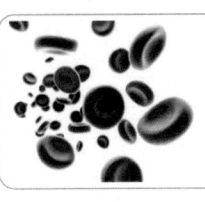

Researchers have identified a simple gene variant related to human red blood cells that helps protect certain people against malaria

The discovery sheds light on how our bodies have evolved to fight against a deadly disease that has plagued our species for millennia, and could open up the way to new treatments

Gene Variant Reduces the Risk of Malaria

The discovery sheds light on how our bodies have evolved to fight against a deadly disease that has plagued our species for millennia, and could open up the way to new treatments

Malaria is caused by five species of single-celled organism belonging to the genus Plasmodium
- Which spread through the bite of mosquitos and then invade the host's red blood cells, or erythrocytes, to reproduce
- It's this rapid growth and traumatic popping of the red cells that causes the disease's symptoms, which include high fever, sweating, chills, and aches, and for some, death
- In 2015, malaria was responsible for taking just under half a million lives across the globe. Most of these were caused by P. falciparum

Yet two of its target blood cell receptors - based on types of glycophorin produced by the genes GYPA and GYPB - have attracted researchers' attention
- Back in 1977, researchers reported that red blood cells from people with a rare GYPA mutation seemed to resist being invaded by P. falciparum
- Since then, variations in erythrocyte receptors have been studied in relation to patterns of malarial infection in the hope of developing new insights that could lead to better treatments or ways to prevent infection

In this latest study, the genomes of 765 individuals from populations across Gambia, Burkina Faso, Cameroon, and Tanzania were sequenced and compared with genomes from the 1000 Genomes Project
- The researchers identified regions surrounding the glycophorin genes that had duplicated, coming up with 27 variations in copied sections
- The spread of these copy variations across the sub-Saharan populations more or less reflected the results of previous studies that found differences in their blood cell's glycophorins
- One copy in particular, duplication 4 (or simply DUP4), was associated with a resistance to severe malarial infections, lowering the risk of the disease by about 40 percent
- This variant reduces the risk of severe malaria by 40 percent, and has recently risen in frequency in parts of Kenya, yet it appears to be absent from west Africa

It's not completely clear how this variation makes it harder for the parasite to get a grip
- But the researchers think it might have something to do with how the copy swaps GYPB with a hybrid GYPB-A receptor
- Possibly changing the properties of the membrane or interfering with the bridge P. falciparum makes with the cell

The DUP4 variation was only present in some of the African populations
- Raising the question of whether the mutation is recent and hasn't yet had a chance to spread, or if it only protects against certain strains of P. falciparum

Yet after millions of years, we finally seem to be winning the war against malaria thanks to the widespread availability of mosquito netting and insecticides, and cheap vaccines on the horizon

Reference: Ellen M. Leffler, Gavin Band, George B. J. Busby, Katja Kivinen, Quang Si Le, Geraldine M. Clarke, Kalifa A. Bojan. Resistance to malaria through structural variation of red blood cell invasion receptor. Science 16 Jun 2017

Chapter 20 : The latest biochemical research articles

20.5.RNA molecule that shields breast cancer stem cells from immune system

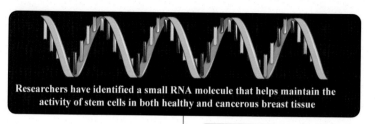

Researchers have identified a small RNA molecule that helps maintain the activity of stem cells in both healthy and cancerous breast tissue

The study suggests that this 'microRNA' promotes particularly deadly forms of breast cancer and that inhibiting the effects of this molecule could improve the efficacy of existing breast cancer therapies

Many tumors also contain so-called "cancer stem cells" that can drive tumor formation

Some tumors, such as triple-negative breast cancers, are particularly deadly because they contain large numbers of cancer stem cells that self-renew and resist differentiation

Scientists searched for short RNA molecules called microRNAs that can bind and inhibit protein-coding messenger RNAs to reduce the levels of specific proteins

To identify factors that help non-cancerous mammary gland stem cells (MaSCs) resist differentiation and retain their capacity to self-renew

Identified one microRNA, called miR-199a

That helps MaSCs retain their stem-cell activity by suppressing the production of a protein called LCOR

Which binds DNA to regulate gene expression

When they boosted miR-199a levels in mouse MaSCs, they suppressed LCOR and increased normal stem cell function

When they increased LCOR levels, they could curtail mammary gland stem cell activity

miR-199a was also expressed in human and mouse breast cancer stem cells

Just as boosting miR-199a levels helped normal mammary gland stem cells retain their activity

The researchers showed that miR-199a enhanced the ability of cancer stem cells to form tumors

By increasing LCOR levels, in contrast, they could reduce the tumor-forming capacity of the cancer stem cells

Breast cancer patients whose tumors expressed large amounts of miR-199a showed poor survival rates, whereas tumors with high levels of LCOR had a better prognosis

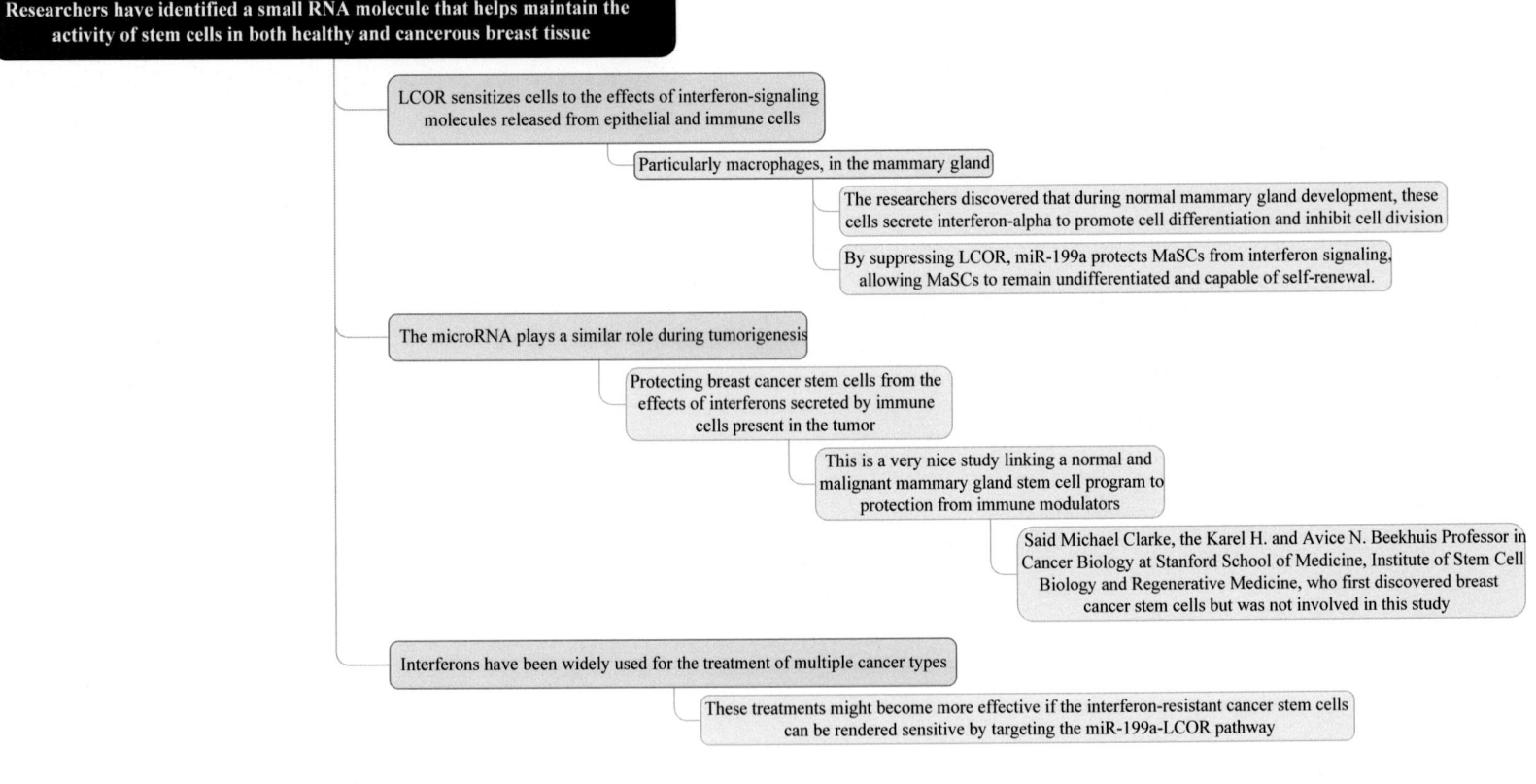

Researchers have identified a small RNA molecule that helps maintain the activity of stem cells in both healthy and cancerous breast tissue

LCOR sensitizes cells to the effects of interferon-signaling molecules released from epithelial and immune cells

Particularly macrophages, in the mammary gland

The researchers discovered that during normal mammary gland development, these cells secrete interferon-alpha to promote cell differentiation and inhibit cell division

By suppressing LCOR, miR-199a protects MaSCs from interferon signaling, allowing MaSCs to remain undifferentiated and capable of self-renewal.

The microRNA plays a similar role during tumorigenesis

Protecting breast cancer stem cells from the effects of interferons secreted by immune cells present in the tumor

This is a very nice study linking a normal and malignant mammary gland stem cell program to protection from immune modulators

Said Michael Clarke, the Karel H. and Avice N. Beekhuis Professor in Cancer Biology at Stanford School of Medicine, Institute of Stem Cell Biology and Regenerative Medicine, who first discovered breast cancer stem cells but was not involved in this study

Interferons have been widely used for the treatment of multiple cancer types

These treatments might become more effective if the interferon-resistant cancer stem cells can be rendered sensitive by targeting the miR-199a-LCOR pathway

Reference: Toni Celià-Terrassa, Daniel D. Liu, Abrar Choudhury, Xiang Hang, Yong Wei, Jose Zamalloa, Raymundo Alfaro-Aco, Rumela Chakrabarti, Yi-Zhou Jiang, Bong Ihn Koh, Heath A. Smith, Christina DeCoste, Jun-Jing Li, Zhi-Ming Shao & Yibin Kang. Normal and cancerous mammary stem cells evade interferon-induced constraint through the miR-199a–LCOR axis. Nature Cell Biology volume 19, pages 711–723 (2017).

20.6.Genetic Switch Decides Between Genome Repair and Cell Death

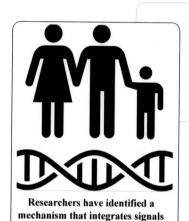

Researchers have identified a mechanism that integrates signals from the ongoing repair process and the cell death machinery

Within seconds after an harmful incident, different mechanisms start

- In a schizophrenic way, the cell starts repairing as well as preparing for apoptosis
- They identified an uncharacterized mechanism that integrates signals from the ongoing repair process and the cell death machinery
- A protein called UFD-2 forms large complexes at the breaks and verifies whether to proceed with the repair or whether it's time to die
- In the process, UFD-2 is a point of intersection that both receives and gives signals

The experiments were performed with the nematode Caenorhabditis elegans

- They were exposed to ionizing radiation to induce double strand breaks and then examined
- The results are important to further understand how and why a cell decides to repair or to die
- Cells lacking UFD-2 fail to undergo apoptosis
- In humans such a situation could lead to a higher risk of a damaged cell becoming a cancer cell

All the proteins that play a part in this mechanism can be found in humans as well and the findings could be highly relevant to better understanding how DNA damage leads to cancer

- DNA damage is also an important driver of the aging process
- Although apoptosis protects from cancer, excessive cell death can lead to tissue degeneration and aging
- The senior author Thorsten Hoppe originally identified UFD-2 as a key regulator of protein degradation
- Here, UFD-2 forms regulatory centers that coordinate DNA repair and cell death
- Hoppe hopes for resulting advances in tumor therapy:
  - The knowledge we gained from this study provides new perspectives for fighting cancer pharmaceutically
  - It might be possible to manipulate the well-balanced process of apoptosis and protein degradation to make clearance of tumor cells more efficient

Reference: Leena Ackermann, Michael Schell, Wojciech Pokrzywa, Éva Kevei, Anton Gartner, Björn Schumacher & Thorsten Hoppe. E4 ligase–specific ubiquitination hubs coordinate DNA double-strand-break repair and apoptosis. Nature Structural & Molecular Biology volume 23, pages 995–1002 (2016)

20.7.Researchers Find Brain Hormone That Triggers Fat Burning

Biologists at The Scripps Research Institute (TSRI) have identified a brain hormone that appears to trigger fat burning in the gut. Their findings in animal models could have implications for future pharmaceutical development

They experimented with roundworms called C. elegans, which are often used as model organisms in biology

These worms have simpler metabolic systems than humans, but their brains produce many of the same signaling molecules

Leading many researchers to believe that findings in C. elegans may be relevant for humans

They deleted genes in C. elegans to see if they could interrupt the path between brain serotonin and fat burning

By testing one gene after another, they hoped to find the gene without which fat burning wouldn't occur

This process of elimination led them to a gene that codes for a neuropeptide hormone they named FLP-7 (pronounced "flip 7")

They found that the mammalian version of FLP-7 (called Tachykinin) had been identified 80 years ago as a peptide that triggered muscle contractions when dribbled on pig intestines

The next step in the new study was to determine if FLP-7 was directly linked to serotonin levels in the brain

Study first author Lavinia Palamiuc, a TSRI research associate, spearheaded this effort by

Tagging FLP-7 with a fluorescent red protein so that it could be visualized in living animals, possible because the roundworm body is transparent

Her work revealed that FLP-7 was indeed secreted from neurons in the brain in response to elevated serotonin levels

FLP-7 then traveled through the circulatory system to start the fat burning process in the gut

20.7.Researchers Find Brain Hormone That Triggers Fat Burning

Biologists at The Scripps Research Institute (TSRI) have identified a brain hormone that appears to trigger fat burning in the gut. Their findings in animal models could have implications for future pharmaceutical development

Next, the researchers investigated the consequences of manipulating FLP-7 levels

While increasing serotonin itself can have a broad impact on an animal's food intake and movement and reproductive behavior

The researchers found that increasing FLP-7 levels farther downstream didn't come with any obvious side effects

The worms continued to function normally while simply burning more fat

Srinivasan said this finding could encourage future studies into how FLP-7 levels could be regulated without causing the side effects often experienced when manipulating overall serotonin levels

For the first time, researchers had found a brain hormone that specifically and selectively stimulates fat metabolism, without any effect on food intake

The newly discovered fat-burning pathway works like this

A neural circuit in the brain produces serotonin in response to sensory cues, such as food availability

This signals another set of neurons to begin producing FLP-7. FLP-7 then activates a receptor in intestinal cells

And the intestines begin turning fat into energy

Reference: Lavinia Palamiuc, Tallie Noble, Emily Witham, Harkaranveer Ratanpal, Megan Vaughan & Supriya Srinivasan. A tachykinin-like neuroendocrine signalling axis couples central serotonin action and nutrient sensing with peripheral lipid metabolism. Nature Communications volume 8, Article number: 14237 (2017)

20.8.Analog DNA circuit does math in a test tube,DNA computers could one day be programmed to diagnose and treat disease

Researchers have created strands of synthetic DNA that, when mixed together in a test tube in the right concentrations, form an analog circuit that can add, subtract and multiply as the molecules form and break bonds

While most DNA circuits are digital, their device performs calculations in an analog fashion by measuring the varying concentrations of specific DNA molecules directly — Without requiring special circuitry to convert them to zeroes and ones first

The researchers describe their approach in the August issue of the journal ACS Synthetic Biology

- Unlike the silicon-based circuits used in most modern day electronics, commercial applications of DNA circuits are still a long way off
- They can do some limited computing, but we can't even begin to think of competing with modern-day PCs or other conventional computing devices
- But DNA circuits can be far tinier than those made of silicon
- And unlike electronic circuits, DNA circuits work in wet environments, which might make them useful for computing inside the bloodstream or the soupy, cramped quarters of the cell

The technology takes advantage of DNA's natural ability to zip and unzip to perform computations — Just like Velcro and magnets have complementary hooks or poles, the nucleotide bases of DNA pair up and bind in a predictable way

The researchers first create short pieces of synthetic DNA, some single-stranded and some double-stranded with single-stranded ends, and mix them in a test tube

- When a single strand encounters a perfect match at the end of one of the partially double-stranded ones
- It latches on and binds, displacing the previously bound strand and causing it to detach, like someone cutting in on a dancing couple
- The newly released strand can in turn pair up with other complementary DNA molecules downstream in the circuit, creating a domino effect.

The researchers solve math problems by measuring the concentrations of specific outgoing strands as the reaction reaches equilibrium

Analog circuits are also better suited for sensing signals that don't lend themselves to simple on-off, all-or-none values — Such as vital signs and other physiological measurements involved in diagnosing and treating disease

The hope is that, in the distant future, such devices could be programmed to sense whether particular blood chemicals lie inside or outside the range of values considered normal — And release a specific DNA or RNA -- DNA's chemical cousin -- that has a drug-like effect

They are beginning to work on DNA-based devices that could detect molecular signatures of particular types of cancer cells, and release substances that spur the immune system to fight back — Even very simple DNA computing could still have huge impacts in medicine or science

Reference: Tianqi Song, Sudhanshu Garg, Reem Mokhtar, Hieu Bui, and John Reif. Analog Computation by DNA Strand Displacement Circuits. :ACS Synth. Biol. 2016, 5, 8, 898-912

Amino acids

1. b	2. a	3. a	4. c	5. d	6. d	7. b	8. b
9. c	10. c	11. b	12. a	13. c	14. d	15. a	16. c
17. b	18. c	19. b	20. b	21. b	22. a		

Structure of proteins

1. b	2. d	3.a	4.b	5.d	6.c	7.c	8.c
9.d	10.c	11.b	12. b	13. d	14. d	15. b	16.a
17.d	18. b	19. d	20. c	21. d	22. b	23. a	24. a
25. a	26. b	27. a	28. a	29. a	30. a	31. b	32. d
33. c	34. a	35. d	36. d	37. d	38. b		

Globular proteins

1.b	2. d	3. d	4. a	5. c	6. a	7. c	8. d
9. d	10. c	11. a	12. a	13. a	14. a	15. c	16. b
17. b	18. a	19. d	20. b	21. d	22. c	23. c	24. b

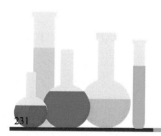

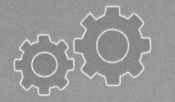

Fibrous proteins

1. c	2. a	3. a	4. d	5. a	6. a	7. c	8. c
9. b	10. c	11. c	12. b	13. a	14. b	15. a	16. a
17. c	18. d	19. d	20. c	21.a	22. a	23. c	24. a
25. a	26. b						

Enzymes

1. c	2. b	3. b	4.c	5. c	6. d	7. d	8. b
9. a	10.b	11. d	12. b	13. a	14. b	15. c	16. d
17. c	18. b	19. c	20. c	21. c	22. a	23. b	24.c
25. c	26. a	27. b	28. a	29. a	30. b	31. b	32. b
33. b	34. b	35. c	36. c	37.d	38.c	39. a	40. b

Oxidative phosphorylation

1. a	2. c	3. a	4. b	5. a	6. c	7. b	8. d
9. d	10. d	11. b	12. a	13. a	14. d	15. d	

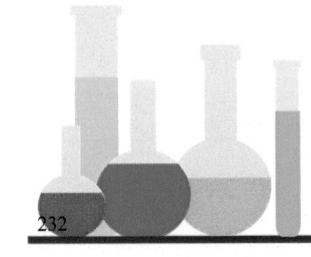

Metabolism of Carbohydrates

1. a	2. a	3.d	4. b	5. c	6. a	7. a	8. d
9. a	10. b	11. b	12. c	13. a	14. c	15. c	16. b
17. a	18. c	19. a	20. d	21. c	22. c	23. b	24. a
25. d	26. a	27. d	28. a	29. a	30. c	31. d	32. b
33. b	34.d	35.a	36. c	37. a	38. c	39. d	40. b
41. c	42. d	43. c	44. d	45. b	46. d	47. a	48. c
49. b	50. d	51. d	52. c	53. b	54. d	55. d	56.c
57. d	58. a	59. b	60. d	61. d	62. b	63. a	

TCA Cycle

1. c	2. a	3.c	4. b	5. c	6. b	7. c	8.d
9. c	10. a	11. b	12. b	13. d	14.a		

Glycogen metabolism

1. a	2. c	3. b	4. d	5. c	6. c	7. c	8. c
9. a	10. b	11. b	12. c	13. d	14. c	15. b	16. c
17. b	18. c	19. c	20. d	21. c			

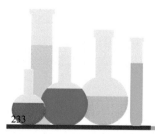

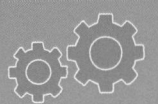

Pentose phosphate pathway

1. b	2. c	3. b	4. b	5. a	6. a	7. b	8. 1
9. a	10. d	11. a	12. d	13.a	14. c	15. a	16. a
17. b	18. d	19. c	20. d	21. c	22. b	23. c	24. c
25. c							

Lipids and Membranes

1. b	2. a	3. d	4. b	5. a	6. a	7. b	8. c
9. c	10. a	11. c	12. b	13. b	14. a	15. c	16. a
17. d	18. b	19. c	20. b	21. b	22. c	23. a	24. d
25. c							

Dietary Lipid Metabolism, Ketone Bodies, Ecosanoids, Cholesterol, Lipoprotein, and Steroid Metabolism, Amino acids: Disposal of Nitrogen

1. b	2.c	3. a	4. d	5. a	6. d	7. b	8. a
9. c	10. b	11.a	12. c	13. d	14. b	15. b	16. a
17. c	18. a	19. b	20. d	21. d	22. c	23. c	24. a
25. b	26. b	26. c	27. b	28. d	29. b	30. a	31. c
32. d	33. a	34. b	35. d	36. a	37. b	38. d	39. a
40. c	41. b	42. d	43. b	44. a	45. d	46. c	47. c
48. a	49. d	50. c	51. a	52. b	53. a	54. c	55. b
56. c	57. a	58.d					

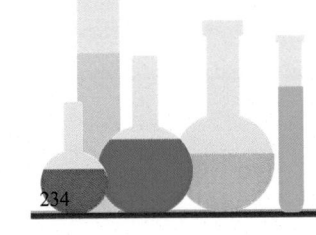

Protein synthesis

1. b	2. d	3. b	4. a	5. c	6. b	7. d	8. c
9. b	10. b	11. a	12. a	13.d	14. c	15. d	16. d
18. a	18. c	19. b	20. c	21. a	22. d	23. b	24. a
25. b	26. b	27. c	28. d	29. a	30. c		

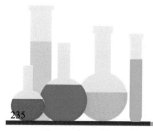

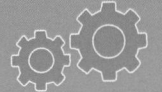
David LN, Michael MC. (2017). Lehninger Principles of Biochemistry Seventh Edition.

Denise F. (2017). Lippincott Illustrated Reviews: Biochemistry (Lippincott Illustrated Reviews Series) Seventh, North American Edition. 2017.

Fruton JS. (1999) Proteins, Enzymes, Genes: The Interplay of Chemistry and Biochemistry, Yale University Press, New Haven. A distinguished historian of biochemistry traces the development of this science and discusses its impact on medicine, pharmacy, and agriculture.

Gray MW, Berger G, Lang BF. (1999) Mitochondrial evolution. Science 283, 1476–1481.

Griffiths AJF, Gelbart WM, Lewinton RC, Miller JH. (2002) Modern Genetic Analysis: Integrating Genes and Genomes, W. H. Freeman and Company, New York. International Human Genome Sequencing Consortium.

Harold FM. (2001) The Way of the Cell: Molecules, Organisms, and the Order of Life, Oxford University Press, Oxford.

Judson HF. (1996) The Eighth Day of Creation: The Makers of the Revolution in Biology, expanded edn. Cold Spring Harbor Laboratory Press, Cold Spring Harbor, NY. A highly readable and authoritative account of the rise of biochemistry and molecular biology in the twentieth century.

Kornberg A. (1987) The two cultures: chemistry and biology. Biochemistry 26, 6888–6891. The importance of applying chemical tools to biological problems, described by an eminent practitioner.

Lodish H, Berk A, Matsudaira P, Kaiser CA, Krieger M, Scott MR, Zipursky SL, Darnell J. (2003) Molecular Cell Biology, 5th edn, W. H. Freeman and Company, New York.

Long M, de Souza SJ, Gilbert W. (1995) Evolution of the intron-exon structure of eukaryotic genes. Curr. Opin. Genet. Dev. 5, 774–778.

Pace NR. (2001) The universal nature of biochemistry. Proc. Natl. Acad. Sci. USA 98, 805–808. A short discussion of the minimal definition of life, on Earth and elsewhere.

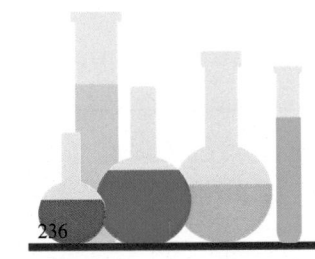

Mind Maps in Biochemistry is new as the best mind maps to enable undergraduates and postgraduate students to understand the fundamental principles of Biochemistry.

Mohamed J. Saadh
Hala M. Sbaih

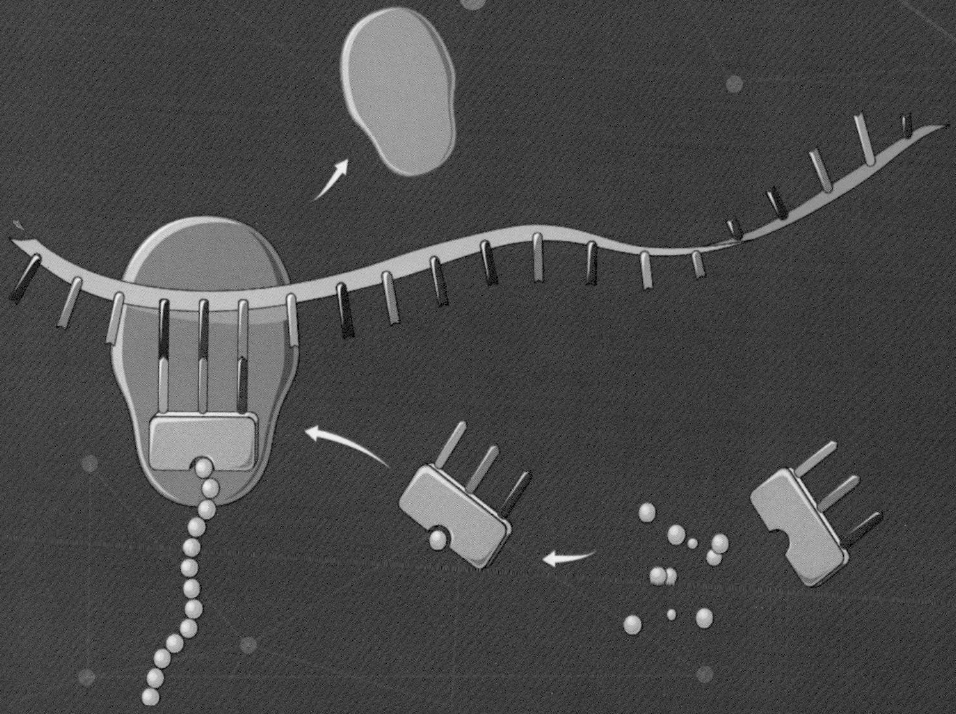

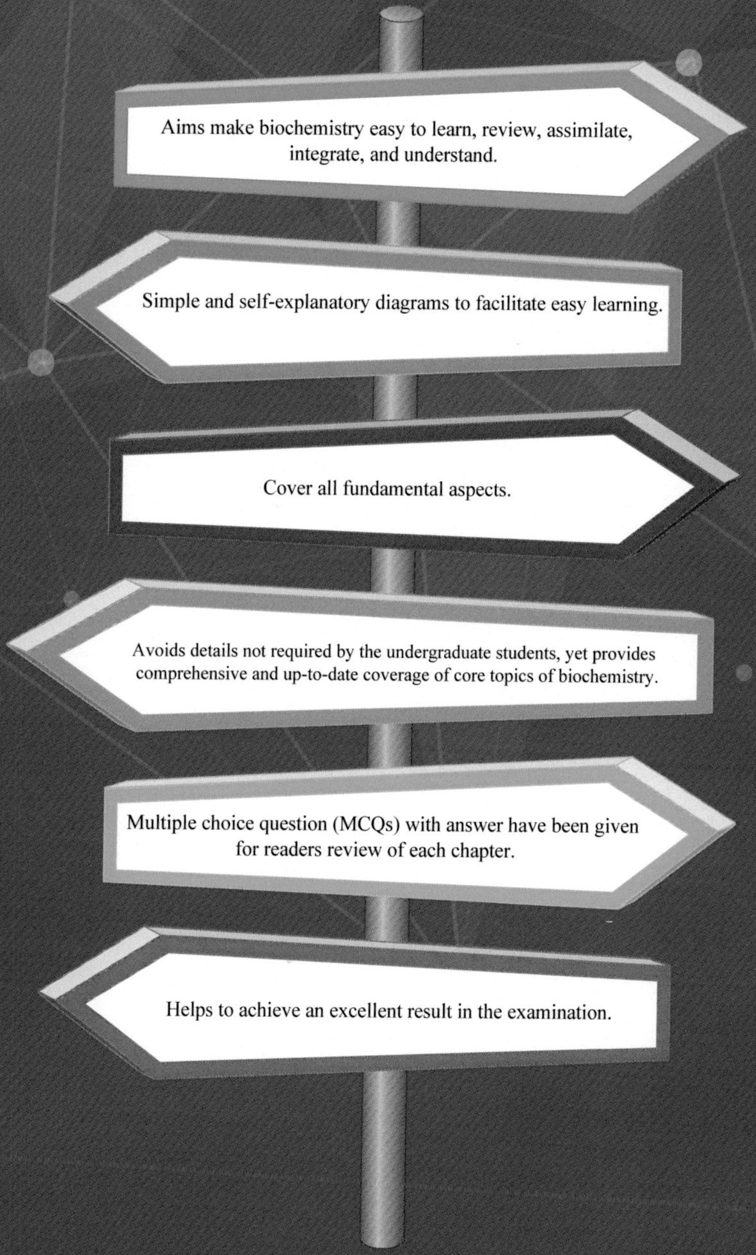

Printed in the United States
By Bookmasters